T0133321

A FAMILY PRACTICE

A FAMILY PRACTICE

THE RUSSELL DOCTORS AND THE EVOLVING BUSINESS OF MEDICINE, 1799–1989

**William D. Lindsey,
William L. Russell,
and Mary L. Ryan**

The University of Arkansas Press
Fayetteville
2020

ISBN: 978-1-68226-127-9
eISBN: 978-1-61075-686-0

24 23 22 21 20   5 4 3 2 1

Designed by Liz Lester

⊗ The paper used in this publication meets the minimum
requirements of the American National Standard
for Permanence of Paper for Printed Library
Materials Z39.48-1984.

Library of Congress Control Number: 2019947837

CONTENTS

FOREWORD

Access to health care has been a basic human concern for millennia. Over the last decade in the United States, this concern has been heightened by empty promises and ill-conceived policies promulgated by politicians and political parties, often to the detriment of their constituents' financial and physical well-being, not to mention the nation's economy. At the interface of a politician's promises and a patient's expectations are our nation's health-care providers. Years of effort (often decades) devoted to studying, preparing, and practicing for the "art of medicine" are rarely appreciated by those outside the health sciences.

Today, many patients, politicians, and media outlets take for granted the seemingly miraculous advances the medical community has made in treating diseases and injuries. Furthermore, many deem access to these "miracles of modern medicine" a basic human right. This is not unexpected, given the fact that many citizens view virtually anything encountered during their "pursuit of happiness" as a basic human right. Such expectations are commonplace in today's America but not in America of bygone days.

In the early days of the republic, health care was certainly not viewed as a right but rather as a service—a much-needed service that not all could access easily. Physicians and their services were often a rare commodity, particularly on the frontier. In those days, a doctor's availability was almost as doubtful as his quality. An apprenticeship of a few months' duration or attendance at a handful of "medical lectures" was often enough to earn students the title of doctor. A few extra lectures or an additional month of observation might qualify one as a surgeon—a far cry from the extensive preparatory measures required today.

As medical science progressed, so too did the quality of its practitioners. For the first 150 years of our nation's history, scientific progression was painstakingly slow and so was the knowledge dispensed by its doctors. In the first half of the 19th century, "heroic" medical practices, such as bloodletting, cupping, and administration of powerful purgatives, were state-of the-art health care for treating diseases like tuberculosis, typhoid fever, and whooping cough. Today such procedures are perceived as barbarous acts of charlatanism, especially when compared to the current state of medical practice in our country. The history of medicine in the United States has been a fascinating roller-coaster ride of remarkable discoveries. These have included the discovery of ether anesthesia, vaccines, antibiotics, and cancer chemotherapy. There have been significant reforms such as the Flexner Report, the Pure Food and Drug Act, and the Food, Drug, and Cosmetic Act. New forms of information distribution, from medical journals to the National Library of Medicine and internet access to medical information, have revolutionized how medicine is practiced, as have establishments like our nationwide network of hospitals and clinics and the National Institutes of Health. As detailed in the pages of this unique narrative, patriarchs of the Russell family constituted a rare unbroken lineage of American physicians who were riders on this amazing roller coaster. Their stories provide a fascinating insight into the realities of American medical practice, most notably in the rural South from 1821–1989.

Fast forward to 2020, and advances in medical science have virtually eliminated many diseases and maladies that plagued patients of the Russell clan. Today, advanced, non-invasive imaging technologies, robot-assisted surgical procedures, an understanding of the human genome and its role in health and disease, and a wellspring of novel and effective pharmaceutical agents are just a few staples of 21st century medicine that serve as foundational underpinnings for the perceived "right" to health care. These standards of modern American medicine currently serve as a lodestone to the rest of the world, and ironically, such successes may ultimately lead to the system's own self-destruction.

Because of our unique American health-care system and those professionals dedicated to its continued progress and success, the world is literally "beating a path" to our door. A case in point is the burgeoning influx of "undocumented" sick and ailing end users coming across our southern border on a daily basis. Diseases like measles, tuberculosis, and typhus, once considered eradicated, are now on the verge of sparking new epidemics. Outpacing this incursion of uninvited "new patients" for practitioners of various specialties and subspecialties is a rising elderly American population and an ever-growing day-to-day demand for patient care. Couple this with tremendous student debt accrued during medical school, insurance vexations, tremendously long hours in the clinic or operating room, and malpractice concerns, and it is no wonder that physicians spend less than fifteen minutes with a typical patient during an office visit. To paraphrase Charles Dickens, "It is the best of times, it is the worst of times" to be a physician.

Given the realities of modern medicine, we now find ourselves on the brink of a significant physician shortage in the United States. Some would argue that, throughout the course of our nation's history, there has always been a shortage of competent physicians, an argument strongly supported herein by the Russell family narrative. What people also have difficulty understanding is that medicine is a business; at least it has been that way since this nation's founding. Being a physician is demanding enough, being a successful physician/businessman is even more challenging, but being a successful physician/businessman/father in the 19th and early 20th centuries was downright hard.

The evolution of the American physician/businessman is exemplified in *A Family Practice: The Russell Doctors and the Evolving Business of Medicine, 1799–1989*. While the Russell pedigree is not unique to American medicine—many of today's physicians often come from a "long line of doctors"—tracing the lives and legacies of four generations of Russell physicians makes this an authentic American epic, not unlike the medical equivalent to Alex Haley's *Roots*. Even more fascinating are the authors' voluminous sources, both genealogical and historical, drawn upon in weaving together this saga of sojourning surgeons.

For well over two centuries, the fabric of the history of medicine in the United States has been woven with the published "threads" of physicians, nurses, pharmacists, scientists, and other traditional and non-traditional health-care providers. Yet, numerous unpublished "yarns" remain to be spun and woven into the colorful cloth of medicine's storied tapestry. The fibers for the Russell family "thread" have now been gathered, processed, and shuttled into the literary loom, providing a lasting stitch in the "white coat" of medical historiography.

BILL J. GURLEY, PH.D.
Professor of Pharmaceutical Sciences, College of Pharmacy
University of Arkansas for Medical Sciences

ACKNOWLEDGMENTS

Anyone writing a book of this magnitude covering four generations and almost 200 years of a family's history depends on the work of many others, and the authors of this book are no exception. In trying to uncover the story of the Russell family, we depended on many primary resources, including approximately 150 letters, two scrapbooks, and boxes full of photos and other items that had been collected by various family members and preserved for generations. Especially valuable was the genealogical research that William L. Russell Jr. started in the early 1970s and continues to this day. He interviewed family members, outlined the family tree, and identified where family members lived at different times during their lives, what they did for a living, etc. Ava Russell Norwood preserved family letters that were passed down to her granddaughter Sara Lee Suttle, who preserved them, as well as two scrapbooks and other items that provided impetus for Mr. Russell to investigate many areas of interest. Other family members who participated in the early years of the research included Mrs. Ruby Kitchens, Mrs. Grace Norton, Gary and Sandy Pack, Wanda Rae Dailey, Marvin Vaughter, Clayton Russell, Dr. Phillip Russell, and Dr. George W. Russell. George's three children—George Seaborn Russell, Paul Russell, and Anne Russell Zorn—played an important role in providing photographs and information about their father.

Research projects such as this are very dependent on the work, past and present, performed by staff in libraries and archives, as well as in historical and genealogical societies, courthouses, and county government offices. We are extremely grateful to the many staff members at these places who assisted in our research.

We owe special thanks to the staff of the University of Arkansas for Medical Sciences (UAMS) Library, including CaLee Henderson, Tim Nutt, Suzanne Easley, April Hughes, Margaret Johnson, and Edwina Walls Mann in the Library's Historical Research Center, who assisted in ways too numerous to mention; Susan Steelman, who assisted with literature searches; Cindy Caton and Belinda Rogers, who quickly provided us with books and journal articles not owned by the library, and Libby Ingram and the Circulation staff, who provided access to materials in the library; Loretta Edwards and Fred Bassett, who provided technical support; Nancy Sessoms and Joe Lamb, who helped identify information about Ralph Russell's *Handbook of Home Medicine*; and Jan Hart, Library Director, who assisted in many ways. Others at UAMS who were helpful include Dr. Bill Gurley, UAMS College of Pharmacy, whose advice led us to W. J. P. Russell's Civil War story, and Dr. John Shock, retired founder of the UAMS Jones Eye Institute, who helped answer questions about the history of eye surgery.

Also in Arkansas, Jessie Burchfield and Melissa Serfass at the University of Arkansas Little Rock (UALR) Bowen School of Law Library; the late Karen Russ at the UALR Ottenheimer Library; Kathleen Fowler at the Arkansas State Library; staff at the Arkansas State Archives; staff at the Bobby L. Roberts Library of Arkansas History and Culture, the UALR Center for Arkansas History and Culture, and the Butler Center for Arkansas Studies, Central Arkansas Library System; Mickey Clements, Genealogy Department at the Fayetteville Public Library; Bentley Hovis, Pulaski County Treasurer's Office; Linda Johnson, Doug DalPorto, and other staff at the Pulaski County Circuit Clerk's Office; Tony Wappel, Judy Drummond, and other staff at the Washington County Office of Archives and Records Management; Special Collections staff at the Mullins Library, University of Arkansas at Fayetteville; Kaye Holmes, Venus Allen, Jim Burgess, and others at the Greene County Historical and Genealogical Society, and staff in Greene County government offices; staff at the Franklin County Courthouse; County Judge Toby Davis, Bill Wyatt at the Perry County Highway Department, and the staffs at the Perry County Circuit Clerk, County Clerk, and Tax Assessor's offices; the Lafayette County Public Library; Lawrence McElroy and other staff at the Cane Hill Museum; Harold Ott, Bedford Camera, Little Rock; and Dr. Sam Taggart of Benton, who gave us useful advice on information resources.

In Georgia, Jay Ergle, Kennon Kewe, Ann Carey, and Susan Clay at the University of Georgia Main Library, the University of Georgia Special Collections Staff, and Mazie Bowen and others at the Hargrett Library; Renee Sharrock and Brenda Seago at the Greenblatt Library, and Historical Research Coordinator Sarah Brasswell, Medical College of Georgia, Augusta University; Julie Gaines, Head of the Augusta University/University of Georgia Medical Partnership Campus Library, Athens; the Gwinnett County Historical Society staff, including Jim Nicholls, Harriett Nicholls, Bobbie Tkacik, Rachel Schmalz, Bill Baughman, and Susan Gilbert; Gwinnett County, Clerk of Superior Court, Real Estate Division, Lawrenceville; staff at the Fairview Presbyterian Church, Lawrenceville; Lynda Noland, Macon; and Emily Corbin, archivist at the Columbia Theological Seminary Library, Decatur.

In Alabama, Craig and Susan Boden, and staff of the Etowah Historical Society and the Nicholls Genealogical Library in Gadsden; Peggy Balch and Ted Gemberling, University of Alabama at Birmingham (UAB) Lister Hill Library of the Health Sciences; staff at the Reynolds-Finley Library, Birmingham Public Library; Jim Snider, independent researcher; and Norwood Kerr, Alabama Department of Archives and History, Montgomery.

In Illinois, Wendy Winkelman, Union County Treasurer's Office; Brandi Boyd, Union County, County Clerk's Office; staff at the Union County Clerk's Office; Barbara Caspar, Jonesboro City Clerk/ Collector; and Karen Hallam, librarian, Jonesboro Public Library.

In Texas, Sherrie Archer and Cindy Cooper, Library of Genealogy and Local History, Van Zandt County Genealogical Society; Mary Ritchie and Karen Asher, Van Zandt County Appraisal Office; historian Elvis Allen, Wills Point; David Kapitan, *Wills Point Chronicle;* Pat Mitchell, Wills Point Depot Museum; Brenda Petillo, Wills Point Chamber of Commerce; staff at the Wills Point City Hall; and Kelly Gonzalez and Cameron Kainerstorfer at the University of Texas (UT) Southwestern Health Sciences Library in Dallas.

In Pennsylvania, Chrissie Perella, archivist, Historical Medical Library, The College of Physicians of Philadelphia; Timothy Horning, University of Pennsylvania Archives; Stephanie Roth, Special Collections Research Center, Ginsburg Health Sciences Library, Temple University; and Michael Barber.

In Maryland, Terry Hambrecht, MD, Senior Technical Advisor to the National Museum of Civil War Medicine, Rockville, who gave us much valuable information about W. J. P. Russell, especially his Civil War activities; Stephen Greenberg and Jeff Reznick, National Library of Medicine, National Institutes of Health; and Michael Rhode and Andre Sobocinski at the US Navy Bureau of Medicine and Surgery (BUMED) Communications Directorate Office of Medical History.

In South Carolina, Rebekah Cockrell at the Walnut Grove Plantation; staff of the Spartanburg County Regional History

Museum; and Katie Phillips at the Waring Historical Library, Medical University of South Carolina.

In Louisiana, Millie Moore and Mary Holt at the Tulane Health Sciences Library, and Debbie Sibley and Jennifer Lloyd at the Louisiana State University (LSU) Health Sciences Library, New Orleans. In Massachusetts, Pat Boulos at the Boston Athenæum, and Jack Eckert at the Francis A. Countway Library of Medicine, Harvard University, Boston. In North Carolina, Dawne Lucas at the Health Sciences Library, University of North Carolina at Chapel Hill, and Karin F. Smith, Deputy Register of Deeds, Transylvania County. In Tennessee, Jennifer Langford at the University of Tennessee Health Sciences Center Library, Memphis. In Mississippi, Misti Thornton, Rowland Medical Library, University of Mississippi Medical Center. In Washington, D.C., the US National Archives and Records Administration (NARA) and independent researcher Vonnie Zullo. In Utah, staff at the Family History Library, Church of Jesus Christ of Latter-Day Saints, Salt Lake City. In Rhode Island, Elizabeth Delmage, Naval Historical Collection, Naval War College, Newport. In New York, Chris Hoolihan and Julia Sollenberger at the Edward G. Miner Library, University of Rochester Medical Center. In Iowa, Dr. William Feis, author and professor of history at Buena Vista University, Storm Lake, whose advice, articles, and book on Civil War military intelligence were very helpful.

A special thank you goes to the Hathi Trust (www.hathitrust.org) and the member libraries that have provided many historical items to be digitized and made available online. This is a great service that deserves special recognition for facilitating research throughout the world.

We especially appreciate Mike Bieker and David Scott Cunningham at the University of Arkansas Press, who were support-ive from the very beginning of this project and helped us navigate the publication process. Thanks also to Jenny Vos, Molly Rector, and Shirley Rash, who gave indispensable assistance in the final stages of the process, and to anonymous reviewers who provided valuable feedback about the manuscript.

Most importantly, thanks to Dr. Stephen Schafer for his assis-tance and moral support throughout the project and for obtaining some research funding, and thanks to many other family members and friends who provided moral support and encouragement during the four years that it took to write this book.

A FAMILY PRACTICE

INTRODUCTION

'The time has come,' the Walrus said,
'To talk of many things:
Of shoes—and ships—and sealing-wax—
Of cabbages—and kings—'

—LEWIS CARROLL,
"The Walrus and the Carpenter"

'

This book talks of many things—if not cabbages and kings, then Vi-Be Ni tonic, orange groves, and spying for the Union army. It is a sweeping saga of four generations of doctors connected by blood, Russell men seeking innovative ways to sustain themselves as medical practitioners in the American South in a time span running from the early nineteenth to the latter half of the twentieth century.

The thread that binds the stories in this saga is one of blood, of medical vocations passed intergenerationally from fathers to sons and nephews. This study of four generations of Russell doctors is an *historical* study with a biographical thread running through it. It emphasizes historical points and employs historiographical techniques as it develops its multi-generational *historical biographical* study.[1]

This study *has* to employ a wide-ranging optic because it is examining lives whose birth years run from 1799 to 1915, of men who lived in places as diverse as the Carolinas, Georgia, Illinois, Louisiana, Mississippi, Alabama, Arkansas, Texas, Pennsylvania, and New York. Geographically, Arkansas is another thread tying together these disparate stories, since, with the exception of the founding figure of this medical dynasty, William James Russell (1799–1872), every man in the chain lived at some point in Arkansas.

William James Russell's son William James Park (W. J. P.) Russell (1830–1892) moved his family to Northwest Arkansas following the Civil War, after time in a Union prison in Tennessee on charges of

engaging in cotton-running schemes that involved top Union officers. Strong indicators suggest that he was a Union spy—though he
and wife Avarilla Octavia Dunn Law kept this secret closely guarded
throughout their lives. Their choice to move to the western border of
Arkansas abutting Indian Territory in 1866 may well have had something to do with concern to distance themselves from the places in
which W. J. P. Russell had spied for the Union during the war.

W. J. P.'s sons Seaborn Rentz (1859–1928) and Ralph Morgan
Russell (1867–1916) were reared in Arkansas and educated at Cane
Hill College in Washington County, the state's first institution of
higher learning, before their parents relocated to Texas, where W. J. P.
established a practice shared briefly with his sons. After a few years,
Seaborn returned to Arkansas and spent the rest of his medical career
in the state, working in Greene and White Counties before moving to
Perry County and finally to Little Rock, doctoring there as a general
practitioner and surgeon for the final twenty-five years of his life.

When his parents left Arkansas in 1885, Ralph headed to medical school at Bellevue Medical College in New York. While in medical school, Ralph married his cousin Mary Woodliff of Gadsden,
Alabama. After graduation in 1888, he opened a practice in Gadsden
and then Birmingham, where he established the Russell Medical
Institute following several months of study in 1895–1896 at King's
College Medical School in London. Ralph lived the rest of his years
in Birmingham, where he died at forty-nine from a stroke.

The final two doctors represented in this study, Benjamin Franklin
Norwood (1886–1942) and George Washington Russell (1915–1989),
grew up in Arkansas. Ben was the son of W. J. P. Russell's daughter Ava Leona Russell, who married Benjamin Franklin Norwood
Sr. of Stamps, Arkansas. George was Seaborn's youngest son and
was born and raised in Little Rock. Both were career naval medical
officers—Ben as a surgeon and George as a psychiatrist. Naval service provided both with opportunities to live in far-flung places and
do further study. Military assignments brought Ben and wife Anne
Parker Robinson to New York City, where he died unexpectedly, and
George to Pennsylvania. Following his military retirement in 1946,
George studied at the University of Pennsylvania Graduate School
and then directed the Bucks County Mental Health Guidance Center
in Doylestown, Pennsylvania, before moving with wife Jeanette

Roberts and their children to the Poconos and establishing the Russell Psychiatric Clinic, which he directed for his final twenty-five years.

So, geographical and blood ties connect the four generations of doctors studied here. In addition, thematic connections link their stories. This multi-generational line of practitioners exhibited marked concern to find innovative ways to make their practices economically robust, often under trying conditions that thwarted this goal. The patriarch William James Russell established a tradition of surgical specialization that became the lynchpin of the practices of his son W. J. P. and W. J. P.'s sons Seaborn and Ralph—even as each also branched out into other areas.

With W. J. P. Russell and his sons, the surgical focus became the centerpiece of an interesting traveling practice, a peripatetic medical show of sorts, as they took their surgery on the road, moving from area to area performing corrective surgeries for ophthalmic conditions such as strabismus and for other congenital problems like cleft lip and clubfoot.

The Russell doctors also augmented the often erratic income they garnered through their practices with canny investments and supplemental business ventures—an approach used by many doctors over the course of medical history in the US. When it comes to creative ways to generate income through para-medical schemes, perhaps the most interesting of the Russell doctors is Ralph, whose Birmingham Institute marketed his own remedies, including Vi-Be Ni tonic and the Electrozone, a device for which he made fantastic medical claims. The Institute was connected to a mail-order business built around Ralph's *Handbook of Home Medicine*, a compendium of diagnostic and therapeutic information standing within a long tradition of self-help books in American medicine.

Handbook of Home Medicine was mailed to customers, who were invited to inform Ralph through "symptom blanks" of their medical issues and to receive his advice—accompanied by drugs manufactured by his staff, though, as we'll see, Ralph's claim to have "staff" at his Birmingham operation was quite an overstatement. In key respects, by developing his Institute, Ralph was continuing his father's peripatetic practice in an inventive new way—albeit one that raises questions about where the line should be drawn between quackery and *bona fide* practice.

In the last generation of Russell doctors, with cousins Ben and George, we find less need to fashion secure economic moorings for their work, since by their generation, requirements for medical practice, including educational ones, had been firmly established. This assured that the discipline of medicine became, by the twentieth century, a highly regarded professional enterprise that was remunerative for many medical practitioners. Ben and George did not have to go to the lengths of generations before them to assure that they had solid income.

Strong interest in sound medical education also links the generations of Russell doctors. Though it appears that William James Russell lacked formal medical education—as almost all practitioners of his period did—he had a sound classical education and did a preceptorship with Dr. Andrew Barry Moore, who had studied under the famous early American physician Benjamin Rush. He trained with noted surgeon Dr. Charles Harris, as well. Of the doctors on whom this book focuses, only Seaborn appears to have lacked any formal medical education, though it is clear that he was well trained by his father in the preceptorial way in which most doctors were trained before formal medical education became a precondition for practicing medicine. It appears that Seaborn did take courses at the College of Physicians and Surgeons in Little Rock but did not complete the requirements for a degree.

Another dominant motif of this study: In each generation, these men had strong women backing them—wives sharing their lives and sacrifices and keeping their families together as their husbands worked to build prosperous practices. This multi-generational study of a *group of men* practicing medicine is simultaneously a study of *some exceptionally resolute women* who were co-investors in the practices their husbands established.

One final introductory note: This study is co-authored by three people—William L. Russell, Mary L. Ryan, and William D. Lindsey. The text uses the first-person plural pronoun repeatedly not to employ a royal "we" but because it was authored collaboratively by three hands. Bill Russell has decades of experience researching the Russell family, his own family. A retired professor of communications, he has accumulated a wealth of family documents, including a precious cache of letters and other material that provided a primary leg on which this book stands.

Mary, who worked for over forty years in health sciences libraries, provided other crucial legs of this study through assiduous digging in archival holdings and gathering, reading, and annotating any number of studies of American medical history. She and Bill Russell also conducted on-the-ground research over a period of several years in various places, including Wills Point, Texas; Birmingham and Gadsden, Alabama; Lawrenceville, Georgia; Spartanburg, South Carolina; and Philadelphia, Pennsylvania.

Bill Lindsey, a retired college administrator and professor of historical theology, connects to the other Bill through Seaborn Russell's first wife, Alcie Bachelor, who is Bill Russell's great-grandmother and a cousin in Bill Lindsey's family tree. Several years ago, the two Bills collaborated on a study of Alcie's father Dr. Wilson R. Bachelor entitled *Fiat Flux*.[2]

The co-authorship of this book has provided three distinctly different perspectives on the Russell doctors studied here. At times, we have seen their lives differently and read various documents outlining those lives through different optics. We did not always entirely agree with each other's interpretations of evidence.

In our view, the diversity of perspectives and backgrounds enriches this study. It also assures that the scope the study employs is broad and reflects the diverse interests and perspectives of three collaborators, as it moves from musings about medical history and distinctions between quackery and real medicine, to what was happening in Nashville during the Civil War, to lovesick letters written by an overworked naval doctor who spent his days in World War II patching up wounded soldiers and his evenings burying bodies at sea. We hope you will agree that our collaborative approach has made the book an intriguing and worthwhile read.

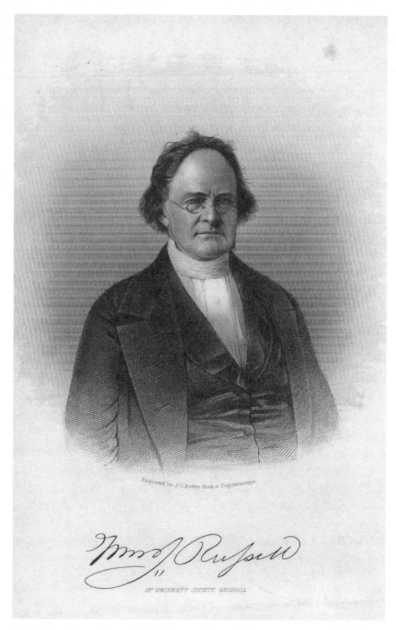

Engraved by J.C.Buttre from a Daguerreotype

OF GWINNETT COUNTY, GEORGIA.

Dr. William James Russell of Gwinnett County, Georgia, circa 1855, by John
Chester Buttre, 1821–1893. *Courtesy of the Boston Athenæum.*

CHAPTER I

William James Russell
(1799–1872)

Native talent struggling with the dark adversities
of fortune, and rising superior to her frown, has
ever commanded the admiration of the world.

—JOHN LIVINGSTON,
Portraits of Eminent Americans Now Living:
With Biographical and Historical Memoirs
of Their Lives and Actions[1]

Birth and Early Life

As with so many stories, William James Russell's begins with a rags-to-riches theme of overcoming daunting adversity by hard work. In the words of John Livingston,

> He never knew a father's care, nor received a father's blessing, nor inherited a patrimonial estate. His father died some months antecedent to his birth. An orphan from infancy, he became the architect of his own fortunes and character.[2]

Livingston adds,

> As we have already noticed, he was born in a state of orphanage, and destitute of those pecuniary facilities for entering successfully upon the duties and trials of life, which the more affluent possess; yet young Russell, impelled by an ardent and aspiring spirit, and thirsting for knowledge and distinction, went forth in his fourteenth year, to battle it with the difficulties and adversities of life. To obtain a competent education

was his fixed purpose. Without means, yet buoyant with hope, he was therefore during several years alternately engaged in the business of *teaching* and being *taught*. The proceeds of one year's toil in the schoolroom, was expended the next in the prosecution of his studies.[3]

William James Russell was born 24 August 1799 near Concord in Cabarrus County, North Carolina. His father William was the son of James Russell, an immigrant from County Antrim, Ireland, who came to North Carolina from Pennsylvania in the early 1760s. William died 13 February 1799, six months before his son was born.[4]

And there is more adversity: We know from Cabarrus County records that a nasty dispute arose about the paternity of William James following the death of his grandfather on 20 February 1799. The dispute centered on whether he had a legal right to an inheritance from his grandfather since his paternity had been called into question by some of James's heirs. Court minutes indicate that an arbitration committee ruled in October 1801 that William James was a legitimate son of William and thus a legitimate heir of James entitled to a portion of the grandfather's estate. That portion—£127 3p and 240 acres of land in lieu of 600 silver dollars—was allotted to him in October 1803 and April 1804.[5] As the estate was being settled, young Russell was placed in the care of James Scott on 23 April 1801 and then William Means on 10 October 1802.[6]

All this happened before William J. Russell reached five years and after his mother Sarah McCree Russell had remarried on 19 March 1803 to Major John Alexander and moved to South Carolina with him and her son. Alexander was made William's guardian following the marriage.[7] An officer in the American Revolution, he was from Spartanburg County, South Carolina, and an elder of Fairview Presbyterian Church in contiguous Greenville County.[8] These biographical details provide the context for Livingston's observation (reported to him probably by Russell himself) that William J. was not set up by the circumstances of birth and upbringing to find an easy path to education when he chose a medical vocation. As Livingston's biography adds, such medical schools as existed in this period in the US were in New York and Philadelphia, and Russell's finances did not permit him to attend these.[9]

We are emphasizing this rags-to-riches motif because it will recur

in the generations who followed William James in practicing medicine. In different respects, his descendants who were doctors, down
to the generation of his great-grandsons, would also struggle to find
educational and economic footing in a world in which it was not easy
for a practitioner to make a living.

In addition, rumors about the character of William J. Russell's
mother would bedevil him in his adult life even after he had established
himself as a well-regarded doctor. In 1832, his wife Sophia Park Russell
was called before their church, Fairview Presbyterian in Lawrenceville,
Georgia, and charged with having slandered her mother-in-law by suggesting that Sarah had given birth five months after her marriage to
William Russell—a charge without foundation since a tombstone in
the Old Rocky River Presbyterian Cemetery near Concord in which
William Russell is buried indicates that the couple, who married in
August 1797, had a daughter born 4 May 1798 who died two days later.[10]
More adversity to overcome: Russell's obituary in his hometown paper
will sum up his life story by stressing this same theme.[11]

Education

No surviving documents make clear what influenced William J.
Russell to undertake a medical vocation. By his first wife Elizabeth
Williamson, Russell's stepfather had a son Thomas Williamson
Alexander (1790–1840), some years older than William J., who had
chosen to study medicine, and that family connection may well have
set the course for Russell as he entered the same career.[12]

Livingston's account states that, as a boy of fourteen, Russell began
his formal schooling, as well as his teaching career, the latter providing
him resources to further his own education. Several pieces of information allow us to infer that Russell began studying and teaching at
a school connected to a local doctor in Spartanburg County, South
Carolina. This was Andrew Barry Moore.

A. Education: Andrew Barry Moore,
Spartanburg County, South Carolina

Andrew Barry Moore (1771–1848) was the first educated physician in
Spartanburg County of whom we have record.[13] Moore was born 11

February 1771 at the Walnut Grove Plantation of his father Charles
and died there on 23 January 1848.[14] Uncorroborated family traditions
state that Charles was a man of some formal education who may have
studied at either Trinity College in Dublin or Oxford University. In
1770, he established one of the first schools in the county, the Rocky
Spring Academy, near Walnut Grove. He taught in this school, and
his son Andrew was educated there.[15]

In a March 1889 letter to J. B. O. Landrum that Landrum transcribes in his *History of Spartanburg County*, Thomas J. Moore states
that the graduates of Rocky Spring and Minerva Academies, the
county's first two schools, readily entered highly regarded colleges.
After being educated at Rocky Spring (and perhaps also Minerva),
Andrew B. Moore graduated from Dickinson College in Carlisle,
Pennsylvania, in 1795. He then studied medicine under noted doctor
Benjamin Rush in Philadelphia before returning home to practice
medicine and mentor students in Spartanburg County.[16]

At the time William J. Russell studied and taught at Rocky
Spring, the academy operated under the auspices of the Spartanburg
Philanthropic Society, established in 1794. However, even after this
society assumed control, Andrew B. Moore retained a close connec-
tion to the school since it was situated on his father's plantation, where
Andrew lived and practiced medicine after his father's death in 1805.[17]
His medical office at Walnut Grove has been preserved and is main-
tained as a museum by the Spartanburg County Historical Society.

The artifacts from Moore's practice held by the museum provide
a glimpse into how doctors did business in this region in the early
19th century. They include forceps Moore used to extract teeth and his
porcelain bleeding bowl. Moore's journals from 1800–1815 state that
the cost of a tooth extraction was two dollars, with an additional fifty
cents if one wanted rum to dull the pain of the procedure.[18] The journals indicate that though he charged his patients in pounds, shillings,
pence or dollars and cents, he was frequently paid in whiskey, cloth,
pen knives, saddlebags, locks, and the services of a cobbler.[19]

B. Education: The Preceptorial Method

After his stint of teaching and studying with Dr. Moore, William J.
Russell returned to Cabarrus County, North Carolina, in 1818 and

placed himself under the tutelage of Dr. Charles Harris. As Livingston explains,

> Here he continued some two or more years, when he was taken into co-partnership by his instructor in the practice of medicine, Doctor Harris giving him one-fourth of the proceeds, by which he was enabled to defray his expenses, and still continue his studies when not engaged in the active duties of his profession.[20]

The academy in which Russell studied as he apprenticed himself to Harris was associated with Reverend John Robinson's Poplar Tent Presbyterian Church. Charles Harris and John Robinson were co-instructors in the school.[21] The preceptorial method by which Russell learned medicine was far from unusual in this period. In fact, for a lengthy period of time, education by apprenticeship was the norm for those learning to doctor in the colonies and the states formed from them after the American Revolution. As William Frederick Norwood indicates, in colonial America medical preceptorship followed the rubric used in other apprenticeships, a seven-year period being the rule of thumb.[22] After the Revolution, the term began to shift to three years.[23] Martin Kaufman notes that the vast majority of American physicians were trained through apprenticeship until well into the nineteenth century.[24]

The aspiring practitioner often signed a formal contract of apprenticeship.[25] As Norwood notes, the distinguished early American physician, Benjamin Rush, with whom Andrew B. Moore had studied, was apprenticed for five-and-one-half years to John Redman of Philadelphia, a Leyden graduate who had studied at Paris and Edinburgh and was a consulting physician at the Pennsylvania Hospital.[26] Upon the completion of apprenticeship, the apprentice received a certificate from the preceptor.[27]

The preceptorial system continued after medical schools began to be established, and, indeed, through much of the nineteenth century in many areas of the United States. Of those students who entered medical school in the colonial and early statehood periods, only a minor portion ever graduated.[28]

This American system is distinct from the British and European systems during this period. As John Duffy notes, physicians in 17th-

and 18th-century Europe were university-trained; this assured that almost all practitioners came from backgrounds of affluence and prestige.[29] As a result, European and British doctors tended to treat people of their own social class, guaranteeing them a reliable, stable income.

By contrast, the fluidity of American society made it impossible to maintain the sharp distinction between physicians, surgeons, and apothecaries that characterized the British and European systems.[30] In America, doctors were not only expected to treat a wide range of illnesses and assist at childbirth and deathbeds but also perform surgery and compound and dispense medicine. As Duffy indicates, few highly educated doctors were to be found in the colonies.[31] He adds:

> Following the American Revolution, the ties with England and Europe were understandably loosened, and Americans were reluctant to seek medical training abroad. As of 1800, only four medical schools were in existence to supply America's growing need for doctors.[32]

As with medical training in general in this period, surgery was taught in the United States primarily through apprenticeship.[33] The hands-on method of learning by watching and doing might, in some cases, be augmented by access to physicians' libraries, which often included European textbooks—though the possibility for students trained by preceptorship to have access to such resources was slimmer for those in frontier areas where books were less accessible.[34]

Because of the key role that surgery played in the practices of William J. Russell and his son and grandsons, a brief overview of the history of surgical training in American medical schools in the eighteenth and nineteenth centuries is in order. Surgery was taught formally at the first medical school in the colonies, the College of Philadelphia (later the University of Pennsylvania), established in 1765. One of the school's original faculty members, John Morgan, believed in the advantages of specialization, stating that if surgeons and physicians had specific assignments, "each would become more skillful and dexterous in his respective parts." In Morgan's view, surgeons should spend their time practicing surgery while physicians "needed time to study . . . patients and their illnesses."[35]

Surgery was also taught at King's College (now Columbia University) by John Jones in the late 1700s. Jones was perhaps the best-known surgeon in the colonies. His 1775 volume *Plain Concise Practical*

Remarks on the Treatment of Wounds and Fractures, the first medical book published in the United States, was invaluable to the Continental Army's field surgeons during the Revolutionary War. Jones emphasized that surgical skill was both manual and medical, requiring students to become familiar with all branches of medicine while gaining in-depth knowledge of anatomy by dissection and experience.[36]

Later, the American surgical tradition would be enhanced by William Gibson, who studied with leading British surgeons before becoming professor of surgery at Philadelphia in 1819. Under his preceptorship, students learned through lectures and by observing surgeons at work at the Pennsylvania Hospital and the city almshouse. Gibson's *The Institutes and Practice of Surgery* became a standard manual for training American surgeons.[37]

Also significant was the work of Frank Hamilton, who taught surgery at three medical colleges before teaching at Bellevue Hospital Medical College in New York from 1861 to 1875. Stating that physicians "must cut as well as cure," Hamilton emphasized the importance of careful study of anatomy and of learning medicine in addition to surgery.[38] Hamilton published eight editions of *A Practical Treatise on Fractures and Dislocations* between 1860 and 1891.

In addition to the seminal texts just mentioned, one should note Samuel Gross's popular study *A System of Surgery* (1859), which by 1872 reached a fifth edition of two volumes, each with over 1,000 pages. Gross placed strong emphasis on the importance of both principles and techniques of surgery, maintaining, "A Work on surgery . . . without principles, may be compared to a vessel at sea without helm or rudder to guide it to its place of destination."[39]

How and what students were taught about surgery in the late 1700s and first half of the 1800s varied considerably depending on the quality of mentors and access to schools, textbooks, and hospitals, where patients provided hands-on learning opportunities. In the 1860s, the Jefferson Medical School in Philadelphia was fortunate to have two outstanding surgeons on faculty, Samuel Gross and Joseph Pancoast, the latter teaching anatomy.

A student of Gross, J. Collins Warren, commented on his teaching style as follows:

> A most painstaking instructor, Gross hammered on the rudiments of surgery with a clearness and force which commanded the attention of the class and left an impression never to be

forgotten. Instinctively he selected the small details of rudimentary knowledge for which the student mind was craving and dwelt upon them with patient care. . . . By understanding how to keep on the level of his audience, he kept his lectures both popular and instructive. This was in strong contrast to the many prominent medical lecturers of the day. . . . [40]

Due to the growing influence of the French method of teaching surgery, purely clinical schools similar to those prevalent in Europe began to develop in the 1860s, including Bellevue in New York, which Russell's grandson Ralph Russell would attend in 1887–1888. The strong emphasis on clinical practice at Bellevue and similar schools is evident in the insistence of Bellevue's Stephen Smith that too many medical schools taught surgery in an "excessively didactic" way:

They teach theories and systems, but they do not teach practical medicine. They educate the brain, but leave the hand palsied, the eye blind, and the ear deaf. Their graduates go forth to practical life like full-fledged eaglets deprived of wings. [41]

Despite the attempt of prominent US schools to offer strong clinical training in surgery, most still provided very little clinical experience to the end of the nineteenth century. With most teaching hospitals having fewer than one operation per day, surgery was still uncommon. In 1883 there were only 48 operations at the 450-bed City and County Hospital of San Francisco, and only 291 at New Orleans's Charity Hospital in 1890. [42]

The sub-optimal state of medical education in the US from colonial times until the early 1900s resulted in many American students traveling to Europe for schooling, as W. J. P. Russell's son Ralph did, studying at King's College in London after graduating from Bellevue. In the estimation of Thomas Bonner, nearly 15,000 American students studied at German medical schools between 1870 and 1914. [43]

C. Education: Charles Wilson Harris, Cabarrus County, North Carolina

William J. Russell's second medical mentor, surgeon-doctor Charles Harris (1762–1825), "taught at his home probably the first medical school" in North Carolina, according to Kemp Plummer Battle. [44]

One of the first physicians in his region, Harris brought to his practice a strong education.[45] Having studied under Dr. Isaac Alexander of Camden, South Carolina, he completed his formal studies at the University of Pennsylvania School of Medicine, where he studied with Benjamin Rush, who also taught Russell's first preceptor Andrew B. Moore.[46] D. M. Furches, an acquaintance of Harris's family, sums up his contribution to early medical education in North Carolina as follows:

> I knew that . . . Dr. Charles Harris, of that county [i.e., Cabarrus], was the leading physician of this section of the State; that he established the first medical school in the State where young men were taught the science of medicine. . . .[47]

As North Carolina historian John Hill Wheeler notes,

> Devoted to his profession, he [i.e., Charles W. Harris] was unrivaled as a physician and surgeon. His reputation was widely extended, and his skill and success justified this celebrity. He had a medical school, and instructed ninety three young men in the healing art.[48]

A letter his nephew wrote his brother from Harris's Favoni plantation in February 1799 suggests the kind of medical treatments his uncle taught students. The letter states that, feeling unwell, Harris's nephew had prescribed for himself "a regular course of the Rushonion, or Sangradian practice of physic," with positive results.[49] As H. M. Wagstaff explains,

> The Rushonion or Sangradian practice of physic was the practice of copious blood-letting as a cure for numerous human ills. Dr. Benjamin Rush, of Philadelphia, a signer of the Declaration of Independence, was its chief exponent of use in America during the latter decade of the 18th century. . . . [During the yellow fever epidemic of 1793] [h]is method of treatment was to give doses of calomel and jalap, bleed freely, and drench the patient, within and without, with warm water.[50]

John Hill Wheeler's observation that Charles Harris excelled at surgery is an important historical detail to keep in mind as we look at the practices of the generations of doctors whose progenitor William J. Russell was trained by Harris with a strong focus on surgical treatment. The medical education that Harris gave Russell evidently had a multi-generational effect.

We know of Russell's study with Harris from Livingston's biography, which speaks of the "co-partnership" as Russell studied in North Carolina. William S. Harris's history of the Poplar Tent Presbyterian Church in Cabarrus County also states that Dr. William Russell was one of a number of young men "distinguished in the healing art" educated by Reverend John Robinson at Poplar Tent Academy.[51]

Robinson was pastor of the Poplar Tent Church from 1808 to 1818.[52] His teacher, Robert Archibald, who became Poplar Tent's pastor about 1785, was a Princeton graduate (1772) who had studied medicine before being licensed by the Presbytery of Orange in 1775.[53] Robinson had also had medical training in Charlotte from a Dr. Henderson. Robert H. Morrison writes,

> He [i.e., John Robinson] received part of his classical education in the town of Charlotte, in an Academy taught by Dr. Henderson, an eminent physician, in the old College building, and part in the neighbourhood of Poplar Tent, in an Academy taught by a Mr. Archibald.[54]

As William S. Harris indicates in summing up John Robinson's contribution to the history of medical education in North Carolina, "There was a large number of young men educated by this illustrious preceptor, who adorned the medical profession and stamped their usefulness on every walk of life."[55] According to Dorothy Long, a notice in the *Raleigh Register* in 1811 indicates that by that year, Harris and Robinson had educated about ninety students.[56]

Before we leave the topic of Russell's education, it is worth noting that the strong interest in education exhibited by Russell and his descendants extended to female family members.[57] Russell sent his oldest daughter Mary Catherine to Salem College in North Carolina. Established in 1772, it is the oldest educational institution for women in the United States. The college register shows Mary Catherine matriculating on 13 June 1840 but leaving school on 27 May 1842 to attend to her mother Sophia during her last illness.[58]

D. Education: Influence of Benjamin Rush

As noted, William J. Russell's mentors, Andrew B. Moore and Charles Harris, both studied with the eminent early American physician Benjamin Rush (1746–1813) in Philadelphia, where the first clinical instruction in medicine was offered in the United States.[59] For this reason, Rush deserves attention as a strong formative influence on Russell's medical education via Moore and Harris.

As biographer Carl Binger notes, Rush was one of the leading medical teachers in the period of early statehood: From 1790, the year before his appointment as a professor at the University of Pennsylvania School of Medicine, to 1812, the year before his death, the number of students he taught increased from 45 to 332.[60] In addition, Rush took on private apprentices; in 1790, there were six of these, and in later years, their numbers increased from fifteen to thirty.[61] The students and apprentices came from all thirteen of the new nation's states.[62]

Rush entered Princeton in 1759 and had not reached fifteen years when he received the bachelor's degree in 1760.[63] He then apprenticed himself for some six years to John Redman of Philadelphia[64] before graduating from the University of Edinburgh in 1768 with a doctorate in medicine.[65] In 1796, when Andrew B. Moore was studying with him, Rush was elected professor of the practice of physic at University of Pennsylvania's medical school.[66]

As historian William Frederick Norwood notes, Edinburgh-trained physicians exerted strong influence on American medical education in this formative period.[67] Rush was a primary conduit of this influence: he popularized Edinburgh-trained John Brown's theory from *Elementa medicinae* (1780) that illness represents a dynamic imbalance of forces and results from over- or under-stimulation of the organism.[68] Rush's notorious "glorification of bleeding"[69] had much to do with Brown's theory that bleeding restored balance within the organism. This is a questionable conclusion when, as Norwood notes, "As Shryock has expressed it, 'Anyone could see that if the patient were bled long enough he would—sooner or later—relax!'"[70]

As Alex Berman observes, Rush's emphasis on bleeding and the "heroic" approach to treatment proved strongly determinative for American medicine well into the nineteenth century.[71] Nor was bleeding the sum total of heroic treatment: As David Dary indicates, the "dreaded triad of heroic medicine" included purging and dosing patients with emetics, too.[72] In Rush's own practice, sweating and blistering accompanied bleeding, purging, and vomiting.[73]

Fielding Garrison points out that among illnesses Rush sought to treat with "copious blood-letting" was yellow fever. Garrison also notes the influence of English physician Thomas Sydenham (1624–1689) in the extent to which Rush relied on bleeding.[74] Through Rush, who had overweening influence in early American medical journals including *Medical Repository* and *Philadelphia Medical Museum*, the heroic practices of bleeding, purging, sweating, blistering, and dosing with emetics became excessively prescribed treatments in American medicine in the eighteenth and nineteenth centuries.[75]

Other aspects of Rush's work also had seminal influence. In the words of biographer Dagobert Runes, Rush was an "indefatigable student of natural science" who made a point of questioning people from all walks of life about matters of natural science.[76] Rush stressed to students that practitioners gain knowledge not only through schooling but also from experience. He encouraged students to pay close attention to what nurses and others skilled in healing, including elderly women, slaves, and native peoples, might tell them about medical matters.[77] This democratic approach with openness to the therapeutic wisdom of the native peoples was to have significant influence in American medical thinking in the nineteenth century.[78]

As his biographer Binger notes, in response to student queries, Rush also developed "a kind of medical mail-order business or correspondence course."[79] In some American medical circles, this mail-order approach to dispensing medical information would prove well-nigh normative for years to come: William J. Russell's grandson Ralph made this a cornerstone of his medical practice in the twentieth century.

In important ways, Benjamin Rush was a bridge between the very different medical worldviews of the eighteenth and nineteenth centuries. As Garrison notes, the eighteenth century was, in terms of medical thought, an "age of theories and systems."[80] The Revolution interrupted the theorizing, however, and disrupted organized medical instruction for North Americans, cutting practitioners off for a period of time from their British and European counterparts.[81]

Five medical schools existed in the United States before 1800— the University of Pennsylvania (1765); King's College, New York

(1767) (later the Medical Faculty of Columbia College [1792]); Harvard (1782); the College of Philadelphia (1790); and the Medical School of Dartmouth College (1797).[82] Of these, two—the College of Philadelphia and King's College in New York—dealt with the fragmentation of theoretical approaches to treatment by entering into open rivalry at the end of the eighteenth century. The dissolution of theoretical consensus in the field of medicine meant that students were now offered a variety of approaches to treatment, some conflicting with each other.[83]

The disruption of medical education during the Revolution, with the disputes about what constituted state-of-the-art practice, opened the door for another significant development as the nineteenth century got underway: This was the adoption of French methods, particularly in the field of surgery. Outside France, interest in surgery had previously been limited—in part, due to popular aversion to autopsies and dissection, which long delayed the development of clinical and pathological anatomy in American medicine.[84]

By the second decade of the nineteenth century, the French methods and stress on surgery began to make significant inroads in American medical practice.[85] Medical journals, which French schools had pioneered following the establishment of the first academic journal in Europe, *Journal des Scavans* in 1665, began to proliferate in the United States.[86] *Medical Repository*, the first American medical journal, began publication in 1797, and by 1850, over 200 journals were being published. These included *Carolina Journal of Medicine, Science and Agriculture* (Charleston), which began in 1825, and *Southern Medical and Surgical Journal*, established in Augusta, Georgia, in 1836.[87]

The movement away from systematic theories and the development of rival schools in American medicine led to heated disputes between several competing medical "sects" as the nineteenth century unfolded.[88] The largest and most influential of these were the Thomsonian, homeopathic, and hydropathic schools.[89]

Thomsonian medicine, which drew on the "eclectic" ideas of Wooster Beach (1794–1868), who founded the Reformed Medical Society of the United States in New York in 1829, promoted the use of herbs and roots as an alternative to "heroic" treatment.[90] Building on this foundation, New Hampshire farmer Samuel Thomson (1769–1843), who learned much of his lore from a local herbalist, established a system that relied heavily on "steaming, peppering, and puking" patients with botanic agents—in particular, lobelia, an emetic long used by native peoples. Because of the ease with which it could be used in home contexts, the Thomsonian system was considered ideal for the medical needs of the new republic as it expanded westward.[91]

As Ronald Numbers and Myrl Ebert explain, in the 1820s and 1830s, the Thomsonian approach began to be promoted widely beyond New England, with agents fanning out through the South and West offering "family rights" to Thomson's guidelines. In 1806, Thomson began offering these "rights" for sale at $20. A family buying "family rights" received Thomson's instruction booklet *Family Botanic Medicine* and enrollment in his Friendly Botanic Society.[92] Again: a century later, William J. Russell's grandson Ralph would employ some of these same marketing techniques.

By the 1820s, Thomson had produced a more substantial booklet, *New Guide to Health*, which was sold in tandem with his autobiography. A German edition was compiled for immigrants in the Midwest in the first part of the 1800s. By 1840, Thomson had sold approximately 100,000 family rights and estimated that some three million people had adopted his system. In far-flung places like Arkansas, where doctors were scarce and people were eager for home guides to treatment, Thomson's *New Guide* had become by mid-century something of a bible for many.[93]

As Numbers notes, the Thomsonian rallying cry "Every man his own physician!" appealed to the Jacksonian temper of the times, as did the suggestion that the initial outlay of money for Thomson's guide and supplies would allow families to avoid doctor bills.[94] By the 1840s, as Thomsonianism waned and homeopathic treatment waxed, the do-it-yourself trend of family treatment remained an established part of American medical life as homeopaths also hawked "domestic kits" stocked with herbals and guides to their use for home treatment.[95]

The stage was set, then, as William J. Russell launched his medical career in Georgia, with its population after the Revolution due to in-migration of land-hungry settlers from the Carolinas, Virginia, and the Middle Colonies. There, he would find a ready market for medicine he had learned from Moore, Harris, and Robinson, in which Rush's influence was strong. This influence would have caused Russell's practice to rely on the heroic approach. It would perhaps also have predisposed him to use of herbal remedies later popularized by Beach and Thomson, treatment in which we know from his lectures that Rush, too, had an interest.

Russell's medical practice also definitely emphasized surgery, an emphasis bequeathed to him by Harris, whose tombstone inscription indicates that he was preeminent in the practice of surgery.[96] When Russell established his practice in Georgia, this surgical emphasis would have placed him on the cutting edge of medicine in his period as surgical treatment expanded in American practice in the first decades of the nineteenth century.

Move to Georgia

In the spring of 1821, as an unmarried man not yet twenty-two, William J. Russell moved to Georgia. He was following his mother and stepfather, who had left South Carolina for Georgia the preceding year. Russell's motivation for the move was to set up a medical practice there. Livingston writes,

> Having passed several years of private study under the care of the best medical instructors which the country afforded, and having seen much practice in the department of both medicine and surgery, he determined to offer himself at once to the public as a practising physician.[97]

Georgia was an obvious choice for a young man with medical training in the Carolinas looking for a market for his practice. The invention of the cotton gin in the late 1790s spurred the extension of a slave economy to the old Southwest, with Georgia playing a leading role in this as it claimed territory that later became Alabama and Mississippi.[98] The market for land (and slave labor) was brisk in Georgia after the Revolution, such that, as Edward Baptist notes, "Georgia men" became a byword for the extension of the slave system, with its close ties to a global economic network enriching members of the American owning class and many others internationally.[99]

After the Revolution, Georgia counties issued land grants to veterans from within the state and honored applications by veterans from other states who wanted to settle there. These land incentives coupled with the development of the cotton gin and the expansion of a slave economy spurred migration into the state.[100] At the same time, the Carolinas were experiencing economic difficulties, causing an exodus of families, including wealthy slaveholders, with many of these families choosing Georgia as their new residence.[101] In choosing Georgia, Russell was choosing not only a promising market for his medical services but also a place in which kinfolk and former acquaintances were settling.

Russell initially settled in Morgan County in middle Georgia in June 1821. Livingston notes that he chose this area because it was "sickly" and suited to his purpose of establishing a practice.[102] After Russell was prostrated for a year by bilious fever, a seasonal fever common in lower-lying areas, he decided that "health and comfort were to be preferred to wealth and disease" and relocated to North Georgia, where the climate was considered healthier.[103]

Settling in Gwinnett County

Livingston presents Russell's decision to relocate to North Georgia as motivated by his desire to find a healthier place to live. It is important to note, however, that Gwinnett County, where he chose to settle in 1823, had just been founded, and as its seat Lawrenceville was being established, there were also significant economic opportunities for an enterprising young doctor.

After Gwinnett was established in 1818, Lawrenceville was laid off in 1821 by Elisha Winn, whose son-in-law William Maltbie named the town.[104] Kinship ties would bind the Winn-Maltbie-Russell-Alexander families together after Russell's arrival in Lawrenceville.

After Winn purchased lots to start Gwinnett's courthouse town and William Towers sited the courthouse in 1821, Lawrenceville began to develop. James Flanigan notes,

> The county officials began to buy lots on which to erect homes; prospective merchants attended the auction sales and stores, built with logs, were constructed around the square. A lawyer came along and looked for a place to hang out his shingle. A boarding house, among the first dwellings erected, did a rushing business.[105]

In relocating to Lawrenceville, Russell was moving to a courthouse town just being set up in a section rapidly being settled, where auspicious prospects waited. As a young doctor just establishing himself, he would place himself on the ground floor of the new community's professional life, where, as Flanigan also notes, doctors and lawyers began renting offices as soon as Lawrenceville began.[106] He obviously undertook the move from Morgan to Gwinnett County not merely for health reasons but also due to canny calculation about Lawrenceville's future. He wanted to position himself as a leading doctor of the town by arriving as it was being built.[107]

It should also be noted that Russell was setting up his practice as the profession of medicine was being officially established in Georgia. Steps had been taken by 1785 to create a medical college in the state. In 1804, Savannah doctors secured a charter for the Georgia Medical Society. In July 1808, the *Augusta Herald* published a call for a statewide medical association, but no permanent organization was founded until 1822 when the Medical Society of Augusta was established. In 1829, this society collaborated with Dr. Milton Antony to set up the Medical Academy of Georgia.[108] Russell's decision to open his practice in the early 1820s as Georgia developed medical organizations was calculated to position him as a leader in the state's developing medical community.

As James Cassedy indicates, it was common in this period for physicians to help establish new communities in the South and West or to settle in such places soon after they were founded.[109] The need for doctors was especially pronounced on the growing edge of the frontier in the first half of the nineteenth century.[110] Cassedy also observes that it was not uncommon for doctors to dabble in politics or speculate in business ventures in new towns: "Not a few had businesses on the side—banks, stores, interests in railroads."[111] As we'll see, Russell will fit this description as he toys with the idea of a political career, invests in a cotton mill, and, so it appears, speculates in railroad investments.[112]

The wisdom of Russell's calculations is apparent as Lawrenceville quickly became not only a courthouse town but an educational, professional, and market center, as well. In 1828, Elisha Winn was instrumental in helping start Lawrenceville Academy with Reverend Dr. John S. Wilson, who had arrived in Lawrenceville in 1824 as pastor of the newly founded Fairview Presbyterian Church, of which Russell was a charter member.[113] Russell was also involved in the establishment of the academy: His name appears in a 23 December 1826 act of the state legislature naming trustees for schools in Gwinnett County.[114] Lawrenceville Academy was a boys' academy. In 1838, a female school was opened and named Lawrenceville Female Seminary.[115]

Establishing a Medical Practice and Raising a Family in Lawrenceville

What we learn about William J. Russell's life following his move to Lawrenceville we glean largely from sources other than Livingston, who passes over the 1823–1854 period in relative silence, noting that Russell acquired "a handsome competence" in these years but did not become "so rich as some others would have been, having his various advantages, and lucrative business, with a less charitable heart."[116]

Livingston does note[117] Russell's marriages in 1825 and 1845. On 14 November 1825 in Morgan County, Russell married Sophia A. Park Davenport, daughter of James Daniel Park, a Revolutionary War veteran, and Phebe Hogue. Sophia was the widow of Burkett Davenport, who died in November 1824 following their marriage in March 1824.[118]

Around the time of his marriage, Russell built a house at 106–108 Oak Street in Lawrenceville, in which he and Sophia raised their family as he doctored in a home office, a typical arrangement. Local historians have suggested that the house may have been the oldest house standing in Lawrenceville in the early 1980s when attempts were made to place it on the National Register of Historic Places. Unfortunately, the house was destroyed by fire not long after these efforts began.[119]

William J. and Sophia raised three children there: Mary Phebe Catherine (1827–1907), who married Bryant E. Strickland, son of Milza Strickland and Sarah S. Watkins; William James Park (1830–1892), who married Avarilla Octavia Dunn Law, daughter of James Franklin Law and Polly Ingram; and Wallace Randolph Chamberlain (1833–1883), who married 1) Julia English and 2) Martha Gray. Two other children—Sarah Amanda (1826–1827) and Richard Henry Harrison (1837–1843)—died in childhood.[120]

In February 1826, Russell was elected to the Fairview Presbyterian board of trustees.[121] Church minutes show him encountering trouble when the session censured him in August for fighting.[122] Brawling appears to have been an endemic problem in early Gwinnett: Court

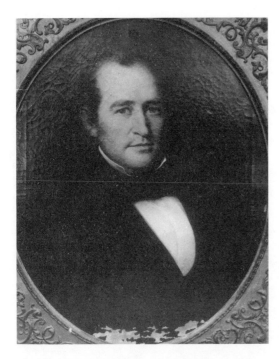

Dr. William James
Russell, circa 1830.
*Courtesy of George S.
Russell; copy in the
Historical Research
Center, University of
Arkansas for Medical
Sciences (UAMS).*

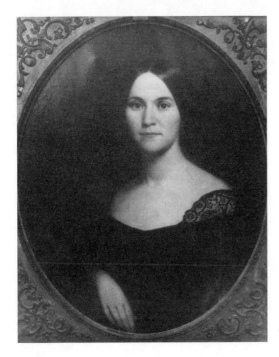

Sophia Park Russell,
circa 1830. *Courtesy
of George S. Russell;
copy in the Historical
Research Center,
University of Arkansas
for Medical Sciences
(UAMS).*

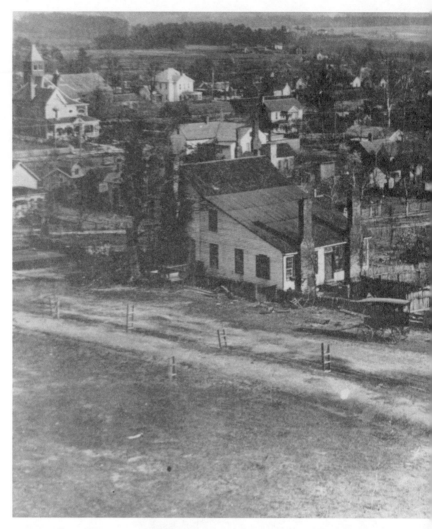

Home of Dr. William James Russell, far left with double fireplace
chimneys, circa 1907. It was built in the late 1820s in Lawrenceville, Georgia.
Courtesy of the Gwinnett County Historical Society, Lawrenceville, Georgia.

records there and in its parent county, Jackson, show leading citizens hauled before the court repeatedly on charges of assault.[123] Even
Lawrenceville founder Elisha Winn, a pillar of the Methodist church
whom his son Richard remembered as "of a decided and positive character" and "a gentleman by nature" who never used indelicate language, was
not immune to engaging in violent assault, as Flanigan's history notes.[124]

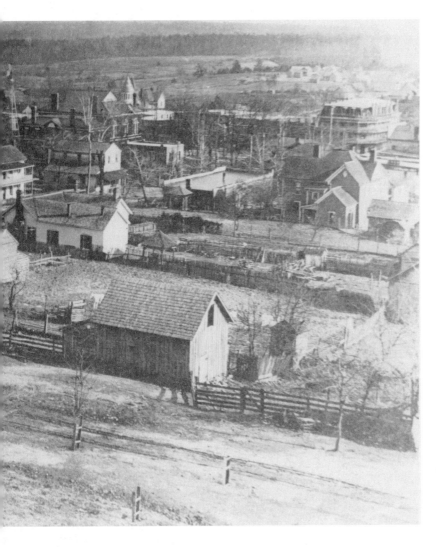

At the time Fairview was being organized along with Lawrenceville, North Georgia was very much a frontier area. As a sketch of Fairview's history notes,

> The church served as a moral compass, a social center. It provided the discipline needed to bring order to life at the frontier. As Franklin Talmage notes in his book, 'The History of the Presbytery of Atlanta,' churches of the time were critical in the development of the civic and moral character of their communities. People often lived far from law enforcement

officers, travel was slow and challenging, opportunities for irresponsible and intemperate behavior abounded.[125]

In frontier society, churches functioned parallel to and sometimes supplemented the legal system in monitoring behavior and punishing social and civil infractions. As Dickson D. Bruce states,

> The moral thrust of religion on the frontier was found mainly in strictly administered church disciplines covering all aspects of secular and religious life. The frontier churches have accurately been called 'frontier moral courts' because, for their members, they were substituted for secular legal institutions in a broad range of disputes.[126]

As Marian Silveus notes, "Practically every phase of an individual's conduct was considered a proper field for regulation [in Presbyterian sessions]."[127] Fairview session minutes are full of cases of members charged with intemperance, drunkenness, fornication, adultery, profanity, slander, fighting, shooting a slave, etc. Gwinnett and Jackson court minutes suggest that brawling and fighting were pronounced problems on the Georgia frontier, where a code of honor required avenging slights; the code has, in fact, persisted in southern culture, making the region susceptible to entrenched violence surpassing levels found in other regions.[128]

Session minutes tell us that Sophia Russell joined Fairview on 8 March 1828.[129] Her name appears again in Fairview minutes when the session charged her in May 1832 with having slandered her mother-in-law by stating at a party at her house in April that Sarah Alexander had borne a child five months following her first marriage.

As we have noted, this claim appears to be incorrect. Though Sophia denied the accusation, she refused two summonses to answer these charges before the session, and in July 1834, she was excluded from Fairview.[130] She then joined Lawrenceville's Methodist church. William J. Russell appears also to have left Fairview at this time, though it is not clear that he joined the Methodists along with Sophia.

As Sophia was undergoing her session ordeal, Russell was involving himself in politics: He represented Gwinnett in the state legislature in 1833 and was elected a nullifier when the state constitutional convention was held that year.[131] Livingston notes that Russell had served four years on the county court by 1854, without specifying when this service occurred. Flanigan indicates that Russell was a judge of the inferior court from January 1845 to January 1849.[132]

The *Southern Recorder* on 3 May 1836 shows Russell representing Gwinnett at the Milledgeville anti-Van Buren convention that month, along with his half-brother Samuel F. Alexander and Lawrenceville founder Elisha Winn.[133] In the same month, another paper, the *Columbus Enquirer*, notes that the Gwinnett representatives endorsed Tennessee Whig Senator Hugh Lawson White for president and John Tyler of Virginia as White's running mate. As Livingston notes, White was Russell's cousin through his mother Sarah.[134]

If Russell had aspirations to a career combining politics with doctoring, these appear to have been dashed by the death of Sophia on 16 March 1844. As her detailed obituary (unusually voluble for a woman in this time and place, perhaps written by her grieving husband) in Milledgeville's *Southern Recorder* explains, she had suffered from breast cancer and had undergone surgery a year before her death. The cancer had, however, "shot its roots, and spread its fatal influence far into the system beyond the reach of the surgeon's blade" and could not be cured.[135]

The obituary also tells us that two weeks before her death, Sophia had gone with daughter Mary to Jefferson Hall in Greene County, where an unnamed specialist thought to have skill in treating cancer saw her. She died under his care, and her body was returned to Lawrenceville for burial in the city cemetery beside her son Richard, who had died of scarlet fever on 2 February 1843, aged five.

Death of Sophia, Marriage to Iantha Huff, and Medical Practice

Sophia left three children aged ten to seventeen. On 22 April 1845, William J. Russell remarried to Iantha Missenia Huff, daughter of John Ausborn Huff and Malinda Martin.[136] Twelve years later, he began another family of children: Clara May (1857–1925), who married Edwin Jones Henry; Alma (1858–1860); Maudelin Aline (1861–1886), who married John Wade Marshall; Paul Wilmer (1862–1863); Paul Edgar (1864–1919), who married Anna Maria Matthews; Arthur Wynton (1866–1935), who married Annie Elaine Kinningham; and Mott A. (1870–1951), who married Minnie Harris.[137]

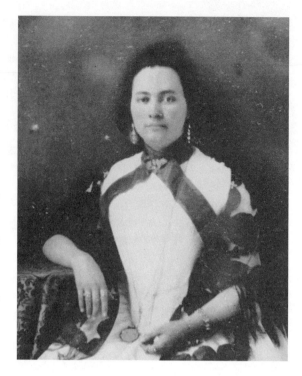

Iantha Missenia Huff Russell, wife of Dr. William James Russell, circa 1855. *Courtesy of Lynda Noland and Michael Barber; copy in the Historical Research Center, University of Arkansas for Medical Sciences (UAMS).*

After having brought William J. Russell to Lawrenceville and the establishment of his practice, Livingston falls silent about the details of that practice, other than to note that Russell was an esteemed doctor who accumulated a "handsome competence" despite his treatment of many indigent patients. Concrete information about *how* Russell practiced medicine—how his practice was organized, whom he treated, what kinds of therapeutic measures he took for which illnesses—is sparse.

From an article in the *Athenian*, we know that by 10 February 1829, Russell had a practice shared with his stepbrother Thomas W. Alexander. We know from several indicators that, as was common, Russell was also tutoring aspiring doctors, including his son. When W. J. P. graduated from Philadelphia College of Medicine in 1850, the graduation notice states that Dr. W. J. Russell was his preceptor.[138] In addition, both the 1850 and the 1860 federal censuses show in Russell's household a younger doctor who appears to have been reading medicine with him. In 1850, this is Jesse Lowe. Since we know from other sources that Russell was in partnership with James M. Gordon at this time, it appears Lowe was apprenticing, though he had graduated from the Medical College of Georgia in 1845.[139] In 1860, Andrew J. Shaffer is in Russell's household; he may have been both a student and partner and would take over the practice following Russell's death.[140]

Russell and Lowe appear as collaborators in a case the Georgia Supreme Court heard in May 1860, *Fundy v. the State of Georgia*. This concerned a murder on 3 October 1859, when John Fundy stabbed Hardin Colson at Ambrose's store in Lawrenceville. Both Russell and Lowe were called to examine the body, and both gave testimony.[141]

Also in 1860, we find Russell collaborating with both Lowe and John Winn Maltbie on another medical case mentioned in the diary of Lawrenceville resident Lucretia Douglas, portions of which are transcribed in Flanigan's *History of Gwinnett County*.[142] On 2 October 1860, Douglas states that she had been consulting local doctors about a tumor that had troubled her since 1845 and had turned to Maltbie for assistance. She asked Maltbie if she could bring in Russell as a consultant, and Maltbie agreed. Russell told her that nothing could be done. The same entry mentions that Lowe was also assisting with treatment.

We know from a letter Russell sent Governor Joseph Emerson Brown during the Civil War that another of his students was Andrew Jackson Flowers (1833–1881) of Gwinnett County. The letter (undated but archived with Brown's correspondence 1861–1865) states that Flowers was trying to secure a position as a Confederate physician and was "a young gentleman who was raised in this county and read medicine with me."[143]

In addition, an 1872 biographical sketch by Richard D. Winn of James M. Gordon (1821–1854) states that Gordon "began the study of medicine under Dr. William J. Russell" before he went to the medical college in Augusta to complete his education.[144] Winn adds that, having graduated, Gordon began a practice in Lawrenceville with Russell, which continued until he moved to Savannah in 1854. While practicing with Russell, Gordon lived about two-and-a-half miles outside town, though their practice was at Russell's house in Lawrenceville.[145]

During the period in which Russell and Gordon were practicing together, Gordon published an interesting account of a case on which the two collaborated, which casts some light on their shared practice. The account, entitled "A Remarkable Case of Volvulus and

Strangulation of the Intestines Within the Abdomen," appears in the *Southern Medical and Surgical Journal* in August 1845.[146]

Gordon reports that in May 1845, he and Russell were called to treat a young planter suffering from severe abdominal pain. He had previously consulted a "Thompsonian [*sic*] physician" who was unable to help him.[147] Russell and Gordon tried a regimen of "local revulsives" applied to the spinal column to relieve the patient's pain, augmented with opiates and antispasmodics. They also tried cathartics and an enema, but nothing availed. The unfortunate young man died, and autopsy showed that he suffered from volvulus and strangulation of the intestines.

The case is interesting because it suggests the skepticism of trained physicians about herbal treatments administered by Thomsonians, most of whom lacked medical training. It also demonstrates the extent to which practitioners continued to rely on the heroic approach of Rush, with its reliance on purgatives and emetics. The autopsy shows a methodical thoroughness on the part of the two doctors, too. They were clearly determined to do all they could to discover the cause of death.

Gordon's autopsy notes are clinically astute, indicating that Russell had trained him well in medical terminology and the art of surgery. The 1850 federal census lists Russell as a surgeon and physician of Lawrenceville (the census puts "surgeon" before "physician"); this is in contrast to a doctor living in the next household, Richard Parks, who is listed solely as a physician, and to Jesse Lowe, who is listed also (in Russell's household) only as a physician.[148]

Gordon was active in publishing accounts of his practice (still shared with Russell) in the *Southern Medical and Surgical Journal* in the latter half of the 1840s. In 1847, he published notes on a case of midwifery[149] and, in 1849, a study of the treatment of ranula.[150] His midwifery notes make the following interesting observation:

> In a plethoric subject, with fullness of the vascular system, we employ *blood-letting*, carried to a sufficient extent to protect the brain from the injury it might otherwise sustain from congestion. . . .[151]

This is followed with a caution that, though bleeding might be useful in plethoric cases, it was not a miracle cure and could, in some cases, be actively harmful.[152] As these cautions indicate, though that other long-customary prop of the "dreaded triad" of heroic medicine, blood-letting, was still in vogue, its shortcomings as a cure-all for any and all conditions were also being increasingly recognized. Since Gordon had been trained by Russell and was in practice with him, one can assume that his cautions about the use of bleeding reflect Russell's views.

Another interesting tidbit in the same journal is a February 1849 letter of Gordon pleading with fellow doctors to support the journal, which was published by the faculty of the Medical Academy of Georgia after its establishment in 1828 (the name was changed to Medical College of Georgia in 1833). Gordon's letter noted that subscriptions were diminishing and encouraged his colleagues to subscribe to the journal.[153]

As Russell and Gordon tracked medical developments in Georgia during this period, one wonders what they made of the discovery of the anesthetic properties of ether in the early 1840s by their fellow doctor Crawford Williamson Long (1815–1878) in Jefferson, thirty-five miles east of Lawrenceville. Long concluded that ether anesthetizes after he attended "ether frolics" at which he observed its effect on those inhaling it for recreational purposes.[154] In 1842, he began experimenting with its use to anesthetize patients, though he did not publish his findings until 1849.[155]

Long's hands-on experiments at "ether frolics" and Gordon's early death at thirty-three are reminders of how dangerous doctoring could be in this period. As Winn's biography notes, when an epidemic of yellow fever erupted in Savannah during the fall of 1854, Gordon sent his family away but insisted on remaining there to tend the sick. Winn cites a letter Gordon sent his wife Elizabeth, who was the daughter of Russell's stepbrother Thomas W. Alexander, in which he states,

> I have finally concluded to remain and am devoting my whole time and energies to the relief of the sufferers. Should I fall in the epidemic, my friends at least have the gratification to know that I fell in the discharge of my duty.[156]

Gordon died 18 September 1854. His tombstone in Laurel Grove Cemetery in Savannah states that he died of yellow fever.

As a 19 March 1873 article in the *Gwinnett Herald* indicates, runaway horses also posed a danger for doctors as they made their rounds. The article states that Russell's partner Dr. Shaffer had just left a patient when a shaft on his buggy detached and his horse bolted. Fortunately, Shaffer was not injured.[157] Russell's stepbrother Thomas W. Alexander was, in fact, killed on 26 February 1847 when his horse ran away with him, though he was conducting business in Decatur, Georgia, and not on a medical call.[158]

Another tragic example of what could befall nineteenth-century doctors as they visited patients is what happened to Charles Wilson Harris, a nephew of Russell's teacher with the same name. On the night of 19 January 1857, as he was making rounds near Concord, North Carolina, he was thrown from his horse or decided to leave his horse and proceed on foot. Harris fell into a branch, and his body was found the next morning near the stream where he had frozen to death.[159]

When Russell's son W. J. P. entered the Medical College of Georgia in 1849, a member of his matriculating class was Freeman Walker Schley. Schley died in the same yellow fever epidemic in Savannah in which James M. Gordon died; he died twelve days prior to Gordon, with his tombstone also reporting that he died of yellow fever while tending the sick.[160] The *Richmond Dispatch* reported on 15 September 1854 that five other doctors in Savannah had been stricken: Drs. West, Wells, Wayne, Ellis, and Arnold.[161]

Dealing on a daily basis with suffering people could also take a psychological toll. Jesse Lowe, the young doctor whom Russell trained and with whom he collaborated, was committed to the Georgia Insane Asylum in Milledgeville in June 1877.[162]

On the family front in the 1840s and 1850s, a number of indicators suggest that William J. Russell was enjoying a harmonious family life with wife Iantha, who was twenty-seven years his junior. On 12 September 1846, Iantha was admitted to membership by the Fairview Church.[163] In 1858, Russell returned to Fairview after having left the church when it expelled his wife Sophia: Session minutes for 13 November 1858 state that he had applied for readmission after years in which he had absented himself and "had fallen into great irregularities, disorder, and sin":

> Upon his making satisfactory acknowledgement for his course of conduct during these many years for his absence from the communion of the table of the Lord, together with his sin against his heavenly Master but more especially for

the evidence he gave of recent change of heart wrought by
the saving grace of a God upon which he now bases a hope
of his acceptance with God, was restored to the privileges of
the Church again and his name ordered to be placed on the
Church Roll.[164]

These years were evidently also prosperous ones for Russell and his
family: Various records show him holding considerable property,
including enslaved people, prior to the Civil War. From 1830, when he
owned no enslaved people, to 1860, he had acquired twenty enslaved
people and 2,700 acres of land.[165]

An announcement in April 1851 in the Athens paper *Southern
Banner* also indicates that Russell had invested in the Lawrenceville
Manufacturing Company, a cotton mill being established in the
town by a number of leading citizens, including Russell's stepbroth-
ers Thomas and Samuel Alexander, Richard Winn and son-in-law
William Maltbie, and James M. Gordon and his father Few Gordon.
Thomas Alexander's wife Martha is listed as an investor, too.[166] The
company was incorporated by the Georgia legislature on 22 January
1852.[167] This business venture is noteworthy since, in the following
decade, W. J. P. Russell was involved in a scheme of cotton speculation
that led to his imprisonment and trial by the Union army.

There are hints, too, that William J. Russell was interested in railroad projects toward the end of his life. An 8 February 1872 *Atlanta
Constitution* article[168] states that he hosted a dinner at which members
of the Georgia division of the Engineer Corps of the Atlantic and
Great Western discussed a proposal to create a canal linking the eastern and western halves of the continent.[169] Since we know from his
obituary that Russell had been partially paralyzed by a stroke two years
before he died in October 1872,[170] it seems likely that this meeting was
hosted primarily by his partner A. J. Shaffer, who led the discussion of
the railroad project according to the *Atlanta Constitution*. But it also
seems evident that the meeting would not have been held at Russell's
house if he did not have a keen interest in this and perhaps other
railroad projects.

Historians note that the two kinds of business in which Russell
and his son W. J. P. showed a keen interest—cotton brokering and
the extension of the railway system—often converged. It appears that
by the early 1860s, when W. J. P. settled his family in Mississippi, he

was working for a St. Louis firm, Maurice and Company, which had investments in both areas.[171]

The Final Years and Death

William J. Russell's obituary in the Lawrenceville paper *Gwinnett Herald*, along with a codicil to his will, frames the final period of his life for us with echoes of the "dark adversities of fortune" we encounter as we open Livingston's biography. Russell made his will on 4 October 1859, thirteen years before his death. The will distributes his property among his two sets of children and wife Iantha.

But on 15 June 1866, Russell added a codicil, which notes, "I have lost much of my property by reason of my Slaves having been Freed which reduced my property greatly."[172] Russell's obituary adds:

> By his practice he accumulated a large property, but his kind-heartedness and confidence in his friends caused him to lose large sums of money two or three times during his life, by becoming surety for those in whom he confided.[173]

For William J. Russell, as with other southern slaveholding planters, the 1860s—the final full decade of his life—were a period of economic reversal. Census estimates of real and personal worth that had looked large on paper turned out, after Emancipation, to have meant little more than numbers. In the case of slaveholders, wealth was based on a claim of some human beings to a right to hold others in bondage and to exploit their labor, a right that the outcome of the war determined to be illusionary.

As the obituary's statement about Russell's losses also reminds us, the plantation system was based on the extension of credit that involved planters in boom-or-bust cycles in which the wealth they generated with slave-operated plantations proved to be paper wealth that was illusionary in yet another way. When banks and creditors called in notes, what appeared to be a fortune based on slave-based agriculture could quickly dwindle. As Edward Baptist notes in his illuminating study of the slave system, *The Half Has Never Been Told*, such periodic losses were part and parcel of the economic lives of slaveholding planters, particularly in places like Georgia, where the plantation system was rapidly expanding from 1800 to 1860.[174]

It is possible to track the dwindling of Russell's estate prior to his death by focusing on some of his land transactions as the war ended. In November 1865, he sold a lot in Lawrenceville and 740 acres to his partner Andrew J. Shaffer for $5,800 and then another 175 acres in February 1867 for $225.[175] The sale of the 740 acres came less than a year before he made the codicil to his will noting that his property has been reduced: it suggests that he was *anticipating* what would happen—that is, the freeing of his enslaved people—when the war ended a few months before he sold the land to Shaffer.

Judged by figures on paper, Russell was riding high, economically speaking, up to the end of the war. Tax records show him paying taxes on 1,600 acres in Gwinnett in 1864, as well as on 1,171 acres in Cherokee, Paulding, Habersham, Dawson, and Cobb Counties.[176] Any of this land that was under cultivation in 1864 would have been cultivated by the labor of enslaved people. As a measure of real worth, then, the value of the land was intrinsically tied to slaveholding, so that the emancipation of Russell's enslaved people diminished the value of the land and would have been a significant part of the loss he sustained as the war ended. Since we know from his will that one of his preoccupations in these final years was to secure his estate for his children and wife and to divide it equitably, it seems likely that his sale of land to Shaffer in 1865 and 1867 was a strategy to liquidate some assets before they diminished significantly in worth and, in this way, to assure that he had property of substance to bequeath.

The reversal of Russell's fortunes in the period 1860–1870 can also be measured by comparing the estimate of his real and personal worth provided by the federal censuses of 1860 and 1870. In 1860, Russell had $6,000 real worth and $27,500 personal worth. In 1870, the figures had fallen to $250 and $2,000. In 1860, the personal property included, of course, enslaved people.[177]

Along with many of his fellow citizens, William J. Russell signed the oath of allegiance to the United States on 18 July 1867. Shortly after this, his health took a dramatic turn for the worse: in 1870, he suffered the stroke that partially disabled him. This event is alluded to in a notice that the *Gwinnett Herald* published five days before his death, which states that he had been seriously affected by a stroke a year or two previously but was now in very low condition following a more devastating stroke.[178] His obituary seven days later also notes that he had been suffering from paralysis for two years prior to his death.[179]

The obituary eulogizes the esteemed doctor, "one of the oldest citizens of our town and county," as follows:

> There is perhaps no man in Upper Georgia better known, as a physician, than Dr. Russell; having been in active practice for half a century. He moved to Lawrenceville in 1823, and led an active, laborious life up to three or four years ago. We doubt whether there is a man in the State who has done as much hard riding, day and night, to relieve the afflicted, as the subject of this notice. With a wonderful constitution, nothing deterred him—summer's heat nor winter's cold—from going whenever suffering humanity asked his skilled assistance.[180]

William J. Russell died on 7 October 1872 and was buried in Fairview Presbyterian Cemetery with a tombstone providing his dates of birth and death and stating, "He was the Orphans Friend." His will scrupulously provides for each of his children equally. Russell notes that, prior to making his will, he had given his oldest children by Sophia, W. J. P. and Mary, $2,000 each, and was setting aside the same amount for their brother Wallace, with instructions that the rest of his property be divided in equal portions for his second family of children and Iantha. The codicil revokes the provisions for Wallace, stating that in the intervening period, his father had given him the same share he had already given Wallace's siblings.

In the late 1850s, Wallace had gone wandering to California, where family letters suggest that he married a woman whose name the family did not know and had a child. The 1860 federal census shows him living as a single man in a mining camp at Bidwell's Bar in Butte County.[181] When war broke out, he returned to Georgia and enlisted in the Confederate army, serving first as a sergeant and then lieutenant before being captured by Union forces at Cumberland Gap on 9 September 1863.[182] He was then imprisoned at Johnson Island, Ohio, where he remained until 12 June 1865. A number of letters he wrote from there to a Miss Mary Sneed in Tennessee, a relative of his commander Captain Hardeman, are extant and speak of his longing to return to the "sweet sunny South."[183] By 1867, Wallace had gone to Washington County, Arkansas, where his brother W. J. P. settled in 1866.

William J. Russell's widow Iantha married his business partner Dr. Shaffer on 2 October 1873,[184] and the couple continued to live in the house Russell had built in Lawrenceville, where Shaffer continued his practice. In 1875, the Shaffers sold the house to Tyler Macon Peeples, editor of the *Gwinnett Herald*, and his wife Alice Ann Winn. They then moved to Gainesville, where Shaffer established a practice and where he died on 26 May 1887.[185] His obituary in *Atlanta Constitution* notes that he had practiced medicine for twelve years in Gainesville after moving there from Lawrenceville and "had quite a reputation as a surgeon," a skill that Russell would almost certainly have taught him. Iantha then moved to Hawkinsville, Georgia, where her daughter Maudelin Marshall lived. Iantha died in 1908 and is buried in the Orange Hill Cemetery along with her daughter and daughter's family.

Of William J. Russell's children, one son, William James Park (W. J. P.) Russell, followed in his footsteps as a doctor. It is to his story that we will now turn as we trace the generations of doctors who continued the legacy of William James Russell.

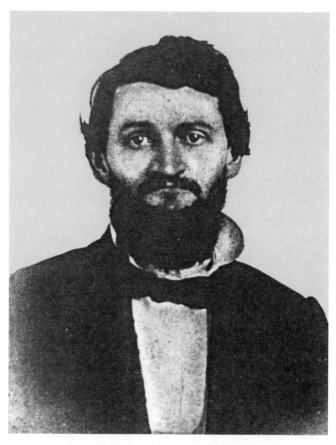

Dr. William James Park Russell, circa 1855. Image of a photographic portrait that hung in Dr. Seaborn Russell's Little Rock office in the 1920s. *Courtesy of Grace Norton; copy in the Historical Research Center, University of Arkansas for Medical Sciences (UAMS).*

CHAPTER 2

William James Park Russell
(1830–1892)

We call the attention of the afflicted to the card of W. J. P. Russell, M.D., Oculist, Aurist and Surgeon. He has taken rooms at Mrs. Dryer's Boarding House, where he can be consulted by those who stand in need of his professional services. Special attention to those afflicted with Strabismus, and he warrants a cure in a few seconds.

—*Tuskegee Republican*, 3 June 1858[1]

Genl if I have offended the majesty of the law in one particular, take me out & have me shot, or inflict on me any other punishment that I may deserve. I claim to be an honorable man & until the contrary is proven, I can not feel that this kind of treatment is fair. Genl excuse me for troubling you about so insignificant a matter, but I would rather face death in any manner than to submit tamely to such an indignity & without I was lost to all honorable feeling I could not do so.

—W. J. P. RUSSELL to Major General William
S. Rosecrans, 17 August 1863[2]

Birth and Early Life

William James Park Russell was born on 17 July 1830 in Lawrenceville, Georgia, as the frontier town was finding its feet.[3] Soon after his birth, he was baptized in the church of which his father was a charter member, Fairview Presbyterian, to which his parents and grandmother belonged.[4] When her son was not yet fourteen, Sophia would die after a protracted struggle with cancer, and his father would marry Iantha Huff, who then raised W. J. P.

No extant sources indicate how W. J. P. was educated before he entered medical school—though we know from his matriculation notice at Philadelphia College of Medicine in 1850 that he had read medicine with his father as preceptor. It is likely he would also have attended Lawrenceville Academy, of which his father was a founding trustee. The emphasis his family placed on obtaining good education for its children can be measured by the fact that William J. and Sophia Russell sent their daughter Mary Catherine to Salem College in North Carolina for education in 1840.

The struggle that peaked as Anglo settlers flooded Texas in the 1830s and Texans revolted against Mexican rule in 1836 appears to have captured the imagination of young men of Russell's generation in Lawrenceville. From the town, James Cochran Winn and Anthony Bates were shot along with some 400 others, many from Georgia, on Palm Sunday 1836 in the Goliad Massacre that spurred the war with Mexico.[5]

When he was seventeen, Russell joined the army: The Army Register of Enlistments shows him enlisting for the war in the 12th Infantry on 1 February 1848 at Columbus, Georgia. The entry identifies him as a student, aged eighteen (he would actually turn eighteen in a few months), from Lawrenceville, with hazel eyes, light hair, 5'11" in height. On 7 July, he was discharged at Fort Moultrie, South Carolina.[6]

Medical School

Having finished his service in July 1848, W. J. P. enrolled in the Medical College of Georgia in Augusta.[7] When Dr. Paul Fitzsimmons Eve (1806–1877), dean from 1836 to 1844 and the college's first professor of surgery, presented a lecture to the matriculating class on 5 November 1849, Russell was one of three students designated to express thanks from their class and to request a copy for publication. The printed copy of Eve's lecture, *The Present Position of the Medical Profession in Society: An Introductory Lecture Delivered in the Medical College of Georgia, November 5, 1849*, is prefaced with the following statement:

MEDICAL COLLEGE OF GEORGIA,
November 10th, 1849.

We, the undersigned, claim the honor to be a Committee delegated to act as the organ of the Class of the Medical College of Georgia, in returning their heart-felt thanks to you, for the very able and eloquent Address delivered before them on Monday morning; and to request a copy of the same for publication, that the positions it assumes may be more generally known.

We are, dear sir, yours very respectfully,

F. W. SCHLEY,
W. J. P. RUSSELL,
A. B. MONTGOMERY.[8]

It was customary for each matriculating class to hear a welcoming lecture preparing them for the challenges of study and practice. Faculty gave these lectures on a rotating basis. Though some of these lectures were published in journals like *Southern Medical and Surgical Journal*, it was unusual for a lecture to be printed as a separate fascicle. That Eve's lecture appeared as a free-standing publication suggests that it was considered especially good—a deduction confirmed by the fact that faculty from other medical schools commented on this lecture in various publications.

Eve's matriculation lecture provides an interesting vista on medical practice of the period. It called on practitioners to help counter widespread skepticism about the scientific basis of good practice, a skepticism fed, Eve thought, by an appetite for nostrums and "secret remedies" (the latter often licensed by the government).[9] Doctors themselves were not blameless here, Eve suggested. The field was riven with factions, leading the public to assume that quackery was as effectual as science-based therapy: as Eve stated,

> When physicians are called to a case of fever and one proposes bleeding, another prescribes purgatives, a third gives tartar emetic, a fourth digitalis, a fifth nitre, it is at once concluded that they differ when in truth, they all harmonize, they are aiming at one and the same result, the reduction of the arterial action and febrile excitement.[10]

Underscoring the point, he added, "Imposters and bad men are to be found in all the walks of life. They are met with in politics, in law, in theology, as well as in medicine. We have quacks even in religion."[11]

A large part of the problem was the American system of licensing, which placed physicians and quacks on the same level. *Anyone* could proclaim himself a qualified doctor in the United States since no license was required to practice "irregular" medicine and no distinction was made "between the regular and the irregular practitioner, between the learned and the illiterate in medicine."[12]

Georgia law actually offered "a premium to empiricism and dishonesty" by declaring that, while formally educated physicians must have licenses, doctors employing the "Thomsonian or botanic" method were exempt from licensing.[13] Recurring throughout Eve's lecture are the terms "nostrum," "quacks," "empirics," "charlatans"; these are juxtaposed with other recurring words—"science," "reason," "education." Eve parses "empirical" as follows:

> The whole system of empiricism is founded upon public credulity, in what is novel, marvelous, or mysterious in treating diseases; and in the popular supposition, that every one can best judge what is good or hurtful to his own system.[14]

As he sketched the context in which the class would be practicing, Eve did not mince words about the role he saw the state playing in contributing to the denigration of doctors and their practices:

> In Georgia alone there are about a thousand churches; in Augusta we have no less than ten; but within her whole territory we are now assembled in the only building appropriated to medical science, and neither this city nor community has ever contributed a cent to this Medical College.[15]

All this, not to mention the proverb that physicians' bills were notoriously the last that most families paid: Medicine was hardly a golden sinecure.[16] Since Eve was a highly regarded physician from a family replete with practitioners, the class would not have taken his words lightly.

The minutes of the trustees of the Medical College provide a concise snapshot of the class who heard Eve's 1849 lecture. 133 students had just completed the school's annual course of lectures, 100 from

Georgia.[17] The following year, 179 students were enrolled, of whom 140 were Georgians.[18]

As the printed copy of Eve's lecture makes plain, W. J. P. Russell was a member of the 1849–1850 class. He did not, however, graduate in 1850. Faculty minutes state that on 1 March 1850, the faculty met to vote on candidates for graduation, and: "The following were rejected: H. A. Urquhart, S. I. Willard, W. J. P. Russell, Samuel Boyd." The following day, the faculty met to re-examine those rejected and again rejected them.[19] Faculty minutes provide no specific reason for this decision. According to medical historian Sarah Braswell, students could be rejected for reasons ranging from academic failure to brawling or drunkenness.[20]

The school's 1850 catalog, *Twenty-Fifth Annual Announcement of the Medical College of Georgia*,[21] spells out requirements for graduation:

> No Student shall be an eligible candidate for the Degree of Doctor of Medicine, until he shall have attended two full Courses of Lectures in this, or one in this, and one in some other Medical Institution, in addition to the usual private reading in Medicine, and shall have delivered to the Dean of the Faculty an original Thesis on some medical subject, one month previous to the annual Commencement. In no case shall a Student of immoral character be admitted to examination.[22]

In the same catalog we read that the school charged $105 per course, $5 for matriculation, $10 for practical anatomy, and $30 for a diploma. As Steven M. Stowe notes, the standard term in medical schools in the South in the 1830s was four months. Around 1830, Georgia's school expanded its term to six months then retreated to the four-month term when other schools did not follow suit. In 1848, many schools began lengthening their terms to six months under the influence of the American Medical Association.[23]

Immediately after his rejection at Medical College of Georgia, we find W. J. P. Russell matriculating at Philadelphia College of Medicine on 3 March.[24] The notice of his matriculation states that W. J. Russell—his father—was his preceptor. The catalog shows 106 students in the class of 1849–1850, of whom 25 graduated in 1850.

Philadelphia College of Medicine had been organized in 1846.

James McClintock (1809–1881), a graduate of Jefferson Medical College known for brilliant anatomical demonstrations, was instrumental in its organization. Prior to this, he had founded the Philadelphia School of Anatomy in 1838. Though leading colleagues in Philadelphia regarded McClintock as an "irregular" practitioner, he had a solid background, having been president of Vermont's Castleton Medical College (1841) and professor of anatomy and physiology at Berkshire Medical Institution in Massachusetts.[25]

In its first seven years, Philadelphia College of Medicine graduated 400 students. The school specialized in anatomical studies and maintained an extensive anatomical museum. In addition, it had a department of pharmacy that taught students to compound medicine.[26]

As Harold Abrahams indicates,

> Following the thought of the London schools of medicine, the Philadelphia College of Medicine recommended the European curriculum of studies, as follows:
>
> First Course: anatomy, chemistry, materia medica, midwifery, dissections.
>
> Second Course: anatomy, materia medica, physiology, obstetrics, therapeutics, toxicology, practical chemistry.
>
> Third Course: surgery, dissecting, theory and practice of medicine, chemistry, hospital attendance, and clinical instruction.
>
> Fourth Course: surgery, practice of medicine, materia medica, anatomy, physiology, pathology, diseases of women and children, hospital attendance.[27]

One of the school's innovations was to offer two terms in one year, allowing faster advancement to graduation. This caused other schools to look askance at it. In fact, as William Frederick Norwood suggests, Philadelphia College of Medicine developed a reputation for being the place for "students who wanted a quick training."[28] The school eventually abandoned the two-term approach, and in 1859, Philadelphia College of Medicine merged with the Medical Department of Philadelphia College, with the merged faculties operating under the latter name. That school then closed in 1861.

On 19 July 1850, W. J. P. Russell graduated from Philadelphia

College of Medicine.[29] As we have seen, formal education was far from the norm for doctors of the eighteenth and nineteenth centuries, particularly in the South. David Baird notes that most early physicians in Arkansas apprenticed themselves to an established practitioner, accompanying him on calls and reading medicine to learn its arts and skills. Only a handful of Arkansas's early doctors studied formally in medical schools.[30]

Noting the role of family ties in inducing young men to study medicine in the early 1800s,[31] Stowe states:

> Becoming an M.D. in the mid-nineteenth-century United States was not an outlandish choice for a young man; it was not like running away to sea. But medicine, straddling the line between trade and profession, filled with economic and therapeutic uncertainties, was anything but the main chance. In the South, before and after the Civil War, the ideal of manly success was to master a flourishing plantation, the traditional seat of a man's economic power, political influence, and social esteem. Nonetheless, thousands of southern men made orthodox medicine their choice during the mid-nineteenth century, and increasing numbers of them (including some men already in practice) decided that formal medical schools were the best place to pursue it.[32]

Marriage, Starting a Family, Establishing a Medical Practice

Having obtained his degree, W. J. P. Russell married Avarilla Octavia Dunn Law, the daughter of James Franklin Law and Mary Ingram, on 14 November 1850 in Gainesville, Georgia.[33] She was a young heiress whose father had just died in May, leaving a will with an interesting stipulation: it stated that Ava's brother James was to receive an inheritance of $1,500, and then specified,

> I give and bequeath to my daughter Avarilla O. D. Law and her children free from the control and liability of any future husband my negro woman Sophia and her two children Jordan and Daniel and all future increase said slave[s] to be at valuation at the time of reception and what they fall short

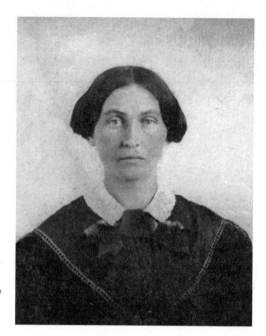

Ava Octavia Dunn Law Russell, who married Dr. W. J. P. Russell on 14 November 1850. *Courtesy of Sara Lee Suttle; copy in the Historical Research Center, University of Arkansas for Medical Sciences (UAMS).*

of Fifteen hundred dollars (if any) to be paid by my executors, and should they exceed in value that amount the difference to be paid by her to my executors.[34]

Though Georgia law followed English precedent in placing women under "coverture" of their husbands (and of fathers or brothers before marriage), James F. Law's will specifically states that Ava was to hold her inheritance "free from the control and liability of any future husband." As Angela Robbins explains,

> Married women traditionally relinquished all property rights and income to their husbands under coverture. Under the law, a married woman's legal identity was one with her husband, and she could not act separately from him. She could not enter into contracts, particularly to buy or sell property, independently of her husband; creditors could seize her separate estate or inheritance to cover her debts; and any income she earned belonged to her husband.[35]

Throughout her marital life, Ava appears to have controlled property independent of her husband. She contributed to their family economically by investing her own resources held separate from her husband's with his apparent blessing—an unusual arrangement in the American South at the time.

It is possible that following their marriage, the young couple initially intended to settle near Ava's family since W. J. P. bought a lot outside Gainesville on 25 March 1851.[36] Later the same year on 25 October, he sold 140 acres in Hall County that appear to have come to him from Ava's father. The stipulation of Law's will about a separation between his daughter's property and that of a future husband applied to movable property including enslaved people; real property from the estate would have been placed by law in W. J. P.'s name as Ava's husband.[37] The couple held onto land in Hall County up to the year before W. J. P.'s death when they sold their final 300 acres there on 8 August 1891.[38]

Soon after they married, W. J. P. and Ava began a pattern that would continue throughout their marriage: While Ava remained at home or with her mother, W. J. P. sallied forth to explore lucrative options for his practice. Within only a few years after their marriage, he began to establish a traveling surgical practice that he would share with sons Seaborn and Ralph as they came of age. An 1852 deed in Polk County, Georgia, gives us a glimpse of how this familial division of labor began to unfold within two years of the marriage: in December 1852 for a nominal sum, W. J. P.'s father had deeded his son a tract of land in Polk County, where (the deed specifies) W. J. P. was then living.[39]

Polk is in extreme northwest Georgia on the Alabama line. While W. J. P. was there—obviously scouting options for establishing a practice—Ava was with her mother in Gainesville, some thirty miles northeast of Lawrenceville, where her son William was born in 1851. In 1853, when son Charles was born, she had joined W. J. P. in Van Wert (Polk County).[40] After this, the family appears to have settled in Calhoun in northwest Georgia, where Russell bought several lots in 1853 while continuing to hold his property in Polk County. Calhoun had multiple attractions: it was the seat of a newly founded county, and was on the Western and Atlantic railroad line, which had just been laid through the town.[41]

It appears, then, that W. J. P. spent the first years after his marriage following patterns his father had followed, seeking as a venue for his practice a newly founded town, preferably a county seat, with a cotton-planting class poised to play a key role in its development. With the railroad also running through Calhoun, it must have looked like a good prospect—akin to Lawrenceville when his father settled there. The railroad is not insignificant. As we have seen, it appears that the elder Russell had an interest in railroad investments, and there is a discernible pattern in the life of W. J. P. as he moved from place to place, a pattern of almost always following the westward expansion of the railroad.

On 18 May 1855, a daughter, Mary Sophia, was born to W. J. P. and Ava in Calhoun.[42] Gordon County records show the family selling its Calhoun lots the same year—evidently with an eye to exploring another locale for Russell's practice: The couple's next child, a son named Virginus Law Russell, was born in Van Wert on 5 May 1857.[43] Formerly the county seat of Paulding County but by 1857 in Polk County, Van Wert is twenty-five miles from Alabama. In 1858, ads for Russell's surgical practice began appearing in *Tuskegee Republican*, indicating that he had begun extending his practice into Alabama within a year following Virginus's birth—and that he had chosen Van Wert with that objective in mind.[44]

We know another piece of information about Russell's practice at this time from a biography of Roberson Jasper Pierce (1837–1911), a doctor of Marion County, Arkansas: Russell was mentoring Pierce. Pierce's biography in Goodspeed's *Reminiscent History of the Ozark Region* states that he began studying medicine in Georgia in 1856 under Dr. Russell, a graduate of Philadelphia College of Medicine.[45]

The next Russell child, Seaborn, was born in Canton in Cherokee County on 7 September 1859.[46] At the time of Seaborn's birth, it appears that W. J. P. and Ava still held their residence in Polk County. A December 1867 Georgia Supreme Court case, *Scott v. Russell and Allen*, tells us that James N. Scott sued Russell for debt there on 28 April 1858. In 1862, Polk's Superior Court ruled in favor of Scott. H. W. Allen had given security for a promissory note Russell made to Scott. When Russell could not be found to make good on his debt because he had left Georgia, the case ended up in the state supreme court.[47] But as the supreme court record specifies, Russell was still in Polk in April 1858 or still owned property there when Scott sued him. In September 1858, the *Southern Banner* of Athens printed a notice from

A. Tabor warning people against trading for a promissory note given by Dr. W. J. P. Russell because Russell had failed to back the note— another indicator that he was in financial trouble.[48]

Yet another indicator of trouble appears in a 9 November 1857 legal action in Polk County in which Russell relinquished his interest in "all the Books Kept by myself & Dr J. J. Boring for the year of our Lord one thousand eight hundred and fifty Seven." The indenture notes that Russell was indebted to William J. Wardlaw, Boring's father-in-law, for $1,500 and, to satisfy the debt, was relinquishing his interest in account books he shared with Boring, who was in practice with him at the time.[49] The document trail indicates that Russell was faltering financially, and this perhaps spurred the decision to leave Georgia after Seaborn's birth to seek new venues for his practice—first in Alabama, then Texas.

Leaving Georgia, Launching Surgical Career

An entry in a diary kept by Seaborn commenting on his own birth tells us that his parents were together in Georgia in September 1859 at the time he was born, though we know from the ad W. J. P. placed in Tuskegee in June 1858 that he was there at that time to drum up business.[50] In the same year he placed an identical ad in the *Southern Banner* of Athens.[51]

The first of W. J. P.'s Tuskegee ads appeared in the *Tuskegee Republican* on 3 June 1858.[52] The announcement advertises the services of W. J. P. Russell, a surgeon specializing in ocular and aural treatment, who was in Tuskegee for consultation.

A week later on the 10th, the *Republican* again states that Russell could be consulted at Mrs. Dryer's, and was an oculist, aurist, and surgeon specializing in treating inflammation of the eyes, granular lids, watery eyes, ptosis, ectropium, entropium, pterygium, strabismus, cataract, talipes, hare-lip, torticollis, wens (tumors), enlarged tonsils, deafness, and chronic discharges from the ear. On top of this, he offered to insert artificial eyes painlessly.[53]

Such notices were common in this period: For instance, on 23 March 1853, the *Hinds County Gazette* (Raymond, Mississippi) declares that Dr. S. H. Mitchell, oculist and surgeon, would be available for surgery for strabismus, with vouchers from fellow doctors as to his

W. J. P. RUSSELL, M. D.,

Oculist, Aurist and Surgeon,

TREATS with success the following Diseases and Deformities:

INFLAMATION of the Eyes,
GRANULAR Lids,
Stopping of tear passage, (Watery-Eyes,)
PTOSIS, (drooping of Upper Eye-Lid,)
ECTROPIUM, } deformities of Lids,
ENTROPIUM,
PTERIGYUM,
STRABISMUS, (Cross-Eyes cured in a few seconds,)
CATARACT, (a form of Blindness,)
TALIPES, (Club-Foot,)
HARE-LIP,
TORTICOLLIS, (Wry Neck,)
TUMORS, (Wens,)
ENLARGED TONSILS,
DEAFNESS,
CHRONIC discharges from the Ear.
ARTIFICIAL EYES inserted without pain, possessing all the movement and appearance of the natural Eye.
No charge for Examination.
☞ Rooms at Mrs. DRYER's, Tuskegee, Ala., for a few days.   [june 3tf.]

Dr. W. J. P. Russell's ad in the *Tuskegee Republican* (Tuskegee, Alabama), 10 June 1858, page 2, column 6.

skill.[54] Similar "traveling-clinic" announcements continued in southern newspapers throughout the century. On 3 April 1878, the *Arkansas Gazette* advertised the services of one Dr. Connaughton ("Letters containing One Dollar will be answered and none others") who would be available for a limited time to treat cataracts, club-foot, pterygium, hair-lip, and other infirmities.[55]

The surgeries that Russell advertised in the Tuskegee paper in June 1858 (which were, for the most part, ones he and his sons would perform as they continued their portable practice throughout the second half of the century) were also common specializations for surgeons with established clinics. Advertisements for clinics indicate specializations similar to those advertised by Russell in his Tuskegee announcement and by other traveling surgeons of the period.[56]

For example, an interesting July 1871 advertisement in the *Arkansas Gazette* for the infirmary of Dr. J. W. McClure, surgeon oculist of Springfield, Arkansas, states,

> Sure cure; oldest Oculist in the west; twenty-one years experience; can make those of 60 see to read in 15 minutes; healthy town; boarding $10 per month; chalybeate springs to build up the general health; Practicing Physicians, Ministers of the Gospel, and indigent widows and orphans' prescriptions free. Come and be cured.[57]

McClure notes as well that he specializes in sore eyes, granular lids, cataract, cross-eye, pterygium, and inserting artificial eyes.

It is perhaps not accidental that most such ads announcing the services of *itinerant* doctors, in particular, were specifically for *surgeons,* ones specializing in specific surgeries. In contrast to other aspects of medical treatment, surgery was a "portable" skill easily taken on the road. In communities in which doctors' primary practice was treating infectious diseases, bandaging wounds, and assisting at childbirth and death, these "portable" skills would have been in high demand as specialized procedures most small-town or rural doctors, and even many urban ones, could not provide.[58]

Traveling medical shows in which surgeons quickly cured crossed eyes, cleft lips and palates, or clubfeet were also welcome theater in small towns in the nineteenth century. A surgeon's announcement appeared in a newspaper, stating that he would be in a hotel lobby for several days for patients suffering from such afflictions to consult with him;[59] he then performed surgery on the spot, and the long-suffering patient was instantly relieved of the malady. The results would have been, in many cases, dramatic and instantaneous—with low overhead for the traveling doctor and tedious convalescent care delegated to others, so that this kind of practice had economic benefits for an enterprising surgeon willing to move about in search of promising new fields for his discretely limited operations.

At the time that W. J. P. Russell began advertising his specializations in 1858, there was lively interest in several of these surgeries. In the absence of documentary evidence, how much detailed knowledge Russell would have had about important nineteenth-century developments in the surgeries in which he specialized is an open question.

It is likely that his choice to pursue a surgical career was rooted in his father's tutelage.

Philadelphia College of Medicine required surgical education in the final two courses students took, as well as in anatomy in their first two courses. We know from Harold J. Abrahams that textbooks used at the college when Russell was there included Robert Druitt's *The Principles and Practice of Modern Surgery*, Robert Liston's *Practical Surgery* and *Elements of Surgery*, William Gibson's *Institutes and Practice of Surgery*, George McClellan's *Principles and Practice of Surgery*, and Alfred Velpeau's *New Elements of Operative Surgery*, among others in the surgical field.[60]

It seems likely, then, that W. J. P. Russell had received solid grounding in surgery from both his father and his training in Philadelphia. Given this, it is not difficult to understand his decision to market himself as a surgeon specializing in reparative surgeries when he began shifting his career in the latter part of the 1850s.

The Civil War Years

At some point in late 1859 following Seaborn's birth in September or in early 1860, W. J. P. and Ava headed to Texas, where they are enumerated on the federal census on 19 June 1860 in Bosqueville in McLennan County in the household of B. O. W. Whatley.[61] Seaborn was with them, while their other children were with Ava's mother in Gainesville.[62]

No extant documents provide information about this Texas move. An obituary of Whatley's son Lucius says that his parents moved from Newton County, Georgia, to Texas in 1858.[63] The 1860 census tells us that Burwell Ornan Wilson Whatley (1808–1889) was a prosperous planter with sixty-nine slaves when he relocated to Texas; it lists W. J. P. Russell as a doctor but provides no clue as to why he, Ava, and Seaborn were living with the Whatleys. From the time the Russells left Georgia through the Civil War and in the years immediately following the war, there are a number of such mysteries regarding their movements, with little documentation to allow us to decipher their movements.[64]

If the couple was dreaming about starting a new life in Texas, those dreams quickly faded with the coming of war in April 1861. By

May 1862, the Russells had relocated to Corinth, Mississippi. Several documents state that the family came to Corinth prior to its first battle, 29 April to 30 May 1862. In addition, in a Bible register in which she recorded family dates, Ava indicates that daughter Ava Leona was born 22 June 1862 in Corinth.[65] At some point between 19 June 1860, when we know that they were in Texas, and May 1862 when the family had moved to Corinth, W. J. P. was in New Orleans, a precious tidbit we know because that city's *Times-Picayune* reports on 21 December 1860 that "Russell W J P dr" had an unclaimed letter in the local post office.[66] What Russell was doing there in the latter part of 1860 we cannot say with certainty any more than we can know why he moved his family from Texas to Mississippi soon after the move to Texas. There are, however, tantalizing clues about what may have brought the Russells to Mississippi.

A number of records indicate that, following the first Corinth battle, W. J. P. entered the service of the Union army as a spy providing intelligence to General Henry Halleck while Russell was working for a St. Louis-based cotton firm, Maurice & Co. After General William Starke Rosecrans took command of two divisions of General John Pope's Army of the Mississippi in the summer of 1862, Russell began working for Rosecrans and his Chief of Police William Truesdail, going with them and the Army of the Cumberland to Nashville after Corinth had been occupied by Union troops.

This information (though not any explicit disclosure of Russell's spy work for the Union—he and Ava seem to have withheld this information even from their children) appears in two affidavits as W. J. P. applied for a pension in 1889 for his service in the Mexican War. On 26 March, Russell gave an affidavit stating that he had never performed military service after the Mexican War but had been employed as a detective under Halleck at Corinth and as assistant chief of police under Rosecrans and General James A. Garfield until the battle of Stones River in early 1863.[67]

This affidavit is followed by an undated one Ava gave at roughly the same time. Ava states, "Wm. J. P. Russell entered the service of the United States Army just after the battle of Corinth Miss, about May 1862 under Genl. Halleck, commanding Department as a Detective." She says he subsequently served under Rosecrans at the battle of Corinth and was promoted to the position of Assistant Police Chief under Truesdail, after which he served under Garfield following the battle of Murfreesboro. Significantly, Ava also avows that her husband was paid for his services out of the funds of the secret police: she knew this because he told her so.[68]

There were two battles of Corinth, and these affidavits appear to be referring to both. As previously mentioned, the first occurred 29 April–30 May 1862, at which point Corinth fell to Halleck and the Confederates retreated.[69] Corinth's second battle took place on 3–4 October 1862. Ava's affidavit pinpoints when W. J. P. began providing intelligence for the Union. Since she states (and W. J. P. corroborates) that her husband entered Union service "after" the battle of Corinth in May 1862 and "was then under Genl. Rosencrans at the battle of Corinth and was promoted by him to assistant chief of police with Wm. Truesdail as his chief," his intelligence work obviously began with the first battle. By the time the army had arrived and laid siege to the city in April 1862, W. J. P. Russell had, we may deduce, made connection to someone in the army, leading to his retention as an intelligence agent.

But what were the Russells doing in Corinth in the first place? In September 1863 at the court-martial of Elisha H. Forsyth, who stood accused of engaging in cotton running with Rosecrans, Truesdail, and W. J. P. Russell, Russell testified that he had been engaged in buying cotton for Maurice & Co. when he arrived in Corinth. Another deponent, Ferdinand Emmel, bookkeeper of the Union Cotton Co., formed by the merger of Maurice and other firms, which was at the heart of the allegations in this trial, corroborated this testimony, stating that Russell was buying cotton for Maurice & Co. when Emmel first met him in Mississippi in the summer of 1863.[70]

Truesdail kept a ledger from 1 November 1862 to 1 May 1863, showing his payments as Chief of Police of the Army of the Cumberland to all those he employed.[71] The ledger shows several payments to W. J. P. Russell for unspecified service: $435 for service from 1 October to 30 November 1862, $93 from 10 November to 9 December 1862, and $600 for 1 December 1862 to 26 February 1863. As historian William Feis, author of studies of Grant's secret service and Truesdail's police operation, states,

> What this [information from Truesdail's ledger] tells me is that Dr. Russell . . . did intelligence work of some sort as only

those civilians engaged in spying or scouting were paid this much and the Union armies loved to use native Southern Unionists—especially those who were elite and respected members of Southern society like a physician. And they paid them well. The total amount he earned ($1128) would be a little over $21,000 today. A heck of a lot better than the $13 a month paid to Union enlisted men, who would have to serve around 7 years to make that much. Getting at what he actually did to earn that, however, would take some digging and might be a long shot. Being a Southerner who worked for the Union was not a popular thing in the postwar South, so it is likely that Dr. Russell never committed his service to paper or told his story widely.[72]

Note that these payments corroborate Ava Russell's assertion that Russell was paid out of secret police funds. In addition to the payments listed in Truesdail's ledger, a congressional account of a 10 June 1872 itemization of payments made by the Assistant Quartermaster of the Army of the Cumberland, John W. Taylor, shows W. J. P. Russell being paid for "special service rendered General Rosecrans's command" from 10 August to 10 October 1862. Two such payments are listed in this document: $98.64 for 10 August–10 September and $92.07 for 10 September–10 October.[73]

As Feis's *Grant's Secret Service* indicates, the identities of those engaged in intelligence work were carefully concealed by army commanders, who deliberately did not commit specific information about the activities for which they were paying spies to paper. Feis notes that when Brigadier General Grenville M. Dodge took over Truesdail's intelligence operation in 1863, Dodge went toe to toe with General John A. Rawlins and his quartermaster when these officials insisted that regulations required that payment vouchers state operatives' names and services they had provided. Dodge stated, "There are citizens living in the South who give me the most valuable information [who] will not sign a voucher for fear of consequences in the future."[74] As Feis notes,

> If a person residing in the Confederacy spied for the Federal army and then signed a voucher—a far from confidential document—he or she risked having the nature of their services revealed, which could lead to threats and violent

retribution from their fellow Southerners both during and after the war.[75]

"Paying secret service personnel also presented a vexing problem, especially since scouts and spies took enormous risks and expected to be well compensated in return": To prevent exposing his spies, Dodge took control of payments, keeping vouchers but refusing to send duplicates to headquarters per regulations.[76] After the war, he retained all copies of secret service vouchers instead of sending them to the War Department. These documents are currently filed in Dodge's personal papers in the National Archives.[77]

As Feis also stresses, Dodge's operation was built on foundations established by Rosecrans and Truesdail. At the time the army laid siege to Corinth, there was a dearth of spies and scouts to provide information, in part, because Grant and Halleck had had little time to recruit personnel in the first part of 1862 and, in part, because of a lack of money to pay agents.[78]

Grant relied heavily on Rosecrans to develop a secret intelligence service, due to Rosecrans's proven organizational skills and Halleck's recommendation.[79] The development of a robust intelligence operation was a key goal for Rosecrans when he took command of the Army of the Mississippi and then of the Cumberland, and it was for this that he commissioned Truesdail to establish a police unit, "a comprehensive intelligence outfit . . . whose duties included information collection, counterintelligence, and investigations of disloyalty in the city [of Nashville]."[80]

Though a spy working for Tennessee governor Andrew Johnson, Ogilvie Byron Young, informed Johnson in a December 1862 letter that Russell had told him he was serving on the medical staff of General Sterling Price prior to his capture at Iuka,[81] there is not a scrap of evidence to support what Young claimed.[82] Indeed, as his January 1889 pension application states, Russell never gave military service after the Mexican War.

Russell's descendants *assumed*, however, that he did give Confederate service: They passed on a story that he had been a Confederate medical officer. In addition, the previously noted Georgia Supreme Court case, *Scott v. Russell and Allen*, states that in the original debt case in Polk County in 1862, Russell could not be found because he was in the

Confederate army.[83] Young's December 1862 report to Andrew Johnson, who distrusted Rosecrans and Truesdail and was employing spies to report about them, suggests that Russell himself may have helped craft the smokescreen about being a Confederate medical officer to put people off the track of his Union intelligence work.

Russell went with Rosecrans and Truesdail to Nashville in the latter months of 1862. In early 1863, after he received his final payment from Truesdail, W. J. P. was arrested and imprisoned in Nashville in connection with charges that he had engaged in cotton-running activities.[84] We learn of his arrest from the case files of Dr. John Rolfe Hudson and wife Araminta of Nashville, who were tried in spring 1863 for Confederate spying. The Hudsons were arrested after a 1 March 1863 report by Union spy Harry Newcomer charged them with spying for the Confederacy. Newcomer stated that Mrs. Hudson had asked him to help get Dr. Russell, a family friend, out of prison.[85]

Testimony in the Forsyth trial suggests a plausible reason for Russell's arrest early in 1863: On 22 September 1863 A. J. Drumwright of Murfreesboro testified that in late February or early March, he had let a wagon to "one Dr. Russell, a man engaged in cotton business" to haul cotton. Drumwright also stated that he had a similar arrangement with Forsyth: the testimony links the two and implies that they were jointly involved in cotton running.[86]

At some point prior to July 1863, Russell was released from prison and then imprisoned again on 15 July. He sent a letter to Rosecrans on 17 August asking to be released.[87] Both this letter and an order from General Stanley's chief of staff in Russell's Union Provost Marshal file indicate he was tried twice prior to 17 August.

When W. J. P. wrote Rosecrans, Stanley was actively pursuing allegations of cotton running by army personnel in Nashville. On 15 August, the *Nashville Daily Union* reported that Stanley had opened an official investigation three days before.[88] The Forsyth trial was conducted under the auspices of this commission, and Russell was a key witness after it commenced on 7 September.[89] His 17 August letter to Rosecrans reflects his concern that he was being targeted by Rosecrans's provost marshal William Wiles and his cronies due to evidence he had provided and would disclose at the Forsyth trial. Written on letterhead reading "Head-Quarters Department of the Cumberland, Office Provost Marshal General," Russell's letter reads,

Dear Sir, I have been tried twice for the same offence & if I have not refuted the charges in both cases it was because I was not allowed a fair chance to do so, on the 15th ult. I was arrested on the streets of Murfreesboro & thrown into the common jail & confined in a cell with convicted felons (negroes) for no offence on earth. The Prov Marshal Maj Scarret told me he had orders from you to arrest me & confine me. He would allow me to have no communication with any one, & instructed the guard to treat me as the vilest of criminals. Genl if I have offended the majesty of the law in one particular, take me out & have me shot, or inflict on me any other punishment that I may deserve. I claim to be an honorable man & until the contrary is proven, I can not feel that this kind of treatment is fair. Genl excuse me for troubling you about so insignificant a matter, but I would rather face death in any manner than to submit tamely to such an indignity & without I was lost to all honorable feeling I could not do so. It is the first time on earth that I have heard of charges against my character & I am as anxious as any one to have a thoro investigation, I want to come out of this thing honorably or not at all.

I am General with sentiments of the profoundest Respect your obedient servant, W. J. P. Russell.[90]

Stanley's investigation had been set in motion by Andrew Johnson, who suspected Rosecrans and Truesdail, with Wiles, Forsyth, and others, of feathering their nests through cotton speculation schemes that involved seizing cotton from local citizens, taking it across Union lines, and selling it at a profit, while trying to fix the market to their advantage.[91] Johnson called for investigation of Truesdail, and, as Johnson biographer Hans Trefousse notes, he also implicated Rosecrans.[92] Underlying Johnson's suspicion was his negative appraisal of the police department Rosecrans had set up in Nashville. As head of the department, Truesdail reported to Wiles and had a wide-ranging charge to ferret out fraud and corruption in the Department of the Cumberland and to detect rebel espionage and smuggling.[93]

Feis indicates that between November 1862 and June 1863, employing some 130 spies, Truesdail confiscated property worth $438,000 in Nashville.[94] Truesdail professed particular concern about the probability that in this Union-occupied city near the North-South line, spying and counter-spying were occurring, with double agents representing themselves as for one side while they gathered information for the other. "There is a bad enemy in this city," Truesdail wrote Rosecrans in late December 1862, "who are doing evil by their intercourse with the enemy."[95]

Contemporary accounts provide conflicting optics on what was taking place between Johnson and Rosecrans/Truesdail in spring 1863 and reveal uncertainty among Union leaders about what was actually happening in Nashville under Rosecrans. These include a 24 October 1863 *Washington Chronicle* article by an unnamed author entitled "Fall of Rosecrans" that mentioned Russell and implicated him in the cotton-running schemes that the author claims Truesdail had organized with Rosecrans's blessing. The *Chronicle* suggests that Truesdail and Russell were abusing police power to commandeer cotton from locals and run it through Union lines to sell at favorable prices that enriched them and others.[96]

Forsyth's trial began in Nashville on 7 September and Russell testified 22–24 September. Charges against Forsyth were passing counterfeit money, theft, unlawful collection of government revenue, obtaining money under fraudulent pretenses, and conspiring to bribe the government, all in connection with cotton-running schemes of Union Cotton Co.[97] William Wiles was connected to this company not only through the role his Provost Marshal's office exercised in preventing cotton running but also because Union Cotton had been formed by merging several companies, including Wiles & Co., headed by his brother Robert.[98]

W. J. P.'s apprehension about being targeted by Wiles as he prepared to testify in the trial is clearly expressed in an anxious telegram he sent Stanley on 21 August. It states that he was "afraid he was going to be arrested by Taylor, Wiles and others."[99] On the same day, he mailed a letter telling Stanley that he was going to Jonesboro, Illinois, and was in fear for his life. Ava and the children had evidently moved there, and in October, she bought land there. It appears Russell was making plans to join his family in Illinois once the trial ended.

Russell's letter to Stanley was hastily scribbled by a considerably agitated man and is in several places difficult to make out. It reads as follows:

Nashville Aug 21 '63

Maj Gen D S Stanley

I start home this day. My address will be Jonesboro, Ill.
for ten days provided I am not made away with surrepti-
tiously [?]. I really feel that they will have me arrested out of
this Department on some pretext or other that I may not be
here to show [?] of the of [?] of this [?] for Lieut Hutchins
in Ten now under arrest on some previous charge, I know in
[?] He would be delayed so as to give them a chance to fore-
stall the authorities at Nash[ville]. Gen Stanley if I am not
forthcoming at the proper time, you have me hunted out I've
got avowments to damn the whole party, & if you can't find
me call on [? ?] [?] claim from my trunk [?] [?] letters Shine,
Taylor, Wiles, and T—will move heaven & earth to get me
out of the way secretly, for they are afraid to come openly at
me. Gen Stanley [?] this matter to the bottom

Your srvnt [?] [?] WJP Russell[100]

Since we know from the case file that Russell was a key witness in
late September, it appears that he did not join his family in Jonesboro
until after he gave his testimony. A monograph could be written about
this interesting trial and the testimony given by and about W. J. P.
Russell, including the claim of one William J. Spence that Russell was
"an impudent fellow" who threw his weight around as Assistant Police
Chief, but telling that story in more detail would take us afield from
this book's primary narrative. In the endnotes, we have pointed readers
who want to know more about the trial to material well worth reading.

After the War: The Peripatetic Years

A. Illinois and Louisiana

As previously noted, Ava and the Russell children were in Jonesboro,
Illinois, by October 1893, when she bought 280 acres of prime land
near the Mississippi River for $3,000 on the 26th.[101] Ava bought the
land in her name, and tax records for Union County, Illinois, show her
taxed for it in 1864–1865.[102] There may have been a pragmatic reason
for this: with the war ongoing and her husband's intelligence work for
the Union and then the controversy over cotton running, it may have
seemed wiser to put the land in Ava's name.

On 14 July 1864, the couple had another child, Sevie Octavia, with Ava's Bible stating that Sevie was born at Clear Creek, Illinois, near Jonesboro.[103] Because Ava's land was rich alluvial farmland ideally suited to cotton, it appears the primary motivation of the Illinois move may have been to raise cotton as the market was favorable, with Confederate cotton embargoed by the Union and mills in New England and England clamoring for cotton.

A 25 April 1863 letter of General Napoleon Burford to War Secretary Edwin Stanton from Burford's headquarters in Cairo thirty-five miles south of Jonesboro indicates that the Union army was interested in growing cotton in southern Illinois.[104] From a number of sources, we know that the crop in this area in both 1864 and 1865 was spectacular. On 4 December 1864, the *New York Times* reported that there had been a bumper cotton crop there, with many bales stacked on the Cairo wharves for shipping out.[105]

Lincoln was assassinated while the Russells lived in Jonesboro, and according to a story that W. J. P.'s son Seaborn told his son George, W. J. P. took Seaborn to Springfield to see Lincoln lying in state on 3–4 May 1865. Soon after this, tragedy struck the family: on 2 June 1865, W. J. P. and Ava's oldest son William James Russell died as he approached his fourteenth birthday and was buried in the Jonesboro Cemetery.[106]

After their son's death, in a pattern that would become typical when they faced loss of this sort, the Russells sold Ava's land and moved in October 1865 to Alexandria, Louisiana, and then to Shreveport.[107] The Union army took control of Alexandria in spring 1863, and by 1864, there were reports that the army was speculating in cotton there, scouring the countryside for Confederate cotton and confiscating even cotton belonging to Unionists.[108] Connected to New Orleans and St. Louis by river networks, Alexandria and Shreveport were important trade centers in Louisiana, so it is possible that the move to Louisiana had something to do with the cotton business that seems to have been central to the family's economic interests in these years.

B. Arkansas

Nine months after the death of their first son, the Russells' second son Charles died on 11 July 1866 in Shreveport.[109] By September, the family had settled at Evansville in Washington County in Northwest Arkansas, a meeting point for the Benge and Bell routes of the Trail of Tears on the Arkansas-Oklahoma (then, Indian Territory) line.[110] Because of its proximity to Indian Territory, Evansville had played a key role in mercantile activities between Anglo settlers of Northwest Arkansas and Native Americans who had been relocated to Indian Territory.[111]

Since it appears that W. J. P. Russell began to use the initials J. W. after the move to Arkansas, one wonders if one reason W. J. P. chose this frontier border town was because he was living in fear of reprisal due to his wartime activities as a spy. If trouble followed from Tennessee and Mississippi, W. J. P. could easily vanish into Cherokee and Choctaw lands.

It seems likely that another reason the Russells chose Evansville after their son's death was because of W. J. P.'s interest in a livestock business he had begun developing with Frank Norwood, his future son-in-law. Family letters speak frequently of this business: on 10 November 1881, Norwood wrote to Ava Leona Russell, speaking of his intent to come from Hope, Arkansas, to Fort Smith and then to the Choctaw Nation to buy ponies for the horse, mule, and cattle business he shared with Ava's father.[112]

Previously, on 24 April 1881, Ava had written Frank from Boonsboro, Arkansas, stating, "I heard Sevie tell Ma she wished Mr. Norwood would come up here and buy up another drove of Mules this summer."[113] In a letter W. J. P. sent Norwood from Eureka Springs on 27 December 1881, he states that they had been engaged in the livestock business together for some time.[114]

As Baird's history of medical education in Arkansas indicates, there was one doctor for every 356 persons in the state by 1860—so the market for practitioners was good when W. J. P. arrived in Arkansas.[115] Steven Stowe's history of doctoring in the South in the nineteenth century underscores the point: Stowe notes that while federal census data identifying doctors show the numbers of physicians in the South increasing at an unprecedented rate on the eve of the Civil War, especially in states like Texas with booming antebellum populations, the numbers significantly dropped off after the war.[116]

When Russell and his family arrived in Arkansas in 1866, the state's first medical society, the Little Rock and Pulaski County Medical Society, had just been established.[117] Its schedule of fees provides a glimpse of what physicians might expect to earn with a practice in the state's central region: Physicians affiliated with the Society could charge two dollars for office calls, three dollars for day visits, and six dollars for night visits.[118] A move was soon afoot to establish a statewide society, the Arkansas State Medical Association, and an organizational meeting was held in 1870 in Little Rock.[119]

Russell had begun to establish himself as a professional man with a respected reputation soon after the family came to Arkansas: A September 1866 article in the *Van Buren Press* notes that Dr. J. W. Russell had been made vice-president of a Johnson Club just organized in Fayetteville.[120] President Andrew Johnson had issued a formal declaration ending the war on 20 August 1866, and the upcoming congressional elections were to be a referendum on his Reconstruction policies. In an effort to secure support, Johnson promoted a coalition of Republicans and Democrats called "Johnson Clubs" throughout the North and in the border states.[121]

Arkansas was, then, a good bet following the Civil War for a family like the Russells. Everything had been so turned upside down by the war, with the southern economy in shambles, that a quasi-frontier state like Arkansas would have had a definite appeal to a family making a new start, headed by a doctor whose services were sorely required. Northwest Arkansas, in particular, may well have appealed to the Russells not only because it bordered on Indian Territory, where we know Russell was developing business interests after the move to Arkansas, but also because it had leaned in the Union direction—and Russell's close ties to Rosecrans and Truesdail, if they were found out, might not have made for a welcome reception in the Confederate-sympathizing part of the state. The Russells did eventually move to southern Arkansas as they gravitated toward Texas in the 1880s when acute memories of the war began to mellow. We know from a series of announcements that Russell placed in the Little Rock *Arkansas Gazette* in October and November 1868 that he had resumed his traveling surgical practice by then, so it appears he settled in Arkansas with the intent of continuing the peripatetic practice of surgeries he had begun to advertise in Tuskegee in 1858. This was a plan that promised immediate remuneration for a doctor resuming professional life in a largely undeveloped state following the war.

The surgeries Russell advertised in 1858 and again in 1868 were relatively quick and not as invasive as other surgeries. They tended to have dramatic results that would have quickly made the lives of patients significantly better. Nor did they require a big outlay of expense by surgeons since they were done for a limited time in places where no overhead for office expenses was required and the after-care cost was borne by the patient. When such surgeries were not routinely performed by other local doctors, this sort of roving, highly specialized practice was a canny economic bet for a doctor like Russell.

The Russells had definitively decided to strike roots in Northwest Arkansas by the start of 1867, when Ava bought land near Evansville on which the family lived until 1870. Again, as with the land bought in Illinois in 1863, the land was in Ava's name, bought with her funds.[122] Another action also designed to establish the family in their new community followed: In spring 1867, J. W. Russell and wife Ava became charter members of the newly founded Pleasant View Christian Church near Evansville.[123] Earlier in the year, a son Ralph Morgan Russell had been born to them at their new Evansville home.[124] As 1867 ended, W. J. P.'s brother Wallace married Julia English in the Pleasant View church.[125]

Russell's first advertisement in the *Arkansas Gazette* appeared 13 October 1868. It states,

> As a specialist Dr. Russell, whose card appears in another column, stands unrivalled. Making the eye his special study, he has devoted twenty years to its practice. We have letters from parties in different parts of the state, of the highest respectability, of his restoring cases of blindness of years' standing, and remedying deformities of various kinds in an incredibly short time. We have no hesitancy in recommending the Doctor to all who may need his services. Call upon him at once as his stay will be short in Little Rock. He has secured rooms at the Anthony House, and will arrive about the 20th inst.[126]

On 15–16 October, ads for the services of "Dr. Russell, Oculist and Surgeon" appeared again, stating that he was at Little Rock's Anthony House and might be consulted for inflammation of the eyes, granular lids, watery eyes, ptosis, ectropium, entropium, pterigyum [*sic*], strabismus, cataract, talipes, hare lip, torticollis, tumors (wens), and enlarged tonsils. The ads also told patients that Russell inserted artificial eyes painlessly. These are virtually the same ads Russell had run in Tuskegee and Athens ten years earlier.[127]

On 20 October, the *Gazette* informed readers that Russell continued at Anthony House and could be consulted "on all matters relating to diseases of the eye and some cases of deformity." The *Gazette* also stated that Russell came highly recommended, as its readers would see by reference to the voucher provided by prominent citizens of Yell County. This card, printed on the same page and entitled "A Card, Dardanelle, Yell Co., Ark, Oct. 16, 1868," reads,

> Feeling that we are by this means conferring a benefit upon that class of persons whose condition appeals most loudly to our sympathies, on account of their helplessness, to wit: the blind of our state, we take this method of assuring the public that Dr. Russell is a responsible, scientific and successful Oculist.
>
> The Doctor has been in our midst long enough to establish his claims to eminence as an operator. We have seen persons with blindness of years standing place themselves under his treatment and he would discharge them in a few days with good sight.
>
> We have, also, seen him straighten a club foot in one week —have witnessed him straighten cross-eyes in a few seconds.
>
> We might cite case after case in proof of the above statements, but suffice it to say that we believe him capable of doing anything he proposes with any sort of deformity or blindness.[128]

The voucher is signed by J. E. Hart, M.D.; W. P. Varnell; L. D. Parish; S. D. Strayhorn; J. Mort. Perry, Druggist; and W. W. Wishard.

The following day, the *Gazette* carried another notice:

> Dr. Russell has been traveling in Arkansas for more than twelve months and has treated successfully hundreds of cases of blindness, as appears from the testimony of leading citizens in different portions of the state. His rooms are at the Anthony House. He cures cross-eyes in a very few moments, and supplies artificial ones when needed.[129]

Russell remained in Little Rock consulting and performing surgeries until at least the middle of November. On 13 November, the *Gazette* announced that, at the house of Col. Hopkins, Dr. Russell would make an artificial pupil in a case of total blindness of nine years' standing. Local and transient physicians were invited to attend.[130]

The resumption of Russell's peripatetic surgical practice in 1868 presaged a period of more moving about for the entire family. On 24 July 1869, Russell's wife Ava gave birth at Evansville to a stillborn daughter Lilly, as noted in her Bible. And then, in the same recurring pattern after W. J. P. and Ava lost a child, they moved. Between July 1869 and November 1870, they settled in Boonsboro, some thirteen miles northeast of Evansville.

Also known as Boonsborough or Cane Hill, Boonsboro had several attractions that would no doubt have lured the family. It was Washington County's oldest settlement and the site of Arkansas's first institution of higher learning, Cane Hill College, which was also the first academy in the state to admit women. It had the state's first public school and library, as well.[131] In addition to the market the well-established community would have offered Russell for his practice, it had strong educational advantages, then, for a family that prized education for both sons and daughters. With daughters fifteen, eight, and six, and sons thirteen, eleven, and three, and another child, Richard, whom his family would call Dick until he reached maturity, on the way, the community would have appealed to the Russells because of the educational opportunities it offered.[132]

As we'll see when we tell Seaborn's and Ralph's stories, we know from several pieces of testimony that both of those sons—and in all likelihood, the other adolescent Russell children—*did* go to the Cane Hill school in the 1870s. Seaborn's diary mentions this, and a letter written by his son George in 1976 also states this. The biography of Ralph M. Russell in *History of Alabama and Her People* indicates that he, too, attended the Cane Hill academy.[133]

Though the family had shifted its residence from Evansville to Boonsboro by the fall of 1870, it retained property in Evansville. Tax records show that in 1875, Russell stopped paying taxes on property in Range 33 West, Section 12 of Washington County in Vineyard Township in the vicinity of Evansville.[134]

In 1870, Russell was taxed in Boonsboro for seven horses, seventy-five head of cattle, a jack (i.e., male donkey), forty hogs, and $750 worth of other personal property.[135] The noteworthy number of livestock here appears to confirm Russell's continuing interest in trading in horses, cattle, and mules. On 2 June 1870, Russell received his previously mentioned payment for services rendered to

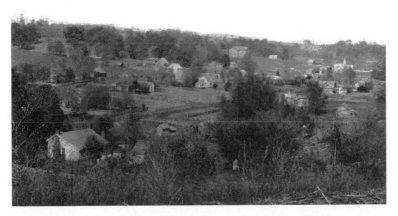

Cane Hill, Arkansas, looking northwest, circa 1895. *Courtesy of The Historic Cane Hill Museum.*

Rosecrans in Mississippi in 1862, a payment itemized in a congressional account prepared by the Assistant Quartermaster of the Army of the Cumberland, John W. Taylor.[136]

On 15 June 1873, the Russell's last child was born. As was also noted in her Bible register when Dick was born in 1870, Ava's Bible states that Eric was born at "Bethesday Camp Ground" in the vicinity of Boonsboro.[137]

The Period of the Family Letters Begins

From April 1878 to January 1892, when W. J. P. Russell died, the Russell family is richly documented in a trove of letters preserved by W. J. P. and Ava's daughter Ava Leona Russell Norwood. At her death in 1935, the letters went to her daughter Ruby Norwood Kitchens, who then passed them to her daughter Sarah Lee Kitchens Suttle of Salem, Oregon. In 1993, Sarah Suttle gave the letters to a cousin in North Little Rock—William L. Russell, a great-great-grandson of W. J. P. and Ava—who transcribed them and, in 2016, donated the collection to the Historical Research Center in the University of Arkansas for Medical Sciences Library.[138]

The first letter in this important set of documents is one that Ava Law Russell wrote from Boonsboro on 14 April 1878 to her younger sister Mary in Georgia. Because of the glimpse it provides us of Ava's character, it is worth quoting in full:

My Dear Sister Mary,

I think its high time to interrupt this period of silence that exists between us for it weighs like a spell of nightmare on my spirits. I have not heard from any of my family in 6 months. Have written twice but received no answer.

We are all at home except Dr. R.—he left a few days ago to go and perform some surgical operation on some person living 50 miles below here. Are you still living in the vicinity of Gainesville and what has become of your dear children? How I would love to see them and you.

Ava and Sevie are grown in size but not in manners and learning. We are just getting through with Measels. Ralph was the last to have them and he is just up. Seaborn is living with us and making a crop for himself on my land free of rent. His father wanted him to become a Surgeon but Seab fancies a farmers life and the company of girls.

Spring is here with its wealth of buds and blossoms and the best prospect for wheat that we've had in several years. Have you never thought of leaving Georgia and going somewhere to make a fortune? Suppose we take our boys to Florida and put us out an Orange orchard? In ten years it would be an independent fortune for us and support us in our old age. Study it out and let me know what you think of it for if we can find a healthy location there is surely money in the Orange trade.

We have a good and pleasant home here but this is a hard country to get money in. We raise all the bread and meat and fruit we can consume but we need money to pay taxes and buy clothing and for other purposes too numerous to mention, and something to bring money in when we are unable to work for it any longer and when our children have left us and set up for themselves. Write and tell about your children. It is most astonishing how little sisters can know of each others children. Of course I know Penn and Eddie and have heard of Ethel—but of their dispositions, tastes, and temper I know nothing. But nothing would delight more than to read a description of each one personally from your pen.

My youngest boy is five years old and I feel like I am growing old—and I hope better in heart. Ava and Sevie have joined the 'Church of God' and are to be immersed in baptism soon, and though they are young and passionate, I pray that they may hold faithful to the end. Where is sister Sallie and her husband? What has become of all the folks—Bros. Jim, Ma,—Bro. Jo was at Hot Springs when we last heard from him 5 or 6 months ago. Did the fire in Hot Springs injure Bro. Sevier much or was he burnt out—if so was he insured?

Now sister please answer soon—Your affectionately,

Ava O. Russell[139]

This letter is interesting from several standpoints. First, it demonstrates the level of education (not to mention independence) of women in the Russell family circle, even when they were living in "a hard country" on what was then virtually the western edge of the frontier in a state not much developed beyond its pioneer period that had just passed through the grand disruption of war. The phrase "of their dispositions, tastes, and temper I know nothing" is a fine one, exhibiting a level of education uncommon for many women of this period in the South.

Then there's the astonishing suggestion that Ava and Mary "take our boys to Florida and put us out an Orange orchard," since "there is surely money in the Orange trade." This, along with the casual allusion to the fact that Seaborn was living rent-free on *her* land, are reminders of the unusual arrangement that Ava's father had made when he left property to her with the stipulation that she was to enjoy the use of that property free of interference from a husband down the road. The letter underscores that Ava was investing along with W. J. P., using her own resources as she did so, to help the family make a living—a decidedly uncommon marital arrangement in the South at this time.

Ava's observations about the difficulty of making a living in Northwest Arkansas also demonstrate the validity of Malcolm Rohrbough's observation that northern and southern Arkansas had developed different societies up to the war, with different economic bases.[140] Where small farms were the core of the economy, money was scarce. For doctors and other professional people, this posed a problem: how to make money by providing professional services. And as Ava says, when there are many other expenses, with a family intent on seeing that both male and female children obtained the best education available, the problem was compounded.

Ava's letter also validates Sarah Fountain's insight that women played a primary role in sustaining family ties as kinship networks spread to distant places in the eighteenth and nineteenth centuries. As Fountain notes in her study of a significant collection of letters exchanged over several generations between families in Alabama and Arkansas, letter-writing was one of the most important tools at women's disposal to achieve that goal and to share information about family health and news of births and deaths.[141]

Finally, there's the reminder that as Ava worked to help provide for her family, assisting with raising and preparing food, nursing the sick, writing letters, clothing and educating her children, her husband was often absent tending to patients or traveling with surgical work. Having borne eleven children, three now dead, and having married off two, Virginus, who married Sarah Braden, and Mollie, who married John Denton Moore, with the anticipation that more marriages would soon follow, Ava may understandably have dreamt of Florida orange groves.

Those orange groves may have appealed to Ava for other reasons, as well: As previously noted, by 1875, W. J. P. had defaulted on his taxes on land that appears to have been bought in his name near Evansville. An August 1878 Washington County tax list notes the sale of some of this as delinquent-tax land. This was only a few months after Ava had written her sister Mary.

That the family may have been experiencing financial difficulty in the "hard country" of Northwest Arkansas is also apparent in another move the Russell family made about 1880: Family correspondence suggests that while retaining their Boonsboro residence, the Russells moved to Eureka Springs, a resort community in Carroll County that was beginning to boom as it was chartered in 1879.[142] As they were making this move, some dispute appears to have developed regarding property they owned in Washington County. An undated accounts ledger of a Fayetteville attorney whose name is not given in the ledger, but who was likely James Russell Pettigrew, notes that he had defended the Russells in a land-claim dispute with Mason Thompson around 1881.[143] It is clear that the family had settled at Eureka Springs by 12 July of that year, which is when daughter Ava wrote Frank Norwood to tell him that her father was going to Boonsboro the following Saturday to bring household furniture to Eureka Springs.[144]

Family correspondence suggests that there were a number of motives for this move. One was to permit W. J. P. to extend his practice in the newly founded community—while both he and Ava speculated in economically promising ventures there. On 27 December 1881, Russell wrote Frank Norwood, noting the two continued their cattle business together and stating,

> I am engaged in the General Practice here but not realizing much out of it as yet as the poor outnumber the rich in the ratio of 20 or even 30 to one. The visiting patrons of this place are some better but still they are not as paying a class as you meet with at vacationing places for pleasure. I am accumulating city property fast and in the near future expect to reap a rich harvest but you know there's many a disappointment. This place is improving very fast now—have 140 new houses going up in sight of where I live and I can't see any of the city proper as I live at the Dairy Spring.

And then he concluded, "I have not made anything over a living here as yet but the prospect is flattering for the future."[145]

In addition to extending his practice to a new town, Russell also continued his peripatetic surgery, as is apparent from an 1883 letter Ava Russell wrote to her daughter Ava from Boonsboro three months after Ava and Frank Norwood married. The letter notes that W. J. P. was at Eureka and would not leave on a surgical tour until after the current court session at Fayetteville.[146]

A number of family letters of the early 1880s provide interesting details about how the family was speculating in lots in Eureka Springs to augment the income Russell brought in by his practice. In a 20 May 1881 letter to Norwood, Ava Leona Russell says that he would hardly recognize Eureka Springs now, due to the "improvement" that had taken place in the town since the preceding fall: "Every house here is more than full and new buildings being errected [sic] continually."[147]

On 18 December, she wrote Frank again from Eureka Springs (noting that he was in Alexandria, Louisiana), stating,

> Ther[e] is quite a boom here now more than ever before. Everybody is building. We have a good time watching the

fights and fusses which are being carried on near here in the reservation of the Dairy Spring. These are parties who persist in holding onto their property which they bought previous to the Survey of the Reserve. The citizens want to keep this as a Park as it is the only place suitable in Eureka—but I don't believe they will make a success as there are several parties who have possession and Pa says they will probably hold their property.

She then notes:

> It is useless for me to describe Eureka Springs. Lots Ma paid $7.50 and $12.50 last Spring she refused $150.00 last week. Pa has 2 nice lots and Ma has four—all of which are very valuable for this part.
>
> Pa has recently engaged in the water shipping business with which he thinks he will do well next Spring. They have built a beautiful stone tank at the basin and have nice seats all around the platform so everything is very nice there. The flight of steps has been replaced where it was when we went up and down so nicely. I never go down there but when I think of dear you and wonder if we will ever have the pleasure of a repitition [*sic*] and only hope we may ere long.[148]

The pattern of both Russells using their separate resources to bring in income continued as both speculated in town lots. In addition, W. J. P. saw opportunity in the new water-bottling business that had developed as the resort grew, with reports that its spring waters had healing properties.[149]

By early 1883, rail service extended to Eureka Springs via the Eureka Springs Railway. On 6 January 1883, Ava wrote to Frank Norwood that the "cars will be running into Eureka by the 15th."[150] Though this would have enhanced the economic prospects of the community, it appears as one reads between the lines in letters of 1882 and 1883 that, as far as the Russells were concerned, the bloom was off this new community and W. J. P. was considering yet another move.

On 20 May 1881, Ava told Frank her Pa was pressing for a move to Texarkana. She opined, "I hardly think he will."[151] Then in December 1881, she noted,

> Pa wants us to consent to move to Texarkana or Louisiana but of no consequence for neither Ma nor I like the South to

a great extent. I think he will win us over by another year if we remain here though.[152]

By next July, she was telling Frank, whom she had hoped to visit in Louisiana,

> Anyhow Eureka Springs is as dead as it can be, almost never saw such a deserted looking place. Everybody has gone except a few visitors. I think we will go home pretty soon if not sooner. Pa has returned and Boas has gone again after Cattle. I did not get to go south visiting. Pa did not come home in time so I was most heartily disappointed.

Even as both W. J. P. and Ava speculated in town lots and W. J. P. invested in a water-bottling business and as he continued his surgical practice, he carried on his livestock business with his son-in-law William J. Troutt ("Boas"), Sevie's husband, and his future son-in-law Frank Norwood, bringing in income by yet another means. By February 1883, the Russells had returned to Boonsboro as a letter Ava wrote her fiancé Frank on the second indicates. Without providing details, the letter states that the family had been "compelled" to return to Boonsboro to take possession of their farm.[153]

By fall 1883, the Russells were on the move again—to Nashville in southwest Arkansas, where they settled in October after W. J. P. and Ava lost another of their children, son Virginus, who died in Eureka Springs on 21 September.[154] By this point, they had launched three more children into adult life—Seaborn, who married Alcie Daisy, daughter of Dr. Wilson Richard Bachelor and Sarah Tankersley Bachelor of Franklin County, on 1 January 1880; Sevie, who married William J. Troutt on 21 July 1881; and Ava, who married Benjamin Franklin Norwood, son of Josiah Moore Norwood and Sarah Auld Norwood of Lafayette County, on 7 March 1883.[155]

This left the couple with three sons to continue raising as they made their move to southwest Arkansas. Part of the motivation for this move appears to have been to permit W. J. P. to continue developing his roving surgical practice with Seaborn and Ralph. Being disencumbered of most of his children as he made this move would have facilitated W. J. P.'s mobility and perhaps made it easier for Ava to hold down the home front.

A letter Ava wrote from Boonsboro to her daughter Ava on 29 April 1883 hints at the relief she may have felt to have most of her

chicks fledged—and also at the price she paid as she maintained a
home while W. J. P. traveled: Ava states that she was happy because
she had had letters from her husband, daughter Ava, and son Ralph,
who was in Hot Springs working for Ava's brother Sevier Law. Then
she adds that she did nursing work and household chores while Sevie
cooked—all of this in addition to "all the milking and churning."[156]

One final note about the collection of letters documenting the
family's activities in this period: As noted previously, these were initially saved by the Russells' daughter Ava Norwood. From 1880 to 1883,
when Ava married Frank, the letters are to a great extent courtship
letters documenting the thrust and parry of a young couple vowed
to but living distant from each other, trying to figure out how (or
whether) to maintain a relationship that would culminate in marriage as they led separate lives in separate places. The correspondence
about Ava and Frank's courtship and marriage concluded with a letter
W. J. P. Russell wrote from Arkadelphia to Frank Norwood in New
Iberia, Louisiana, on 10 February 1883, providing his approval for the
impending marriage:

> Your favor of the 7th January has just been received by
> me and contents made the study of self reflection. The ques-
> tion you ask and the answer you expect is to stir from the
> depths of a parents heart all the fond recollections that cluster
> around the life of an affectionate daughter.
>
> Ava has ever been to me all that a child could be and she
> is now of an age to know what would most conduce to her
> own happiness and I would not throw any obstacle in the
> way of her choice for life, especially as it is the nature of her
> destiny with one I have so long known and so highly approve
> as yourself.
>
> She is the last of my girls and in parting with her I feel
> that the staff I have been so long leaning on has broken. Take
> her Frank and deal gently with her—a purer, more unselfish
> and affectionate child no man ever raised.
>
> May the Lord bless you and her and prosper you in this
> world and save you in His kingdom at last. Your affectionate
> Friend, etc.[157]

The couple married in March 1883.

The Move to Southwest Arkansas

In October 1883, the Russells moved to Nashville in Howard County, Arkansas. It appears they did so with the intent of establishing a new base for Russell's traveling surgical practice in East Texas, where they would move in 1885. Nashville, a county seat in the southwestern corner of Arkansas, was formally incorporated on 29 October 1883, and the Arkansas and Louisiana railroad line opened for business there in 1884.[158]

After the Russells relocated, much of their correspondence concerns W. J. P.'s travels with Seaborn and Ralph as the boys drummed up business and assisted their father with surgeries in Arkansas, Louisiana, and Mississippi. At this point, it appears that W. J. P. was actually doing the surgeries while his sons were under his preceptorship. On 3 December 1883, Ava wrote her daughter to say that W. J. P. had left on 27 November with Ralph and Seab for a "Southern trip" and would go by way of Hamburg in southeast Arkansas, where W. J. P. appears to have had Alexander relatives.[159]

In addition to Seaborn and Ralph, W. J. P. may have hoped to interest Dick in the medical profession. On 9 June 1882, Ava Russell had written Frank Norwood from Eureka Springs, stating that "Pa and Dick have been gone for a month south."[160] As letters after the Russells moved to Texas indicate, Dick did toy with the idea of following in his father's footsteps, but he eventually chose to become a cotton buyer in Wills Point in East Texas, where W. J. P. and Ava spent the final years of their lives.[161]

In her previously mentioned 3 December 1883 letter to her daughter Ava, Ava Russell notes that W. J. P. was encountering difficulty as he sought to bring in income through a settled practice in the Nashville area. He had found the area lacking in economic opportunity, Ava tells her daughter: "[T]he people are sociable and kind tho in rather poor circumstances now as the crops have been cut very short by the drougth [sic] and money is scarce." Hence, his southern tour with his sons. The letter provides a revealing glimpse of Ava's challenges as she kept house and raised the youngest sons as W. J. P. traveled: She tells her daughter that she had written every recent letter as she did chores, "for positively I never begin to write without having to give my attention to something about cooking or sending to town for some article needed or to get something that your Pa needed right away." Then she describes the family's living situation and outlines some of her daily work:

> We are very comfortably situated—have a good frame house with plenty of glass windows and long Piazza and E. and Dick and I cook in a log house nearby whilst Daisy cooks and sleeps in one room—but has a dining room without stove or fireplace. We all cook in a skillet and frying pan and your Pa says that I do a great deal better than he ever thought I would—but when he's here he will help me and the boys are good little fellows—they help all they can and so I have a fine time and not near so hard as I thought I should—tho I do all the work for five of us. We have a garden full of Cabbages and Onions and Mustards. Wish you could steal a few onions out of my garden so that I could see you.[162]

Ava's letter also tells her daughter that one of her chores was to educate Eric and Dick, who were not in school but who "recite 3 lessons each in the forenoon and write a letter in the afternoon daily."

When W. J. P. and Ava moved to southwest Arkansas, Seaborn and his wife Alcie joined in the relocation. As Seaborn traveled with W. J. P., Alcie remained with her mother-in-law, helping to keep house. Ava's December 1883 letter notes that she and Daisy (Alcie's middle name) had recently gone to Franklin County and visited Alcie's parents and that Ava had played the organ at Dr. Bachelor's house. As her letter ends, Ava issues a reminder to her daughter: "Don't neglect your music. Keep it up—home is always pleasant where there's music."

A musical education was not merely an accomplishment that young ladies of a certain class used to *land* a husband in this period; it was also one they were expected to employ to *keep* a husband. In the gendered domestic arrangements of nineteenth-century marriages, home was the sacred preserve of the woman, who was expected to keep it tidy and pleasant for her hard-working husband, the breadwinner.[163] Wives whose husbands strayed were routinely blamed for not having made their households comfortable enough—and playing music was, as Ava's letter suggests, one expectation of a cultivated wife. In addition to all her *other* routine domestic chores. By 14 February 1884, according to a letter Mollie Moore wrote her sister

Ava Norwood from Cowala, Indian Territory, Ava Russell had joined the southern tour with Eric. The letter states, "Bud Seab says Pa, Ma, Ralph, and E. are on the road to Hazlehurst and want to be there in March."[164] By 17 March, the family had traveled into Louisiana and were in East Feliciana, a parish bordering Mississippi in southeastern Louisiana, where W. J. P. wrote his daughter from Clinton. His letter tells Ava that he had just left her mother and Eric five miles outside Port Hudson with "attendants." Russell had left them there because he feared that there would be an accident if the family tried crossing a creek in their wagon after heavy rains. He and Ralph had found a point at which it was safe to cross, and he had sent for his wife, who would arrive at any moment.

The family then made its way to Liberty, Mississippi, about thirty miles from Clinton, where they inquired about cases to be treated. The plan was to arrive in Hazlehurst, another sixty miles, about 24–25 March, as Ava Norwood was expecting her first child there, and her mother wanted to be with her for the delivery.

Family letters indicate that W. J. P. remained in Mississippi into 1885, with Seaborn returning to Arkansas and conveying Alcie and their children to her family in Franklin County. By July, Seaborn was back with W. J. P. and Ralph had gone to Alabama to work on his father's behalf, as a letter W. J. P. wrote his daughter Ava from West Point, Mississippi, on 2 July reveals. Russell's wife was still with him, with both Dick and Eric in tow. The letter indicates that W. J. P. and his sons were finding it difficult to bring in money due to the hard times farmers were having but hoped to do better around Birmingham, Alabama. W. J. P. also notes that Seaborn was in the process of becoming a promising doctor (if he would stick to the work) and that Ralph was heading to New York (for a medical education, though the letter does not spell this out).

The letter ends with a request that Ava direct letters to her father at Kosciusko, Mississippi. Its plaintive notes presage the family's final move to Texas. Money was scarce, farming conditions were poor, more money was to be made around Birmingham with its industrial economy than in the Black Belt counties where the economy was agricultural, and not even the old standby of horse trade was bringing in enough money. Money could be gotten more readily in Texas, particularly in Dallas, where Russell initially set up a practice, and in Wills Point, sixty miles east of Dallas on the Missouri-Pacific railroad.[165]

The Final Move to Texas

By the latter part of 1885, the Russells had made their final shift to Texas. A letter Seaborn wrote his sister Ava from Memphis on 31 August says that he and his father were selling out and heading to Texas with six head of horses. Texas was booming and had just had a fine cotton crop.[166] By December 1885, W. J. P. had set up a Dallas office, according to a letter he sent at Christmas to his daughter Ava. It states that he was finally able to provide a marriage portion for her equal to that of her siblings who had preceded her in marriage:

> As a Christmas gift we send you our obligations for your horse and bed and cow that you should have had as your wedding outfit or marriage portion to make you equal with your elder brothers and sisters. It is but little and we will pass away after a few more years and we wish to place our children on an equal footing in this respect. When you go to housekeeping and will need the articles then we can take up this instrument and give you the money. Have it now to spare if you would rather have the money.

W. J. P. concludes by providing interesting details about his finances:

> You write that you and Frank have saved $800 on the first year—thats doing well—much better in proportion to how I have done. My income has been $5,000 and I have only got through with $1,000 and that is in horses. We have been buying and feeding for the past two months. Feed is cheap—corn 35 cents Oats 25 cents. We will ship a car load of 35 Head to Mississippi tomorrow. I will go myself and sell them. I did intend to send Seab but can't have confidence in him. He can't keep money and may spend mine as he spends his own.

A business card shows W. J. P. sharing a practice with his sons at 1041 Elm St. in Dallas sometime in the period between 1885 and 1890.[167]

Another tidbit of information indicating that W. J. P. had set up a Dallas practice with his sons in 1885 appears in a 1 January 1886 article in the *Fort Worth Daily Gazette* entitled "Morphined Himself." The *Gazette* reports that on 31 December, one B. E. Strickland Jr. had taken an overdose of morphine in the calaboose in Dallas, where he had

---

DRS. RUSSELL & SONS,

ORTHOPEDIC

SURGEONS AND SPECIALISTS.

TREATS WITH SUCCESS ALL THE

➤➤DEFORMITIES OF THE HUMAN BODY.◄◄

Club-Feet Straightened. Hare-Lip cured in three days. Cross-Eyes straightened in a few seconds. Artificial French Eyes to fit any ball. Wry-Neck cured at once.

Affections of the Eye Needing Surgical Operations Solicited, OTHERWISE NOT.

Hemorrhoids removed hyperdermically. Rhinoplastic operations for Scars, Burns, Mercury or Wounds. ☞Skilled Assistants in the House to Supervise Fitting on Instruments.

ROOMS AT 1041 ELM STREET, DALLAS, TEXAS.

——⊕——

Office Hours from ⎰ ⚕Charitable subjects operated on FREE of Charge
10 A. M. to 3 P. M. ⎱ Saturday at 3 P. M.

Dr. W. J. P. Russell's business card when practicing in Dallas, Texas, circa 1885. *Courtesy of Sara Lee Suttle; copy in the Historical Research Center, University of Arkansas for Medical Sciences (UAMS).*

been locked up. He almost died and had been taken to the residence of Dr. Russell to be treated. Bryant Strickland was a son of Russell's sister Mary, though this is not stated in the report.[168]

W. J. P. filed a copy of his medical diploma from Philadelphia College of Medicine with Dallas County on 13 May 1886. This filing is another clear indicator of his intent to practice in Dallas.

A letter that Ava Russell sent daughter Ava Norwood on 6 April 1886 contains information about the family's continuing financial struggles. Writing from 1041 Elm Street, the address on Russell's 1885 business card, Ava says that the family was living in a house of eight rooms, where they hoped her daughter's family might visit them. They intended to remain there at least another month and perhaps all summer.

Ava speaks of religious revivals—evangelists Dwight Moody, Ira Sankey, and Thomas Needham had been in Dallas—which had spurred W. J. P. to renewed religious commitment. Ava also notes a railway strike underway in Dallas as she wrote,

> The strike is affecting all kinds of business here. Banks holding on to their money until they see the end of the strike.

Provisions in some of the towns are scarce—no flour! no coffee! but plenty here—Dallas has large wholesale houses that are well stocked.

As these statements remind us, Ava had her own keen interest in economic matters. She continued holding property in her own name and her land in Washington County, Arkansas, had been claimed by a Mr. English, who had rented it out. Ava writes to tell her daughter that she had written English to tell him that he must vacate the premises or pay rent. Also, a lot she had bought in Eureka Springs had been declared by the state legislature the property of Evans and Company. The title on other lots she had bought in the town had also been voided by the state, confirming the wisdom of what W. J. P. told her as she purchased property: "As Dr. Russell said when I wanted to pay $20 for the little blue house and lot, that I was just throwing away good money for bad—as taxes would eat it up."[169]

There was evidently an ongoing dispute between the Englishes and the Russells. The families were connected by the marriage of W. J. P.'s brother Wallace to Julia English in 1867, a marriage that ended acrimoniously. The *Weekly Democrat* of Fayetteville contains a notice on 25 May 1882 of an impending execution sale following the circuit court suit of J. T. and Nannie English against J. W. and A. O. Russell, which had been decided in favor of the Englishes—so that land belonging to the Russells in Washington County, Arkansas, was to be sold in June 1882 to satisfy the terms of the judgment.[170]

On 28 June 1886, Ava again wrote her daughter from Dallas, telling her that she and Eric were at home alone and that the family had moved from its large house on Elm Street into a cottage with three rooms and a kitchen in which a Mrs. Best helped her pass time in her "Semi Widowhood." It appears that the cottage was at the corner of Cottage Lane and Bullington, according to the city directory for 1886. It also shows W. J. P. and son Ralph with an office at 712 Elm Street.[171] Ava's letter also notes that Dick (now being called Richard by his mother) was considering medicine as a profession and had joined his father and Seaborn on an "operating tour" in the south of Texas, while Seaborn's family remained in Pickens Station, Mississippi.[172]

In August 1886, Ralph married his first cousin Mary Belle (Mollie) Law Woodliff of Gadsden, Alabama, and did not inform his family of the marriage. His parents learned of the event only *post factum*. This is the only marriage of her children that Ava does not record in her Bible register.

By the fall of 1886, the Russells had made their last move—to Wills Point, a prosperous community in Van Zandt County, with 1,200 citizens and four physicians by 1887. Seaborn had already bought forty acres and a house there[173] On 19 November, Ava wrote her daughter Ava, telling her that W. J. P., Seaborn, and Rich had left on a tour the day before and that she had no idea what profession Rich might ultimately choose. After asking her daughter if she thought Frank Norwood might like to join them at Wills Point, Ava adds, "Eric and Dick like Texas pretty well but I don't like it near so well as I do Mississippi—too hot and dry in summer."

The letter ends with news that W. J. P. was "never well long at a time," and Ava was delaying a trip to visit her daughter Mollie in Oklahoma because of concern about her husband's health. In both her January and April 1892 affidavits supporting W. J. P.'s Mexican War pension claim (and then her own widow's claim), Ava notes that he had suffered from chronic dysentery after his military service. A 10 January 1889 statement from Dr. W. O. Williams of Canton, Texas, in the pension file also indicates that W. J. P. was disabled by articular rheumatism.[174]

Also, after conveying news of her husband's health, Ava pens a plaintive statement about Ralph's recent marriage: "I have never had a line from Ralph since he married. He wrote your Pa but said nothing about having married."[175]

W. J. P.'s declining health did not impede his traveling surgical work. On 22 January 1887, he wrote his daughter Ava from Wills Point informing her that, though he was often "so wearied and sometimes sick" that he felt like doing nothing and having his wife wait on him, he had performed three operations on New Year's Day and was heading to Louisiana and Mississippi the next week "to operate on cases that have been advertising in *Home and Farm* for 2 years to find out where I was." One of these was in Concordia Parish and another in Amite County, Mississippi. Eric was to accompany his father as far as Clinton, Mississippi, where he attended college. The letter also contains news of Seaborn, who was becoming a "first rate" surgeon, and Ralph, whose marriage had incurred his father's wrath.

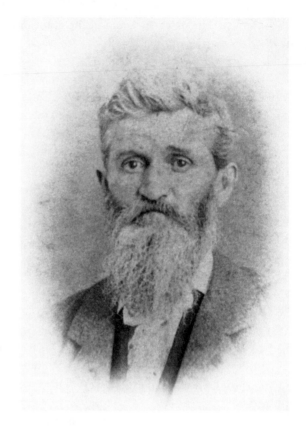

Dr. W. J. P.
Russell, circa
1888. *Courtesy of
Grace Norton;
original in the
Historical Research
Center, University
of Arkansas for
Medical Sciences
(UAMS).*

At some point on this 1887 trip, W. J. P. and Seaborn did surgery in Robeline, Louisiana, according to an article from an unidentified newspaper clipped and preserved by Seaborn's sister Ava in her scrapbook, with "1887" penciled on it.[176] The article states,

> Drs. S. R. and W. J. P. Russell of Dallas and Wills Point, Texas, last Wednesday morning invited the medical fraternity of Robeline and a few other gentlemen to the Keegan Hotel to witness a wonderful surgical operation. The patients were two double hare lipped children, one of them having an abnormal formation something like double front upper teeth. This the Doctors removed and then cut loose the lips and made handsome children of them both in a few minutes.

Despite the fatigue of which W. J. P. had complained in his 27 January letter to his daughter, this 1887 surgical tour extended into autumn, when W. J. P. wrote Frank Norwood from Pine Bluff, Arkansas, on 1 October, stating,

> We have been here several days trying to sell out but find the market overstocked with Texas ponys and money scarcer than I ever knew it in south Arkansas at this season of the year. We did a good business all through Louisiana to Bastrop. After entering Arkansas did nothing to speak of—about paid expenses. Short crops for several years has got the farmers in a bad fix.

His reason for writing was to tell Norwood that Richard was leaving Pine Bluff that day to bring Russell's teams of horses to Minden, Louisiana, which was the best market for horses he had found as they traveled. He could sell the horses there for $225 each and preferred to do this rather than take them back to Texas. Russell asks Norwood to assist Richard in selling the horses since his son was inexperienced and adds, "I don't care much to sell the buggy—can ship it to Wills Point."

As he concludes, W. J. P. tells Norwood that W. J. P.'s wife Ava would join him in Little Rock after he left Pine Bluff, and the couple would travel to Atlanta on 7 October, returning by way of Gadsden, Alabama, where they would visit Ava's sister Chesta, mother of Ralph's wife Mollie, and see Ralph and Mollie. They would remain with Ralph over Christmas as Russell performed surgeries in North Alabama. After their return to Texas, they would begin building at once on their land in Wills Point, eighty acres he had bought in June under Ava's name.[177]

W. J. P. wrote his daughter Ava from Cumberland, Mississippi, on 27 June 1888, stating that he had no further plans to collaborate with or live near Seaborn. Russell tells his daughter,

> Your Ma writes me she is very lonely. I wrote her to sell out as I don't intend to return to Texas. Last winter satisfied me about living close to Seab.

As he wrote this letter, he was on another surgical tour—this time, with son Richard—with whom he was having "phenomenal success not only in our practice but in getting the money." Dick was doing far better with W. J. P. than Dick had done collaborating with Seaborn and a Mr. Renfro who was evidently a drummer assisting the Russells on their surgical tours. Seaborn and Ralph were doing surgeries in Kosciusko as their father toured separately with Dick.

The letter suggests that W. J. P. continued to have misgivings about whether he had provided sufficiently for his daughter at the time of her marriage: Russell states,

> I have your money ready and will send it to you the first opportunity I have to get Post Office Order. It is yours by right—your marriage dowry. I can get on without it and your Ma writes that she has collected enough to pay her debts and some over. I sent her an additional $100 from Kosciusko. She will have enough to live on with her land and my time here will be short so I do not linger with sickness I am content. I want to see Dick start off right and I feel my destiny at an end. I have accomplished my end.[178]

W. J. P. *did*, in fact, return to Wills Point, despite his statement that he would not go back to Texas, and he did continue his plans to build on the Wills Point land located next to Seaborn. In a letter from Wills Point dated 28 October 1889, W. J. P. tells Frank Norwood:

> Found all up and about, began building on the prairie 100 fracas from tract of railroad and just opposite it the day after my arrival. Will have today 4 carpenters and 4 extra men at work. Will have 1 room ready to go in by Saturday next.
>
> All the land is sold on both sides of the road but the strip between yours and road and that would have been sold but that Bennett is holding it for Ma and she is waiting to see if you want it. It will sell in a hurry when Ma turns it loose. If you want it say so at once. We may as well have it as anyone else if you don't want it. The Point is on a boom. Not a house of any kind to rent. Bennett cut hay on your place for Seab, only a few tons. Seab will write in a day or two, is very busy with helping me build.

As this letter and land records indicate, Frank and Ava Norwood also bought land and moved to Wills Point, and W. J. P.'s livestock business continued. He writes,

> I don't approve of having too much land. Would rather have some land and Money. I think 200 acres enough for a small

capital. I am not in favor of extending my purchases beyond
that. Can buy corn for 7px; the money is in Mules.[179]

In his long medical career of almost forty years, the constant chal-
lenge for W. J. P. Russell was to find steady sources of income when his
practice alone was not sufficient. This letter suggests that among the
reasons the family moved so frequently was Russell's perception that
tying his family down with too much land in one spot would hamper
his ability to maximize the profit he might make from his medical
and livestock businesses.

On 10 January 1889, W. J. P. filed his pension claim after a congressional act of 1887 offered pensions to veterans of the Mexican
War.[180] Following his death in January 1892, Ava filed a widow's claim
on 14 April 1892. Her claim was honored, and Ava received a pension
for her husband's Mexican War service to the end of her life.[181]

The summer of 1890 saw W. J. P. off on another surgical jaunt,
the final one of his life. On 4 June 1890, he wrote his daughter Ava
from Lake Charles, Louisiana, stating that he and Seaborn were once
again touring together and that "he is as good to me as he can be."[182]

The final letter from W. J. P. Russell preserved by his daughter
Ava was written on 18 June 1890 from Lafayette, Louisiana. The letter
is addressed to his son Dick. W. J. P. tells Dick of the difficulties he
encountered as a traveling surgeon among the French-speaking people
of South Louisiana:

> We are hammering away amon[g] the French with but little
> success so far but some better than I wrote last. We have a
> first class young man that speaks English and French flu-
> ently. He got a case of X eyes at 50 dollars the first day. Many
> numbers of clubfooted and cross eyed among these people
> and they are well able to pay but they have never heard of
> the like being done before and are superstitious as all Roman
> Catholics are.

And then Russell mentions the farmland around Lafayette—"the
best country I ever saw"—where, with four mules, one man could plant
a hundred acres of rice and recoup fifty dollars per acre. The letter
explains the mechanics of rice farming, as Russell understood them:

> It is just like oats and wheat to raise—takes the same labor
> with the exception of water—Rice has to be flooded after it

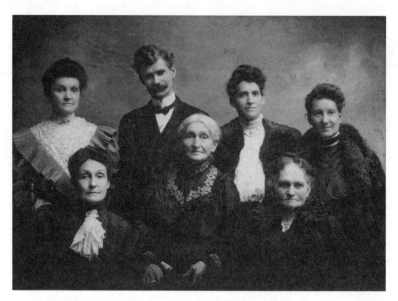

Family photo taken 25 December 1905 in Birmingham, Alabama. Seated left to right are sisters Sallie Law Parker, Ava O. D. Law Russell, and Chesta Law Woodliff. Standing left to right are Ava Russell Norwood, Dr. Ralph Morgan Russell, his wife Mollie Woodliff Russell, and her sister Ollie Woodliff. *Courtesy of Sara Lee Suttle; original in the Historical Research Center, University of Arkansas for Medical Sciences (UAMS).*

comes up and the water drawn off before harvesting. Nothing to do but sit down and wait for it—then go in with a self bindle and cut 20 acres per day worth more than $4.50 per barrel and one acre is good for [illegible]. One man put in 107 acres of sod last year and sold his crop for $6,000. Beats everything I ever heard of. You can buy a rice farm away from the railroad system miles for 5 dollars per acre or less.

Russell closes the letter with instructions to Dick to direct further correspondence to Washington, Louisiana. It demonstrates that, to the end of his life, Russell's practice was plagued by a concern shared by many doctors of this period, particularly in the South, where the economy had been radically disrupted by the war—the concern to make a good living when money was scarce to nonexistent in many areas. That concern had W. J. P. on the road doing surgical tours to his final days.

Ava Law Russell's Bible register tells us, "Dr. William James Park Russell fell asleep in Christ, Jan. 25th 1892, was buried at Wills Point, Texas." A 1975 conversation between Russell's granddaughter Grace Russell Norton and great-great grandson William L. Russell indicates that the cause of death was stomach cancer.[183] Obituary notices for W. J. P. Russell appeared in various Texas newspapers, including the *Fort Worth Gazette* and the *Times-Star* of Terrell, Texas.[184]

In 1894, Ava's physician in Wills Point, Dr. W. H. Coates, filed an affidavit in her Mexican War widow's pension application stating that she had articular rheumatism affecting her knees and fingers and that this had been worse since a severe case of la grippe in 1891.[185] The 1900 federal census shows Ava living with her youngest son Eric at Wills Point as he farmed the land his parents had bought there.[186]

Ava Octavia Dunn Law Russell died 18 December 1907 at the home of her daughter Ava Norwood, who had moved with her husband Frank to Stamps, Arkansas, after 1900.[187] She is buried next to her husband W. J. P. at the White Rose Cemetery in Wills Point. In a 30 May 1975 letter to cousin William L. Russell, Richard Russell's daughter Grace Norton sums up her grandmother Ava (and her grandparents' relationship) as follows: "I faintly remember her as a sweet little lady with a quiet spoken voice—mama always taught us that she was truly aristocratic from a very well to do family and she could calm Grandpa and control him completely. He was a handsome man—deep black eyes and a sharp nose and women were always attracted to him."[188]

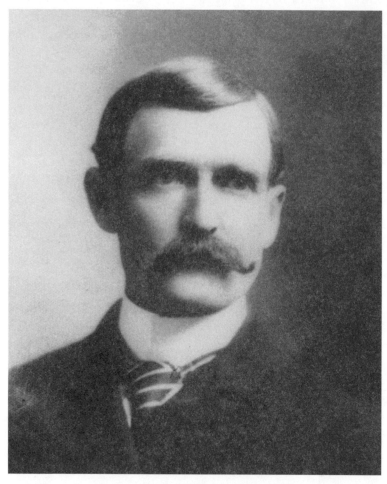

Dr. Seaborn Rentz Russell, circa 1880. *Courtesy of Marvin E. Vaughter Jr.; copy in the Historical Research Center, University of Arkansas for Medical Sciences (UAMS).*

CHAPTER 3

Seaborn Rentz Russell
(1859–1928)

My eventful birth occurred on September 7, 1859 at the little hill village of Canton community site of Cherokee county Georgia now a thriving little city. My Father . . . was enroute to the house of my mothers Father . . . at Gainesville, Hall Co., Georgia with my mother so she could be with her mother. . . . Well I was due to arrive on scheduled time in 2–3 weeks but owing to my Mothers fatigued condition over the long rough roads journey of forty miles that day much to her sorrow and my dear old impatient Dads chagrin, I at once on reaching the modest hill hotel began to make all the trouble possible and never ceased till the earth came on my sight and then they were tied for two weeks.

—SEABORN RENTZ RUSSELL,
diary entry, 7 September 1922[1]

My father was a highly perceptive, highly intelligent man who was devoted to helping people and would still go out on a night to call on poor country people who had not paid him anything on previous medical calls for ten or more years. He was totally impractical, cared nothing for or ever even mentioned money to the point that it occasionally became a financial burden to his family. During the times my mother and father were separated my mother would have to rent out rooms in order

*to have food and to live because he either had no
money or wouldn't send her any or at most only a
few dollars.*

—GEORGE W. RUSSELL, Allentown,
Pennsylvania, to William L. Russell,
Maumelle, Arkansas, March 1976[2]

"Wildness": this is a recurring theme in the life of Seaborn Russell, mentioned in reminiscences of him by his brother Dick and his son George. Wildness is apparent in Seaborn's inability to settle down amicably with his first wife Alcie Bachelor, who bore him six children in ten years before he abandoned them, or his third wife Lounetta Hoobler, by whom he had five children who lived to adulthood, and with whom he had a tempestuous marriage. In between was Emma Sear, about whom he confided in his diary fifteen years after he had married Lounetta that Emma was (with the exception of his mother) the only woman he had ever truly loved, next to whom he wished to be buried.[3] Emma bore Seaborn four children before she died of influenza on 6 May 1900.[4]

An observation made by his son George in the epigraph above notes that his father was "devoted to helping people" and would bend over backward to help people who could not pay for his services. Seaborn's diary confirms his hard work to care for patients. On 11 March 1922, he writes that his family had just moved, and the move would necessitate his occupying new offices—a "morning office" where he would meet patients, with afternoon home visits, and then work at another office into the night. The diary states:

> Find that I will spend mornings on east side until noon and visit bedside cases till 3 PM and then work at 803 W. 7th till 8 PM and then go back on east side till I close work and go to bed.[5]

This is a grueling schedule, with much shifting between locales. When one considers that Seaborn followed this schedule daily (except for Sunday) and was working into the night after his 3–8 shift three years before his death, one can but admire a doctor who gave so heroically to patients, often with no remuneration.

Early Life

The excerpt from Seaborn's diary above captures the unusual circumstances of his birth, as his parents traveled from their home in Van Wert in northwest Georgia to his mother's family in Gainesville, so that Ava could give birth in her mother's home. Shortly after Seaborn's birth, his parents headed to Texas with him and were living there in June 1860 with the family of B. O. W. Whatley in Bosqueville. His siblings were with Ava's mother back in Georgia. From the outset, Seaborn's life was molded by his father's penchant for keeping the family constantly on the move.

In her Bible record of his birth, his mother gives his name as Seaborn Rentz Russell.[6] Later, after his father's death, Seaborn would add William to the name, so that he sometimes appears in records from the 1890s forward as William S. R. or W. S. R. Russell. It seems very likely that W. J. P. and Ava named their son after a Seaborn Rentz who was born in Van Wert in 1858, the son of John Alexander and Josephine Rentz. This family likely had a connection to a Seaborn Jones who lived next to them in 1860 and whose uncle of that name was a US Congressman from Georgia.[7] By 1870, the Rentzes had moved to McLennan County, Texas—just as the Russells did in late 1859 or early 1860.

Following his parents' brief sojourn in Texas, Seaborn spent his early years in Corinth, Mississippi, where his sister Ava was born in June 1862, and in Union County, Illinois, where another sister, Sevie, was born in July 1864. After Illinois, Seaborn went with his parents and siblings first to Alexandria, Louisiana, and then to Shreveport, and, by September 1866, to Evansville in Washington County, Arkansas.

Other than the limited documentation tracking the family's moves during Seaborn's childhood, there is no substantial narrative of his life and those of his siblings, no discussion of how these peregrinations and the deaths of the two oldest children within thirteen months of each other affected the Russell children—though one can imagine that the constant uprooting, coupled with the economic and social upheavals in the South following the war, must surely have given younger family members a strong impression of the transitory nature of everything around them, of the impermanence of time and place and, perhaps, even of the ties that bind people. That transitory perspective may well have made a strong impression on the young

Seaborn, given the testimony of his family members later in his life about his "wildness" and what we know of his marital arrangements.

Arrival in Arkansas:
Education, Marriage, Establishing a Family

It is only after the Russells reach Arkansas that we begin to have clear glimpses of what was taking place in Seaborn's life as he matured to manhood. Several documents tell us that he attended Cane Hill College in Boonsboro. An obituary of James M. Cole of Dardanelle, Arkansas, which Seaborn pasted into his diary on 28 July 1921, has an annotation in Seaborn's hand next to it, reading, "Jim 'Coney' Cole was my school and classmate 1870–1–2 at old Cane Hill College at old Boonsboro, Ark."[8]

In addition, in his March 1976 letter featured above, Seaborn's son George W. Russell states,

> I remember my father talking about Cane Hill College and got the impression that he had been sort of a rounder and had gotten kicked out of several colleges and was finally sent to Cane Hill near the Indian Territory.[9]

It should be noted that "colleges" of the ilk of Cane Hill were more like present-day high schools than colleges proper. Seaborn was, after all, only eleven years old in 1870. Like many such colleges at this period, Cane Hill appears to have operated what might be called a college-preparatory school in conjunction with a more advanced curriculum offered to older students.

By the time he was nineteen, Seaborn was farming his mother's land. Ava's 14 April 1878 letter to her sister Mary Bedell notes that W. J. P. hoped his son would follow in his footsteps as a surgeon, "but Seab fancies a farmers life and the company of girls." At least one attractive young woman had caught his eye by 1878 or 1879: Alcie, daughter of Dr. Wilson Richard Bachelor and Sarah Tankersley Bachelor of Pauline (now Cecil) in Franklin County.

It is not clear how Seaborn and Alcie met. They lived some eighty-five miles apart in different counties, but since both were doctors' children in Northwest Arkansas, their fathers likely knew each other, and the young couple formed an acquaintance. Seaborn and Alcie courted in 1879 and were married on 1 January 1880 in the church

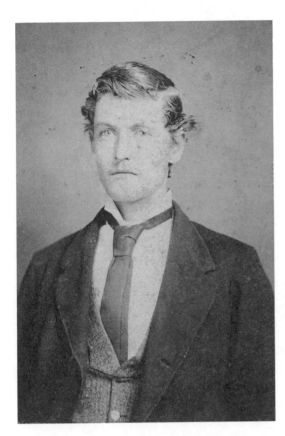

Seaborn Rentz
Russell, age eigh-
teen, photo taken in
Fayetteville, Arkansas.
*Courtesy of George S.
Russell; copy in the
Historical Research
Center, University of
Arkansas for Medical
Sciences (UAMS).*

to which Alcie's mother Sarah belonged in Franklin County, Mill
Creek Missionary Baptist Church.[10] Seaborn was twenty and Alcie
eighteen: she was born 29 October 1861 in Hardin County, Tennessee.

Seaborn's parents appear to have been delighted with Alcie. When
W. J. P. wrote his daughter Ava from Wills Point on 22 January 1887,
he told her, "Alcie is everything we could wish." A 3 December 1883
letter Ava Russell sent her daughter Ava after the family had moved
to Nashville, Arkansas, speaks fondly of Daisy, Alcie's middle name,
and her helpfulness to Ava while Seaborn traveled with his father
doing surgery.[11]

After Seaborn and Alcie married, they continued farming Ava's
land in Cane Hill Township, where they appear on the 1880 federal
census with Seaborn's siblings Ava, Ralph, Dick, and Eric in their
household.[12] W. J. P. and Ava are not found on this census, perhaps
because they were moving from Boonsboro to Eureka Springs as it

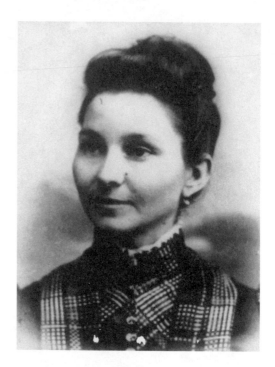

Seaborn Russell's first wife Alcie Daisy Bachelor, whom he married 1 January 1880. *Courtesy of Marvin E. Vaughter Jr.; copy in the Historical Research Center, University of Arkansas for Medical Sciences (UAMS).*

was taken. The 1880 agricultural census shows Seaborn and Alcie growing a wide range of crops, including corn, oats, wheat, sorghum, Irish and sweet potatoes, and apples. Their livestock included horses, mules, cattle, hogs, and chickens. Stating that in the preceding year, he had purchased 250 calves, 50 of which he had later sold, the agricultural listing suggests that Seaborn was carrying on his father's livestock trading business.[13]

On 16 October 1880, the couple's first child, Clara Maude, was born; she was followed by James Wilson on 18 January 1882 and Ada Ava on 5 October 1883. During this time, the couple acquired forty acres near Alcie's parents in Franklin County. Tax lists for 1882–1885 show S. R. Russell paying taxes on this land, for which no deed has been located.[14]

Launching a Medical Career

By November 1883, Seaborn and Alcie had moved with his parents to southwest Arkansas. From family letters, it is evident that Seaborn had decided to follow in his father's footsteps as a doctor. The previously cited December 1883 letter of Ava Russell to her daughter Ava states that W. J. P., Seaborn, and Ralph left on 27 November on a surgical tour of several areas including South Arkansas, North Louisiana, and parts of Mississippi. Hints scattered through family letters indicate that Seaborn was drumming up business for his father and assisting with surgeries.

Noting that Seaborn's wife remained with her in Nashville as he undertook this southern tour, Ava also provides glimpses of the price Alcie was paying while her husband assisted his father. Seaborn and Alcie were striking roots for their own family as they moved south with his parents: The 1884 tax list for Howard County, Arkansas, shows S. R. Russell paying taxes on seven lots, along with a horse, five cattle, seven hogs, and a carriage.[15] As we have seen, by December 1883, Seaborn and Alcie had three infant children, the last only two months old.

From the point of Seaborn's departure on the tour with his father in fall 1883 up to when he and Alcie and their children relocated to Texas in 1885, Alcie entered into the same state of "Semi Widowhood" her mother-in-law had entered. For long periods of time, both women lived entirely on their own, with their children to raise, as their husbands traveled doing surgery.

Family letters indicate that W. J. P. remained in Mississippi on his surgical tour into 1885, while Seaborn returned to Arkansas briefly in 1884 to bring Alcie and their children to her family in Franklin County. Alcie returned to southwest Arkansas early in 1885, where she gave birth to a daughter Sophia on 27 March.

A few months later, however, Alcie had gone again to Franklin County. On 2 July 1885, W. J. P. wrote his daughter Ava from West Point, Mississippi, stating,

> Seab met me here and is going to work for me. His family on back at their Fathers. Am in hopes he will stick to the business and make something—he says he will and he only has to apply himself to do so, he has all the qualities of a first class man.

By the end of August 1885, Alcie and her children were in Mississippi. Seaborn wrote his sister Ava from Memphis on 31 August, telling her the following:

I would have wrote you sooner but did not know where to find you. I was up here from Burnsville, Mississippi on the 23rd on an excursion from Iuka. There was only 1500 people aboard when we reached Memphis and when we left here that night at 9 o'clock there was fully 1,000 men aboard under the influence of liquor.

My wife and babies are now at Burnsville and although among strangers I am well satisfied for them to remain there. I have made all arrangements and have them boarding with a very nice family indeed. Two widows, the widow and widowed daughter of a Dr. Brassland. The daughter is a Mrs. Davis only 28 years old. They have a fine two story house completed and furnished in first class style and they have a fine grand square piano and they both play and both are lively and intelligent and well read women. So you see what kind of a place I have them at—and Ava you ought to write Alcie once in awhile and not expect too much from her for she has had two babys for the last 3 years.

"My wife and babies are now at Burnsville and although among strangers I am well satisfied for them to remain there": Alcie was living among strangers in a boarding house with four small children, one an infant five months old. It is hard to imagine how having access to a "fine grand square piano" and the conversation of "well read women" could possibly solace her as she struggled, in her state of "Semi Widowhood," to care for those children in a place so alien to her, with no family members at hand.

Seaborn's letter ends by telling Ava that he and his father were headed to Texas, a promising market for their surgical and livestock business:

Well sister we are now on our way west—we will sell everything out here and take [train] cars for Texas. We have 6 head of horses and 3 fine ones. Texas has fine crops and they have been picking Cotton for some time. We will strike Texas about Marshall and work northwest. I haven't heard a word from you in a long time and want you to write to me at Texarkana, Texas at once and I will get it.[16]

Alcie continued maintaining the family household as her husband roamed the countryside, not visiting her and their children. W. J. P. wrote his daughter Ava from Dallas on Christmas Day 1885, saying

I am almost in despair about Seaborn. He has been with me 6 months and has been doing a $500 per month business, gets half of all he makes and he has not got money to go and see his wife and little ones. He doesn't drink or gamble and is industrious and is a first rate man for my business but he can't keep money, just throws it around like a millionaire. I have just told him I won't have him with me any longer. But what will become of his little children?[17]

By spring 1886, W. J. P. appears to have overcome his misgivings as he and Seaborn continued working and traveling together while Alcie and her children were in Pickens, Mississippi. As when she was in Burnsville, Alcie would have been among strangers, with no family members nearby.

In August 1886, Seaborn bought land at Wills Point and began making plans to establish a medical practice there with his father.[18] In October, his parents joined him from Dallas, and Alcie and the children also arrived from Mississippi to bring the family back together. On 19 November, Ava Russell wrote her daughter Ava to say that the family was with Seaborn:

We have been here at Seab's for a month or 6 weeks. Pa, Eric, Dick and myself. Seaborn is studying surgery and has induced your Pa to live with him awhile so as to have the benefit of Pa's experience and also his aid in operating on difficult cases.[19]

The letter also mentions that on the previous day, W. J. P. had launched yet another surgical tour, with Seaborn and Dick along.

On 20 January 1887, the *Wills Point Chronicle* published an article noting that Seaborn had opened a practice in the community in collaboration with his father, Dr. W. J. P. Russell of Dallas. The article states,

Dr. S. R. Russell, a specialist in the treatment of the various deformities of the human body, called in our office this week. The doctor has recently located in our midst, having settled two miles northeast of our city. He has wonderful success in the treatment of strabismus or cross-eyes, hair lip, and telipes [*sic*] or club foot, curing cross eyes in a few seconds, and hair lip in three days. He can furnish the best of references from citizens in this and adjoining counties of his successful treatment of the above mentioned deformities, and would be pleased to furnish these references to parties desiring to see them and to secure his services. We saw in our office last Saturday a case of club-foot that has been under his treatment, it being little Cora, daughter of Mr. R. L. Fuller, who lives ten miles north of Wills Point. Dr. Russell showed us a little boy, Willie Oliver, of Upshur County, who is now under treatment for club-foot. Mr. Fuller stated in our presence that his daughter's foot was in as bad condition as this boy's before Dr. Russell treated it, and we must unhesitatingly say that had we not seen with our own eyes the success that has attended his treatment of this case, we should have been skeptical of any report of same. He has showed us most flattering testimonials of his skill in the treatment of cases in his specialties from parties in different parts of the state. In any critical cases, Dr. Russell has the advantage of consultation and assistance of his father, Dr. W. J. P. Russell, of Dallas, who has had 38 years experience in these specialties.[20]

This is the first time Seaborn appears in documents with the title Dr. On 27 January, the *Wills Point Chronicle* notes,

Dr. S. R. Russell and his father, Dr. Russell, of Dallas, left on Monday's train for Gloster Station, one hundred miles south of Vicksburg, Mississippi on professional business and they will be gone about two weeks. The doctor's brother, Master Eric, will accompany them on his way back to Clinton College.[21]

As Ava's 19 November 1886 letter from Wills Point suggests, even after the Russell families gathered again in Texas and Seaborn and W. J. P. made plans for their collaborative practice at Wills Point, Alcie's "Semi Widowhood" continued with Seaborn on surgical tours with his father. When W. J. P. wrote his daughter Ava on 22 January 1887 from Wills Point, he told her,

We are so crowded up here with Seab and his little ones that the boys don't have a chance to write. E. says he will write often when he gets to Clinton. Seab has a good home here and all but 80 acres paid for. He is practicing with me and is a first rate operator. Is much more agreeable than he used to be and Alcie is everything we could wish.[22]

This is the first mention W. J. P. Russell makes in any of his extant letters that he and Seaborn were practicing together. Previous letters speak of Seaborn and Ralph assisting him on surgical tours but imply that his sons' role on these tours was primarily drumming up business while offering help as he did surgery.

It was during their surgical tour in 1887 that W. J. P. and Seaborn performed public surgery at Robeline, Louisiana, on two children with complicated cleft lip problems. The article about this, discussed in the previous chapter, speaks of "Drs. S. R. and W. J. P. Russell of Dallas and Wills Point, Texas," indicating that the two shared a practice in both communities and had held onto their Dallas office even as they began establishing themselves at Wills Point.[23]

In June 1887, Seaborn purchased more land near Wills Point,[24] and by October, he was making plans to liquidate his holdings in Arkansas as he began building a house for his family. Land records from Franklin County, Arkansas, show Seaborn selling his forty acres there in January 1888.[25] On 27 October 1887 the *Wills Point Chronicle* states, "Dr. S. R. Russell, after a long trip to the east on professional business, is at home again."[26]

On 27 July 1888, Seaborn and Alcie's daughter Elsie was born at Wills Point. Now for a time, it seems the misgivings W. J. P. had about Seaborn in 1885 had diminished since he tells Frank Norwood in a 28 October 1889 letter that he and Seaborn had continued their building project at Wills Point and were speculating in land together.[27] Van Zandt County records show Seaborn buying and re-selling a lot in Wills Point in 1888.[28] This transaction bears out W. J. P.'s statement that he and Seaborn were speculating in land around Wills Point in 1888–1889.

On 14 February 1890, when Ava Russell wrote her daughter Ava Norwood from Wills Point to update her on Seaborn's building project, she said that he was preparing to move his family into the house though it was not yet complete. The four-room house had a central hallway and two half-storied rooms above, and though it had a stove, its chimney was not yet operational.

As they moved into this house, Alcie was pregnant with the couple's last child, Seaborn Bachelor Russell, who was born in Franklin County, Arkansas, on 30 September 1890. It appears that Alcie had left Seaborn between June and September, bringing her children to settle beside her parents. The following year, 1891, when her father wrote in his diary at Christmas, he notes that his daughter Alcie and her children were with him.[29]

A letter that Seaborn's niece Ruby Norwood Kitchens sent her cousin Maude Russell on 29 April 1936 provides a glimpse of how the families of W. J. P. and Seaborn Russell settled at Wills Point and of how the dissolution of Seaborn's marriage affected his father. The letter states,

> Well my trip to Wills Point was so sweet. I saw Grandma's house where I was born and Uncle Seab's house where you lived. Were you born there also? Grandma and Grandpa settled on this place about 1887 but I think your father was there first. Uncle Ralph and Uncle Seaborn and Grandpa set up an office in Dallas—I have their card in Mama's things— they did some great work in surgery such as cross eyes, cleft palate, club foot operations and it takes a good one these days even to be successful at that. In one of Grandpa's letters he says Seaborn was thoroughly competent. Seaborn broke Grandpa's heart and one of his letters to Mama shows how crushed he was. Your Mother was so gentle and good and all the family never ceased to speak praise of Aunt Alcie.[30]

On 13 February 1904, Alcie filed a legal writ asking for a separation of property she and Seaborn held jointly. The document states that she and Seaborn had purchased the land on which he built at Wills Point together and that he had abandoned her and their children.[31]

Setting Up a Medical Practice in Arkansas and Relationship with Emma Sear

The termination of Seaborn's marriage to Alcie seems to have coincided with his move to northeastern Arkansas, where he appears on the tax list on 19 March 1891, paying taxes on personal property in Cache Township in Walcott in Greene County.[32] By April 1892, Seaborn was registering credentials to practice in Newport, about fifty-five miles southwest of Lorado, which seems to have been his initial home base after he moved back to Arkansas.[33] That Seaborn was living at Lorado, where Polk's *Arkansas State Gazetteer Business Directories* lists him as "W. S. R. Russell, Physician,"[34] suggests he may have been seeking to develop a roving practice in a circuit in northeastern Arkansas. Following his father's death in Wills Point on 25 January 1892, Seaborn begins to appear in various records as William Seaborn Rentz Russell or W. S. R. Russell.

Lorado was one of the first settlements in Greene County, and as a brief history of it in *Greene County, Arkansas: History and Families* indicates,

> It seems there was always a doctor in residence [in Lorado], with Dr. J. D. Blackwood being the last to practice there. Older doctors who at one time lived and practiced there included Doctors Estes, Russell and Lamb.[35]

At some point either prior to his relocation or after he settled in Arkansas, Seaborn formed a relationship with Emma Sear, whom he claimed as his second wife. No marriage record has been located, and there is no record of any formal dissolution of Seaborn's marriage to Alcie—so he could not have married Emma legally. Information about her background is sparse to nonexistent. On 1 May 1893, the couple had a daughter, Maybelle Emma, born in Paragould.[36] At some point before or after this birth, it appears that the couple had another daughter who died in a house fire while Seaborn was practicing in Lorado, according to information found in a history of the Lorado community based on reminiscences of Winnie Franklin.[37]

The 1893 tax list for Greene County shows Seaborn paying taxes for two horses, six cattle, two mules, five hogs, a carriage, a gold or silver watch, and $325 worth of other personal property.[38] Tax records for 1894 indicate that Seaborn had "gone to Craighead County," bordering Greene on the south.[39] Seaborn continued owning property in Greene County up to 1896, when he appears in the county mortgage registry mortgaging his Lorado house and lot to settle a debt of sixty-five dollars owed to Van Fleet Mansfield Drug Company, which he satisfied within six months.[40] No deed record has been found to indicate when Seaborn purchased the Lorado property.

Another item that allows us to place Seaborn in Lorado and confirm that he was practicing there is a voucher published in the *Charlotte [North Carolina] Medical Journal* in February 1894. The voucher was a statement of praise for a medicine made by Maltbie Chemical Company. Writing from Lorado, Seaborn states

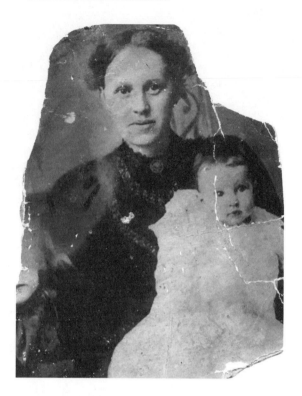

Seaborn Russell's
second spouse (no
marriage record
has been located)
Emma Sear
holding youngest
daughter Mamie
Russell, circa 1898.
*Courtesy of Gary
Pack; copy in the
Historical Research
Center, University
of Arkansas for
Medical Sciences
(UAMS).*

> Your sample of Acetanilid and Caffeine Compound has
> proven very satisfactory indeed, and is all you claim for it, as
> non-depressing Antipyretics are something we have not been
> able to reach before at a reasonable price. Please send me four
> ounces by return mail.

The voucher is signed, "W. S. R. Russell, M.D., Lorado, Ark."[41]

One wonders if doctors who touted the virtues of a pharmaceutical were reimbursed for doing so, perhaps given a price cut when ordering the medicine. It is also worth noting that the Maltbies who owned this company were cousins of the family in Gwinnett County, Georgia, to which Seaborn's grandfather was connected by marriage.

By the time another daughter, Mamie Sear Russell, was born to Seaborn and Emma on 18 December 1898, the couple had moved to Beebe in White County. Records of the Beebe Methodist Church (now First United Methodist Church) show them joining that church in November 1899.[42]

The letterhead used by Dr. W. S. R. (Seaborn) Russell when he was practicing in Lorado, Arkansas, in 1897. Copy in the publication *Letterheads and Documents from Greene County: Businesses, Doctors and Professionals Late 1880s into 1950s Found in Old Probate Records, Book 2*, prepared for the Greene County Historical and Genealogical Society by Cynthia Starling, July 2006. *Courtesy of the Greene County Historical and Genealogical Society.*

In 1900, Alcie appears on the federal census of Franklin County as head of her household next door to her parents, with her name given as Alcie Bachelor and her marital status as a widow.[43] In census entries of this period, "widow" or "widower" was frequently a euphemism for someone separated or divorced. In 1910, Alcie is listed on the Franklin County federal census as Ada [*sic*] D. Russell, divorced.[44] This is the final census on which Alcie appears: she died of liver cancer the following year on 6 August at her home near Cecil and is buried with her parents at Eubanks Cemetery, her father having died in 1903 and her mother the following year.

Emma Sear Russell died at Beebe on 6 May 1900, with one of Arkansas's statewide newspapers, the *Arkansas Democrat*, reporting on the seventh that "Mrs. Dr. Russell" of Beebe had died the previous day of "one of the gravest forms of la grippe" and that the couple's children were also confined to the house with what appeared to be measles.[45] On 21 September the *Democrat* reported that an infant child of Dr. W. S. R. Russell had died and had been brought from Little Rock to Beebe to be buried beside her mother.[46] In a diary entry dated 13 July 1921, Seaborn notes that "little Ava" was buried next to her mother

Emma and that he wanted to be buried beside them since Emma was, apart from his mother, the only woman he had ever truly loved.[47] The three are buried in the town cemetery in Beebe, Emma and Ava in unmarked graves.

Move to Central Arkansas
and Marriage to Lounetta Hoobler Smith

Emma's death inaugurated a new phase in Seaborn's life and practice. Within two months, he had taken a job with a book-selling organization that offered, among other types of books, medical books sold by traveling salesmen. On 14 July 1900, the *Nashville News* (Nashville, Arkansas) stated that Dr. Wm. S. Russell, representing D. Appleton & Co., had spent a day in Nashville that week.[48]

At the same time, it seems Seaborn had relocated to central Arkansas, where he married his next wife, Mary Lounetta Hoobler Smith, who, according to family members, was the caretaker for Emma and the children in Beebe. The couple married in Little Rock on either 23 December 1900 (the date given in Lounetta's Bible register) or on 14 June 1906, the date officially registered in Pulaski County.[49] The marriage record gives Lounetta's name as Mrs. Lounetta M. Smith. Lounetta's Bible register also states that she and Seaborn had a son Charles E. Russell, born 2 September 1901, who died in December 1901.

Seaborn was living at Houston in Perry County by 24 April 1903, when the statewide *Arkansas Gazette* reported that Dr. W. S. Russell of Houston had been injured in a "runaway" accident.[50] On 8 July 1903, Seaborn applied for a license to practice in Arkansas, stating that he was living at Houston and had been practicing medicine for two years in Conway and Perry Counties.[51] Perry borders Pulaski on the northwest, and Conway borders Perry on the north.

It appears that by September 1905, Seaborn was supplementing his income from his practice by working as a railroad physician. As Robert S. Gillespie notes, "railroad doctors" were an important feature of railway companies in the latter part of the nineteenth and early decades of the twentieth century.[52] Rail companies provided doctors as part of employees' benefit packages, and because accidents were lamentably common for railroad workers, these doctors treated those injured at work, sometimes in special "railroad hospitals."

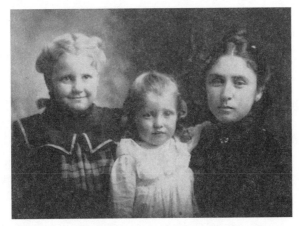

Dr. Seaborn Russell's third wife Mary Lounetta Hoobler
Smith Russell with stepdaughters Mabel and Mamie
Russell, circa 1902. *Courtesy of Gary Pack; copy in the
Historical Research Center, University of Arkansas for
Medical Sciences (UAMS).*

When Seaborn moved to Houston, the Choctaw, Oklahoma,
and Gulf Railroad had just completed running a line through Perry
County.[53] According to county histories, a number of doctors came to
the area with the arrival of the railroad, including a Dr. Russell who
operated the hospital in Houston around 1900.[54]

When he registered his credentials in Jackson County in 1892,
Seaborn indicated that he attended medical school in Philadelphia,
but there is no documentation for this claim.[55] Seaborn's 1903 application for Arkansas licensure states that he had taken courses in the
medical department at Tulane University. Tulane, which kept records
of its graduates in this period but not of those only attending some
courses, has no record showing that Seaborn attended the medical
school at any point.

The catalog for Little Rock's College of Physicians and Surgeons
in 1906/7 lists Seaborn as a matriculant but not a graduate.[56] His listing in the American Medical Association card-index file of deceased
physicians states that he was a "non-graduate."[57] It appears very likely
that if Seaborn did have formal training at a medical school, he did not
complete his course of studies and learned medicine with his father
by the preceptorship method. Seaborn's application for licensure

describes him as a "regular" physician with a specialization in ortho-pedics and optometric surgery.

Seaborn's reason for applying for licensure in 1903 was that Arkansas had just passed its first act requiring such registration. The Arkansas Medical Practices Act of 1903 authorized the governor to create three boards of medical examiners, one each for regular physicians, eclectics, and homeopaths. Each was charged with certifying candidates for practice. Licensure required that candidates pass an exam in areas including anatomy, physiology, chemistry, materia medica, the theory and practice of medicine, surgery, and obstetrics.[58] Both Seaborn's licensure file and the American Medical Association (AMA) deceased physicians index indicate that he was licensed to practice on 18 August 1903.

By November, it appears Seaborn was making plans to relocate to Little Rock—or had already done so. On 10 November, he sold an acre of land in Perry County. The land description in the deed record indicates it was in Houston and that Seaborn was an "unmarried person."[59] Seaborn may have been in debt at this time: the following January, he mortgaged his medical supplies and instruments, household and kitchen goods, a wagon, and a mare and pony to satisfy a debt to R. A. Jones of Perry County.[60]

By 1904, Seaborn begins appearing on lists of registered voters in Pulaski County.[61] Tax records attest to his residence in the county by that year, indicating that he was in Brodie Township in what is now southwestern Little Rock. The 1904 county tax listing shows him taxed for two horses, seven hogs, and two wagons, as well as $270 worth of other personal property.[62] On 22 February 1922, Seaborn wrote in his diary that his daughter Bessie Leona was born 6 April 1903 at the old Gladden place near Mt. Pleasant in Halstead, Arkansas, a small community in southwest Pulaski County, south of Brodie Creek.[63] Bessie's obituary in the *Arkansas Gazette* states, however, that she was born 21 April 1904, the date also given on her tombstone.[64]

Seaborn registered his credentials in Pulaski County in January 1904 and practiced for the subsequent twenty-four years in and around Little Rock.[65] By 23 September 1905, it appears he also had supplementary railway work again. The *Arkansas Democrat* for that date announced that Dr. L. D. Wadley of Runyan & Shinault would leave that afternoon for Stamps to relieve Dr. W. S. Russell, who was in charge of the fumigating station on the Louisiana and Arkansas railroad.[66]

On 20 February 1906, Seaborn bought a five-acre tract from J. M. and Bettie Bruner in Brodie Township, which appears to have been the site of the family's house on Upper Hot Springs Road on Brodie Creek for the next fifteen years.[67] Tax records indicate that Seaborn paid taxes on the Brodie land from 1906 through 1921.[68] In December 1906, he sold the remaining half acre of his Perry County land.[69]

Lounetta and Seaborn had a son, Paul, in 1906. On 22 February 1909, they had another child—Martha Washington Russell. Both were born at home in Brodie, according to Seaborn's diary.[70] The 1910 federal census confirms that the family lived on Upper Hot Springs Road. It lists William S. Russell as head of his household, a physician who is a "county practitioner." In the household were Seaborn's daughters Maybelle and Mamie by Emma and his children by Lounetta—Bessie, Paul, and Martha. Also in the household was Seaborn's widowed mother-in-law Christiann Hoobler.

Curiously, whoever provided information about Seaborn's birthplace and the birthplace of his parents to the census taker was diffident about doing so as the census states merely that all three were born in the "United States." In the column about Seaborn's marital status, the census taker appears to have written the numeral 2 (indicating that Seaborn had been twice-married) and then to have struck through it and written 1. The census indicates that he and wife Mary L., who was twenty-eight and born in Illinois, had been married ten years.[71] The marriage date corresponds to Lounetta's Bible register stating that they married in 1900 and not to their officially recorded marriage date of 1906.

By 20 March 1914, Seaborn was a justice of the peace in Brodie Township, according to a notice in the *Arkansas Democrat*, which gives his name as Dr. W. S. Russell.[72] The 1914 Little Rock city directory lists his residence at 3214 Arch Street.[73] Since this address differs from his Brodie home, it seems that this was one of numerous times when he and wife Lounetta were living separately, a pattern that their descendants report recurred throughout their marriage.

It appears Seaborn and Lounetta were back together when their next child, George Washington Russell, was born at their house in Brodie on 22 February 1915. Lounetta's mother, Christiann Hoobler, died the same day. Seaborn's 22 February 1922 diary entry speaks of the births of his children. He states,

> Old George W. Russell, my real baby boy is seven years old this A.M. God bless his dear good manly soul. He is great company for me now. He and Martha W. Russell who is 13 years old this morning were both born at our old home on 'Upper Hot Springs Road' on Brodie creek just 5 miles west of our city limits on 79th Street Pike. Paul also born there October 4, 1907 and Bessie April 6, 1903 at the old 'Gladden Place' near Mt. Pleasant, Halstead, Arkansas—and Veda May—my real baby daughter was born where we have lived over three years—1622 Lewis Street—June 1920.[74]

George and his older sister Martha were born on George Washington's birthday and were given the names George Washington and Martha Washington Russell as a result.

On 8 August 1918, Seaborn lost the first of his grandchildren born to his two surviving daughters by Emma. The 9 August *Arkansas Democrat* states that ten-month-old Ruth Marie Powell had died the previous day at the home of her grandparents Dr. and Mrs. W. S. Russell of 1900 Wolfe Street.[75] As the death notice indicates, Seaborn and Lounetta had moved to Wolfe Street closer to the city center between 1915 and 1918. An announcement in the *Democrat* on 30 March 1918 shows them advertising for sale the "Dr. Russell home" on Upper Hot Springs Road, a five-room, two-story house with a barn and outbuildings, as well as a servant's house and five acres.[76]

The 1919 Little Rock city directory, however, shows Seaborn living at 1817 Wolfe while Lounetta remained at their house in Brodie.[77] Both Seaborn's diary for 1920 and the city directory for that year show him living apart from Lounetta during parts of that year, too.

There was also evidently turbulence in Seaborn's wider family circle at this time. According to an article in the *Democrat* on 16 April 1919, Seaborn's son-in-law E. R. Powell had been fined for a charge of assault and battery after hitting his father-in-law.[78] The article reports that Powell and Maybelle were separated and that she was seeking a divorce. Powell claimed that her father had interfered in their marital affairs and had forbidden him to see his wife, who was staying at Russell's house. In a fit of rage, he had gone to Dr. Russell's office in the Masonic Temple building and hit him in the face, and Seaborn had pressed charges.

Little Rock Medical Practice and The Final Years

Though Seaborn was licensed in Pulaski County in 1904, we know little about his Little Rock practice before 1920. We have no information about the role he played in treating patients during the 1918 flu pandemic that swept the world and resulted in more than 7,000 deaths in Arkansas alone, with a quarter of citizens in central Arkansas contracting the illness.[79]

Fortunately, for several years in the final decade of his life—the 1920s—there is abundant documentation of Seaborn's life in diaries he kept from 1920–1922. The diaries are now in the possession of George S. Russell and Ann Russell Zorn, the children of his son George, and descendants of Marvin Vaughter, a son of Seaborn's daughter Bessie. These diaries provide detailed information about aspects of Seaborn's practice in the early 1920s, his family life, social activities (including churchgoing), and events in the families of his friends.

The detailed snapshot the diaries give us of Seaborn's practice in the early 1920s shows an energetic general practitioner treating a wide range of medical problems in Arkansas's largest urban community. The diaries indicate that a majority of Seaborn's medical work was done by home visits, not office consultations. In 1920, for instance, he made 418 home visits, including 16 at night, while he had 289 office visits. The following year, he made 627 visits to patients at home, 25 of these at night, and had 329 office visits. As these figures indicate, the home visits increased more than 50% in 1920–1921 while his office visits increased by more than 10% in the same period.

Since Seaborn also studiously registered fees and payments in his diary, they also provide documentation of what general practitioners were charging patients in central Arkansas at the time. Most home visits cost three dollars, with an additional dollar added if the visit was at night, while office visits ranged from two to four dollars, depending, apparently, on their length and the patient's medical issue. The fee for prescriptions, which Seaborn dispensed in both home and office visits, was two dollars. Delivery of a baby cost twenty-five dollars, with an additional five dollars added if twins were delivered. These fees reflect rates mandated by the state medical association in the early 1920s.

Seaborn saw the majority of his patients on a credit basis, and they paid as they were able, often by installment—or they paid in goods (ranging from a chair cushion to a load of wood, a basket of freshly laid eggs, a pail of milk or butter, gallons of preserves, quilts, and a bicycle) or services such as hauling wood. A number of hints in his diaries suggest that Seaborn treated both black and white patients without prejudice.

The diaries show Seaborn dispensing 609 prescriptions in 1920 and 295 in 1921, about a 50% decrease. At the same time, Seaborn's treatment of patients struggling with addiction issues declined from 104 to 7. In January 1921, he was visited by the Narcotics Inspector, who charged him with keeping incomplete records; it appears likely that the decline in Seaborn's treatment of addicts in 1921, and perhaps in the number of prescriptions he dispensed that year, may have been related to the problems he encountered with his narcotic prescriptions—though the bulk of what he prescribed in 1920 and 1921 appears to have been serums and tonics.

Diary entries for both years also show Seaborn consulting with a number of other local doctors, including county coroner Dr. Vaughter (whose son Marvin married Seaborn's daughter Bessie), Dr. McGill, Dr. Hardeman, Dr. Daniel Jones (son of Arkansas Governor Daniel Webster Jones), and Drs. Kirby and Runyan of St. Luke Hospital. On one occasion in 1920, Seaborn reported a colleague for malpractice and neglect of a patient, then made no further mention of this charge. At this time in Arkansas, malpractice accusations were judged by the "vicinity rule" resulting from the case of *Dunman v. Raney* (1915), which said that physicians should be "judged by the practices of other doctors in the vicinity."[80]

Seaborn's 1920–1921 diaries suggest that he treated a wide range of conditions, including asthma, bronchitis, and other respiratory problems; chicken pox; ear and eye infections; erysipelas; gangrene; gastric ulcers, gastritis, and general gastric and digestive complaints; gonorrhea; impotence; influenza; menopausal problems; mumps; rheumatism; tuberculosis; various sores and ulcers; tonsillitis; uremia; and vaginal infections. In 1920, he performed surgeries for gangrene, clubfoot, hemorrhoids, and vaginal abscess, with two abortions. At this time, the 1875 Arkansas abortion law was in effect, allowing only physicians to perform abortions and only when the mother's life was at risk.[81] The following year saw him performing a tonsillectomy, repairing a hip injured in an auto accident, and performing surgery for endometritis. His medical ledger also records a number of cases of mental instability attributed to causes such as grief and shock, manic disorder, depression, and nervousness. One of his patients was committed to the state mental hospital for imbecility.

The diaries note that Seaborn delivered four babies in both 1920 and 1921, including one weighing a whopping twelve pounds and a set of twins. Twenty-nine of Seaborn's home visits in 1920 and fifty-nine in 1921 were to treat ailing babies.

The 1920 diary mentions no automobile-related injuries, but the 1921 diary records six such injuries, including a broken arm and other fractures, internal bruising, and knee and back injuries. One might assume that other local medical registers in this period show a similar increase in such injuries, with growing ownership of cars.

Seaborn's diaries demonstrate the assiduity with which he dealt with patients and suggest that conscientious general practitioners often endured considerable stress as they met patients' needs in this period. On 7 July 1920, he reports that on the preceding day, he had visited patients in North Little Rock, Pulaski Heights, and East Little Rock into the night; these are disparate and widely separated locales of the urban area. Visiting all of them in a single day would have required considerable outlay of time and energy.[82]

On 25 July 1920, Seaborn took his son George with him as he traveled via the "Hood Bros. Special" eighteen miles west of town to visit a patient in need of attention before returning to Little Rock to call on two more patients. Hood Brothers was a Little Rock business that rented cars for day use.[83] After his medical visits, Seaborn and George then went to an open-air sermon preached in the evening by the pastor of their Winfield Methodist Church to an audience of 1,200 revival attendees.[84]

Seaborn's diaries seldom speak of medical problems of his own, but his 1920 diary contains intimations of his growing awareness of his mortality in this final decade of his life. An entry on 21 September 1920 provides a rare glimpse of Seaborn's own infirmity and how it affected his practice: He notes that he was in bed due to a "severe attact [sic] of sciatic rheumatism" and that this was the only day in a year's time in which he had been unable to work due to illness. Then he concludes:

[S]o I have much to be grateful to 'my dear heavenly father' for all his goodness and mercy to me and my dear children and loved ones. Bless his holy, great name, is all my help.

Must come from him but his strong arm is always stretched
out to hold us up and his loving heart yearning to bless those
that trust him. Oh that my children would do so.[85]

An entry on 12 January 1921 further illustrates the dedication
Seaborn gave to his practice—and its arduous nature. Seaborn writes
that Billy Steinkamph [*sic*], "the warmest and dearest German in the
city," had come knocking at his door at 1:30 a.m. to tell him that
"Uncle Billy Parcell" had collapsed and appeared to be dying.[86] Then:

> I jumped into my clothes and rushed out and climbed into
> Mr. Steinkamph's big seven passenger touring car and told
> him to 'let her go' and we shot across the two miles to Uncle
> Billy's in a few seconds and by long continuous heroics, doses,
> and efforts prolonged his life.[87]

The following day, as previously noted, Seaborn had an unpleasant
visit from the Narcotics Inspector, who informed him that he had not
been keeping proper records. Seaborn writes:

> Mr. Mathews, Narcotics Inspector visited me this P.M. and
> found my record of cases treated for habit forming drugs was
> incomplete and I was wrong in supposing it not required.[88]

Ten days later Seaborn states that Mr. Mathews had called on
him again in the evening and "jacked him up" about his neglect of
records.[89] This matter necessitated an outing on 26 January to the
office of Judge Allen, a federal commissioner, with Seaborn being
obliged to give bond due to his failure to keep detailed records of
narcotics prescriptions. Seaborn's diary states that Judge Allen was
"very courteous and pleasant and allowed our mutual friend Mr. M. E.
Durinay to sign a bond for me" and with friends who accompanied
Seaborn.[90] On 22 November, he reports that he had paid Federal Judge
Trieber a fine of $70.23—the first fine ever levied on him at the "ripe
old age of 62" due to the "technicality" of which he had been guilty.[91]

A passage written on 29 January 1921 provides detailed information about a tonsillectomy Seaborn had performed along with Drs.
Kirby and Runyan on his grandson Franklin Long, son of Seaborn's
daughter Mamie.[92] He reports that he had taken "Little Frank" to St.
Luke to see Drs. Kirby and Runyan for a consultation. Following this,

> Gave a welcome and after social amenities were done we
> anaesthisized our Pet and took out both tonsils and a large

mass of Adenoids which completely closed the posterior Nares—also dilated the foreskin to forment 'Tulymasis.' Little Franklin came out from under the ether very slowly. As he struggled so very hard and thereby he had filled the lungs so deeply that 5 hours after you could smell the ether all over my office. But this A.M. he is bright and cheerful and hungry—he took no food yesterday and after bath.[93]

Later in 1921, Seaborn's diary shows his intent concern about treatment of his son George's broken leg. His notes about this case are detailed and worth examining to get a glimpse of how Seaborn doctored. His diary reports that he had called his daughter Mabel on 26 June to meet him at Forest Park, an amusement park. They met there with George and some of his friends, and after the children had ridden ponies, Seaborn left them in Mabel's charge and went to his office. George then jumped out of a swing and broke both bones in his right leg two inches above his ankle.[94] An account in the *Arkansas Democrat* says that George Russell, son of Dr. and Mrs. W. S. Russell of 1622 Lewis Street, had jumped from a merry-go-round and broken his leg.[95]

The day after the accident, Seaborn's diary says that George had waited an hour before his father reached him and began treatment. Seaborn had anesthetized his son, who was in shock, and set the limb, stifling "the awful agony of the broken ends jabbing into the quivering lacerated nerves."[96] George had passed a very bad night.

For days after, George and Seaborn struggled with the effects of the accident. On 28 June, Seaborn reports that George had slept only after taking opiates. Seaborn was concerned that he had not properly set the leg. He states, "[I]f it were not for his weakened condition and the perfect set of broken bones, I would be tempted to Etherage him and redress."[97] The following day, George was somewhat better after Seaborn had cut off some of the splint to relieve pressure on the knee. On 3 July, Seaborn notes that "poor little George" was doing fine, but Seaborn's anxiety about whether the bones were healing properly continued and he mused about doing another x-ray.[98]

On 9 July, George was finally able to sit up. On the tenth, his father took him to Dr. A. G. McGill's office for an x-ray. It showed that Seaborn's anxiety was well founded: the tibia had moved out of alignment.[99]

Seaborn's account on 11–12 July indicates that George had been staying at his office, with Seaborn tending him in a recovery bed. On the eleventh, Seaborn notes that he was concerned that George had spent thirteen days "at this old hot dirty place" with stale air and city water, and he intended to bring George home.[100] The following day, with George at home, Seaborn's anxiety began to abate somewhat, and the diary notes that he was turning his attention to moving his office.[101] On the seventeenth, he again documented the case, noting that he was concerned about changing the dressing for fear of disturbing the new ligature of bones, and on the twentieth, he indicates that he had found a sore on George's leg caused by the pressure of the splint.[102]

Several days later, Seaborn put a steel brace with a foot piece on George's leg, noting that George had had fever in the night but appeared well otherwise.[103] On 3 August, Seaborn notes that despite the brace, George had not walked since the injury. He repeats his concern about George's inability to walk on the sixth, noting that he had consulted specialists and was afraid to allow George to put weight on his leg.

By the ninth, George was learning to use a crutch, and a few days later, he began putting weight on the leg with the brace and splint in front assisting him.[104] On the twenty-first, Seaborn ends the saga of George's broken leg by noting that he and George had spent the night at his new office and that George was still not using his right foot. But one can infer that George was on the road to recovery since the diary says on 16 September 1921 that Seaborn had taken George on the train with him the preceding day so that they could visit Seaborn's sister Mollie Moore in Conway.[105]

One aspect of Seaborn's family life that the diary documents, sometimes inadvertently, is his repeated separations from Lounetta. The 1919 city directory shows Seaborn living at 1817 Wolfe Street, while Lounetta was in Brodie. By 28 June 1920, Seaborn and Lounetta were back together and living at 1622 Lewis Street when their final child, Veda May, was born—though when the Little Rock directory for 1920 was published, Seaborn had apparently moved into his own quarters at 926½ W. 7th Street, near where he would set up a combined residence and office later in 1920.[106]

Then on 4 October, Seaborn explicitly notes that he was moving to another residence on 7th Street, where he hoped to have more privacy.[107] Two days later, the diary records this move:

> Uncle George, Oscar, Paul and I moved all the heavy furniture and all drugs, books, instruments, etc. up street to 1301 to

[*illegible*] building across street from big new building of the American Bakery where I will have rooms and more privacy as well as much more comfort.[108]

The diaries also provide glimpses of Seaborn's relationship with some of his siblings, in particular, with his oldest sister Mary Sophia (Mollie) Russell, who married John Denton Moore. Mollie had moved to Arkansas between 1910–1920, and according to his diary, Seaborn visited her frequently. On 7–8 September 1920, he and George took the train to spend the weekend with his "dear sister Mrs. Mary Sophia Moore at 107 Ash St., Conway," as Seaborn celebrated his sixty-first birthday.[109] The diary entry of 20 March 1921 says that it was Easter Sunday and Seaborn and George had spent the day in "the nice little city of Conway" with his "dearest old Sister Mollie S. Moore and her two cultured and refined daughters Sophia and Ruth and my two smart little Great nephews Edwin and Jimmie Dean." He and Mollie sat on her covered porch and "enjoyed the proverbial 'Feast of Reason and flow of Souls.'" At 8:40 p.m., he and George returned to Little Rock, where he called on a patient, Mr. Miller, at 216 Cross Street, who was recovering from an auto injury.[110]

Mollie is also mentioned in a 23 August 1921 entry in which Seaborn states that he had gotten word from her of the death of their brother Eric and Eric's son Eric Jr. when a train struck their automobile as they were crossing the railroad line near their house in Wills Point. Seaborn pasted into his diary a clipping about the accident, which names Dr. W. S. Russell of 1622 Lewis Street in Little Rock, Arkansas, as a survivor. His diary entry reads,

> Read message from my sister Mollie Moore of Conway that our dear 'baby Brother' Eric Alvin [*sic*] Russell, Sr. and his only son Eric A. Jr. were both killed by a fast train at a crossing near their house in Wills Point, Texas. . . . Oh God help us all—verily in the busy hours of life we are in the *midst* of '*death.*' Alas dearest of all dear brothers must I say farewell for all eternity to these dear 'Time Souls' ushered into the 'Portals of eternity.' Nay, verily we shall meet again soon where no pain nor sorrow nor death ever [illegible]. God help me to so live that when the summons comes I may be found *waiting.*[111]

As his comments about Eric's death and his admiration for his sister Mollie suggest, at this stage of his life, Seaborn exhibited a strong interest in matters spiritual. On 7 November 1920, his diary reports the following unplanned outing to a séance at which his deceased mother imparted a message to him:

> Started to my church for evening service and met up with Mr. Akers, a friend, just at the corner of 5th and Main Sts. who was going to hear a lecture and séance by a verry [*sic*] noted 'spiritualist' of N.Y. and he persuaded me to accompany him to the fraternal hall and found the professor quite interesting and at end of his lecture his wife gave out to members in the audience what she said were messages from the dead, among others one from my loving dead mother, and not knowing what might be possible, I received it as such. God help me.[112]

As the new year opened on 4 January 1921, Seaborn writes that he and daughter Mamie had gone to Liberty Hall to hear evangelist Bud Robinson and his wife preach, "proff" (i.e., prophesy), and, in the case of Robinson's wife, sing. Robinson fascinated Seaborn, and Seaborn went again on 8 January to hear him preach and recount his providential recovery from a car accident. The following day, Seaborn writes that he had been too busy to go to church that morning but had gone in the evening to hear Bud Robinson at Liberty Hall.[113]

The diary states,

> He held the large crowd spellbound for hours while he related the main dark happenings of his unhappy childhood. Born amid the squalid surroundings of a one roomed mud daubed dirt floored log cabin in the lofty Cumberland mountains one hundred miles east of the thriving city of Nashville, Tenn., he was one of 13 children who grew up in that awful place—was 12 years old before he ever spent one night outside that hovel and was seventeen when he escaped and emigrated to west Texas. He was never in school a day in his life, learned to read and write his name at twenty at the age of 55 is the author of several books and easily the greatest evangelist in the Church of the Nazarene.[114]

As William Kostlevy notes, Reuben ("Bud") Robinson was one of a long line of "preacher actors" who have galvanized audiences with their rhetoric. Robinson had moved from the Methodist tradition to the Holiness wing of Methodism that became the Church of the

Nazarene, which sought to incorporate Pentecostal practices into traditional Methodist worship.[115]

The diaries also indicate that Seaborn regularly attended Winfield Methodist Church when his medical duties permitted. Seaborn frequently mentions that George accompanies him to church but never indicates that Lounetta or other family members—except his son Paul, grandson Franklin Long, and once his daughter Mamie—went with him.

On 24 April and 15 May 1921, Seaborn mentions going with George and "Sonnie" (Franklin Long) to the senior high school to hear Rev. Hogg's Sunday evening sermon.[116] On 16 April 1922, Seaborn states that Paul had joined the Winfield Church, and George and Franklin Long had been baptized at the same time. This diary entry mentions that Seaborn had belonged to Winfield for eighteen years.[117]

On Mother's Day 1922, Seaborn's diary combines a notation that he had gone to evening services at Winfield with a reflection on the role of mothers that once again avowed his love for Emma Sear. Noting that he had not been able to attend church in the morning due to office work and visits to patients but had heard his "beloved pastor" preach in the evening about the "Beatitudes of all Sainted Mothers from the Virgin Mary on down the ages to our own Sainted Saintly Mother," he writes:

> How it warmed my heart as my mind went back to my boyhood and I saw the lovely face and form and heard again the gentle voice of the dearest mother. Even grown to a restless ambitious [young man], depraved by both nature and practice and yet held in check and guided in peace, honesty of both mind and purpose by her smart ways of control and advice and later when my dear sainted wife Emma Sear added her dear loving influence to that of Mother's I can only thank God they were mother and wife to me.—W. S. R.[118]

Seaborn's diary also provides evidence of other interests. On 2 November 1920, he notes that he had voted that day—Democratic—but feared that the Republican ticket would win due to its "slush fund" and backing of "Wall Street" and "Big Business."[119] On the fifth, he reports that he had written Municipal Judge Harry B. Hale begging him to modify an order requiring a disabled patient whose legs had been broken in childhood to leave the city by Saturday evening. The patient had been arrested for solicitation. Seaborn asked Hale to think about how the "poor creature" would be able to make a living if he did not modify the order.[120]

As 1920 ended, Seaborn penned a 17 December statement of dismay about the Poindexter Bill, which, in his view, would cause revolution as it sought to stifle strikes. He opposed the bill as undermining everything workers had gained in their struggle against "work slavery."[121]

On 14 March 1922, Seaborn notes that he had just attended a meeting, 1,000 strong, of a group he identifies in an aside as "Little Rock's Klan." He reports that the group had met at "our Hall" (evidently Liberty Hall) and had voted to build an auditorium that could seat 10,000.[122] As Diane Dentice notes, Klan activity began surging circa 1915 after a period of desuetude, and by the early 1920s, new Klan groups were forming in a number of states, including Arkansas.[123] According to Charles Alexander's study of the Klan, it began organizing in Little Rock in the summer of 1921 and, by 1922, was actively recruiting and exerting influence in Little Rock.[124] On 26 March and 5 August, the *Arkansas Gazette* ran full-page ads for the Klan. The announcement on the fifth says that a meeting would be held at the city's park that evening, with a band concert, at which Dr. Harry G. Knowles, pastor of Little Rock's First Christian Church, would expound Klan principles.[125]

A number of Seaborn's 1921–1922 diary entries concern his daughter Mamie, who had separated from her husband Franklin Long. Seaborn's reports about Mamie frequently contain a plaintive note, as when he wrote on 11 and 12 March 1920 that she had gone to Mulberry Station near Fort Smith to visit her half-brother Jim and half-sisters Sophia, Maude, and Elsie, several of Seaborn's children by his first wife Alcie.[126] This is a rare diary entry indicating interchange between his children by Alcie and his children by his next two wives.

Seaborn's daughter Bessie also caused him anxiety. On 13 March 1920, he noted that Bessie had spent a week in bed due to a serious cold and had just now returned to her work at a dress store. The entry concludes: "Hope will be able to so influence her mind with the idea of comfort as to prevent future colds."[127] Then on 13 July, his diary states:

> Paul still out at old man Tom Brown's. I am beginning to miss
> my boy. He is so dutiful and obedient and quiet at home that

we never have to worry about where he is at night—like we
do Bessie sometimes.[128]

Bessie married Marvin Earl Vaughter on 6 April 1921, an event
Seaborn notes in his diary on that date. Seaborn states, "God help
them both for they are both just children—Bessie less than seventeen and while Earl is 22 yet he has had no experience in business or
domestic duties."[129]

As may be obvious, while Seaborn worried about his daughters, he
doted on the sons of his last marriage, George and Paul. "Old George
W." went everywhere with him, including to his office, on visits to
patients, and to church, and was a "perfect little man" of "perfect metal
[sic]."[130] Paul sometimes accompanied Seaborn on his rounds and to
church. On 4 October 1921, when Seaborn reflected on Paul's birth,
he wrote:

> Just 15 years ago old Paul Seaborn Russell was born at our
> house west of this city seven miles. In all these 15 years never
> said a word or was guilty of an act to grieve me or make me
> ashamed to call him my dear son and God help him to so live
> in future life as to carry out these good promises of honesty,
> prudence, and obedience and respect to his elders and cour-
> tesy to the general public—God grant it.[131]

Yet George's children, who say that their father distanced himself
from his father and found him a "religious nut," report that Seaborn
was capable of fits of intense rage and once threw Paul down the stairs.
Seaborn's daughter Martha told William L. Russell in 1974 that her
"father had a violent temper and was a total nonconformist."[132] The
placid surface of family life, propped up by conventional piety, can hide
depths of turbulent feelings.

Perhaps reflecting his growing sense of his mortality, Seaborn
dotted his diary entries in his final decade with obituaries clipped
from various newspapers. His 1920 diary opens with statements noting the deaths of his friends Col. Geo. W. Murphy of Hot Springs and
Sam R. Willcockson of Little Rock.[133] Murphy's obituary is pasted
beside the diary entry. On 7 March 1921, Seaborn wrote that he had
attended the funeral of "poor Rich" at Oakland Cemetery in Little
Rock. Next to the diary entry is an obituary for Richard McFarland.[134]

On 13 July 1921, Seaborn saved the obituary of Mrs. M. T. Webb, wife of the former pastor of Beebe Baptist Church, who was one of four officiants at the funeral of Seaborn's wife Emma. He notes:

> I want *all* my children to have one last look at old dad while you keep my body not less than four (4) days embalmed by my friends Healey and Roth and then to Emma's side.[135]

Healey and Roth was (and still is) a Little Rock funeral home.

Less than a month later on 5 August, Seaborn inserted into his diary a clipping of an obituary for A. D. Grayson, Greene County sheriff, noting that he and Grayson had been intimate friends and that he had been family physician to Grayson and his children from 1891 to 1897.[136]

On 10 February 1921, Seaborn wrote a letter to his grandson Earl O'Rear, son of his deceased daughter Ava and her husband James A. O'Rear.[137] The letter speaks of his difficulty in contacting Earl: He asserted he had tried for some years to make contact but his letters never seemed to reach Earl. The letter includes a lengthy exhortation for Earl to know and cherish his Russell lineage: Seaborn writes,

> Never forget that you are directly descendant from such great statesmen as 'Lord John Russell' who was good Queen Victoria's Prime Minister and chief advisor more than 14 years and directly connected with the noted lives of the illustrious 'Duke of Buckingham' and on the American side we have for a nearby ancestor General William Park of Atlanta, Ga. who was my fathers grandad and was said to have killed in a 'hand to hand' Pistol duel at the Battle of New Orleans 1811–12 the brave British General Ruckelhause and thus ended his attempt to capture the most important Post in the U.S. and gain control of the Miss. River. Also remember both your Great Grandfathers were medical officers and served through the entire Civil War 1861–1866 and could tell pages more. But the history of England gives Russell history so don't fail to remember your middle name means much in lineage to you.

While the Livingston biography of William James Russell mentions Lord John Russell, Seaborn's descent from Lord John Russell is uncorroborated by any sources. Nor did Earl's great-grandfathers W. J. P. Russell and Wilson R. Bachelor serve as medical officers during the Civil War. Bachelor enlisted in neither army, though his Union sympathies seem evident since the federal government appointed him physician in charge of building the national cemetery at Pittsburg Landing (later, Shiloh).[138]

Not long before his death in March 1928, Seaborn sent his daughter Sophia Hoyle an undated letter from his final residence at 5715 Prospect Avenue in Little Rock.[139] The letter addresses his "dearest children," perhaps with the intent of sending some final words through Sophia to all his children by his wife Alcie.

This last testament to his first set of children, whom Seaborn had shamefully neglected, is plaintive in the extreme. He reports in a *sub-rosa* way that he and Lounetta were living apart, noting that "[m]y wife keeps room and board down on W. 12th Street (4 miles from here)," and that, while George was with him, the other members of his third family of children were with their mother. Then he provides news of his health and financial struggles:

> I have been confined to office and most of the time in bed ever since the first freezing weather and was paralyzed in my lower limbs so completely that my hands were affected so I wrote only with such difficulty that I wrote very few notes. You can see how irregular my lines are, but thank God I am better in both feet and hands and lung still very sore but better. I can inflate the cells below the ulcer after six months of self-treatment and little income and honey it sure does hurt me to be unable to feed or house or help my own family for months and George is only help I have had. But he and I just manage to keep him in school up here and he and Sonny both passed. Sonny to fourth grade and George to 7th and now has to go about three miles on street car to P. H. Junior High which makes him hustle. He has to leave here at 7:30 a.m. to make it O.K. but he is determined to have an education and if I could live two more years I would see he was ready for 'Senior High' which is all any boy needs. But in my 69th year and afflicted as I am, I am living on the bounty of God and Our Savior and can't claim a day. But believe God is going to let me live another year and we may get to meet once more on earth. But if not I will meet you up there where parting can never come. Won't it be joyous to meet all our loved ones gone on before? All my brothers except Dick and three gen-

erations of my own blood. But still we are loath to go and leave helpless ones here unprovided for. God pity such.

The letter concludes with greetings to Sophia's children, Joyce, Elsie, and Russell, and her husband, Wheeler Hoyle, and states that, if he lived through "this awful winter," he planned to come with George to west Arkansas on a camping trip and hoped to see her family either at her house or the house of her brother Jim.

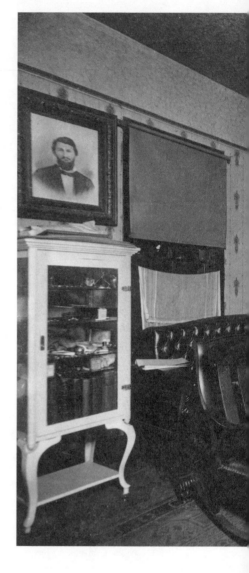

Seaborn Rentz Russell died of pneumonia in Little Rock on 1 March 1928 and was buried next to his second wife Emma Sear and daughter Ava in the town cemetery of Beebe. His younger brother, Richard Dalton Russell, died in October of the same year in Texas. Seaborn's widow Lounetta continued living in Little Rock. She died of a cerebral hemorrhage on 29 August 1958 and is buried at Pinecrest Cemetery in Alexander in Saline County, next to her daughter Bessie Russell Vaughter, who died two years later. When Seaborn died, he incurred a debt of $300 to Healey and Roth Funeral Home. Seaborn's inability to manage money and support his family—a character trait lamented in letters of his parents and in stories told by some of Seaborn's children to their children—remained constant up to the very end of his life.

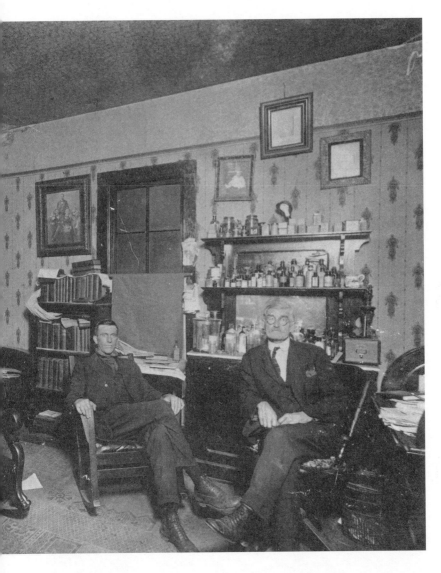

Dr. Seaborn Russell, in his Little Rock medical office with his brother, Richard D. Russell (left), circa 1926. *Courtesy of Marvin E. Vaughter Jr.; original in the Historical Research Center, University of Arkansas for Medical Sciences (UAMS).*

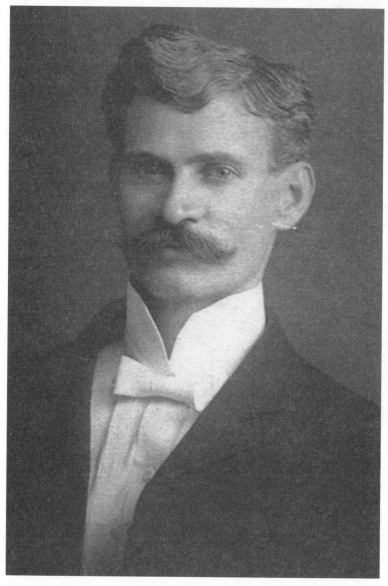

Dr. Ralph Morgan Russell, circa 1886. *Courtesy of Craig Boden; copy in the Historical Research Center, University of Arkansas for Medical Sciences (UAMS).*

CHAPTER 4

Ralph Morgan Russell
(1867–1916)

*Well I am getting up cases for Pa. I get one third
of every case. I have already got one case of cross
eyes and one of club foot and I have only been canvassing for him three days and I have only been
out two days.*

> *Well I think I can make enough money this fall
> and next spring to go to school two years. I believe
> I can graduate in that amount of time. I am going
> to study father's profession. I can comprehend the
> operations in a short time by watching him oper-
> ate for two seasons.*

—RALPH M. RUSSELL, Nashville, Arkansas,
to Ava Russell Norwood, fall 1883[1]

*Vi-Be Ni Malt Tonic, the great liquid food medi-
cine and European hospital remedy for indigestion,
loss of appetite, female weakness, chronic and wasting diseases. For sale at the Centre Drug Store.*

—Advertisement in *Coosa River News*
(Centre, Alabama), 3 November 1899[2]

Of all the Russell doctors, Ralph is perhaps the most elusive to sum
up neatly. As one examines his life and his contributions to his profession, what leaps out is his brilliance. But there is also, as we'll see,
the brittleness that often goes with brilliance, a trait not so evident
in his doctor-kinsmen, his grandfather, father, and brother Seaborn.

An 1895 passport application Ralph made as he prepared to go with wife Mollie and their son Ralph Jr. to London to study at King's College provides a concise summary of his appearance as he neared twenty-eight: he was 5' 11" with a broad, high forehead, blue eyes, a prominent nose and large mouth, light hair, fair complexion, and an oval-shaped face.[3] The same height as his father[4] but a few inches shorter than Seaborn.

The Early Years

Ralph Morgan Russell was the first of W. J. P. and Ava's children born in Arkansas. That much is clear, but extant documentation is unclear about *when* and *where* this birth occurred. Ava's Bible records the date as 1 February 1867 and the place as Evansville in Washington County.[5] But Ralph's biography in *History of Alabama and Her People* states that he was born at "Cain [*sic*] Hill," Arkansas, on 22 February 1867, and this date is on his tombstone.[6] Because the biography was published eleven years after Ralph's death, it is likely that his widow and/or son provided the information. Ralph's death certificate does not record a date of birth.[7] It also gives Texas as his birthplace and states that his parents' names were unknown; the information was supplied by an attending physician whose signature is illegible.

Adding to the confusion, the 1895 passport application, for which *Ralph himself* supplied the information (it is in his handwriting and bears his signature), gives his birthdate as 21 February 1867 and his birthplace as Evansville, Arkansas.[8] On an application Ralph filed in June 1888 in Gadsden, Alabama, to practice medicine in Etowah County, he leaves his date of birth blank but again states that he was born in Evansville.[9] The Evansville birthplace seems well established, and it is easy to understand the confusion about Cane Hill, where Ralph was schooled but not born, when one realizes that the information in *History of Alabama* was supplied by family members after his death. But the discrepancies in his birthdate as given in a number of sources, including his mother's Bible, which might be expected to be the most accurate account, are harder to explain.

Along with his older siblings, Ralph was educated at Cane Hill College in Washington County, Arkansas. His *History of Alabama* biography states that he "received high academic discipline" at "Cave [*sic*] Hill College" before going to Hot Springs for further study.[10] When he was only fourteen, his father also began taking Ralph on surgical trips, presumably to assist W. J. P., a deduction that can be made from a 20 May 1881 letter his sister Ava wrote to Frank Norwood, where she states that her father and Ralph had returned from a trip on 25 April and then gone back onto the road again.[11]

Family letters indicate that in the fall of 1881, Ralph went to Hot Springs, nearly 200 miles south of Boonsboro, to work for his uncles Sevier Clark Law and Joseph Henry Law.[12] Sevier owned a clothing store in Hot Springs and had been its US postmaster since 1874, and Joseph was a banker and former county clerk of Garland County, whom Ralph credited for his business success.[13] However, Joseph died while Ralph was working in Hot Springs.[14]

On 17 October 1882, Ralph's sister Ava wrote to Frank Norwood speaking of "a difficulty" Ralph had experienced in Hot Springs, requiring her father to travel from Nashville, Arkansas, to assist his son.[15] By the following spring, it appears that Ralph had suffered a mishap with his legs—possibly the "difficulty" mentioned in Ava's letter. On 8 April 1883, Ralph's sister Mollie wrote their sister Ava, stating that Ralph had written to tell her he was "sick and has white swelling in the other leg—he says it runs a gallon of water a day."[16] Mollie added:

> You cannot know how I pity our little crippled brother way off there without money or friends and the man he has been working for has him to take care of and you know the child suffers for attention. How my heart goes out to him this day and may God bless him. How much I would love to be with him today and bring him home with me to take care of until he gets well but I can only think of him and shed bitter tears for my favorite brother. He says he went down to the store the other day to try to work but could not and had to go to his room. Mr. Moore says he will send him money to come home and meet him in Van Buren anytime. I will write this eve and see if he wants the money and encourage him to come here where we can take care of him.

The letter also indicates that Ralph's mother was making arrangements to bring him home to Boonsboro while his father was in Eureka Springs. An undated letter of Ava's from Boonsboro in spring 1883 to her daughter Ava states, "I have written Ralph twice but fear he has not gotten my letter as I sent the letter for him by Mr. Lowe too. We wrote we would go for him at any place he would be at."[17] Another letter from Ava in Boonsboro on 29 April 1883 also notes Ralph's problems with his legs.[18]

Ralph continued in Hot Springs, working in a store owned by John Walsh. He then took a position clerking for the law firm of Douglas and Johnson in April 1883.[19] A few months later, he would write his sister Ava to tell her he was making good wages.

By the summer of 1883, the family was growing concerned about Ralph's lack of communication, a recurrent theme in family letters over many years. On 17 June 1883, Mollie wrote her sister Ava from Boonsboro expressing concern about not having had word from Ralph. She tells Ava that, though she had continued writing him, she had not heard from him in a long time.[20] The following day, Ava's mother wrote her: "Do see if you can get Ralph to write to you often. He only writes to any of us semi-annually and I want to hear from him more often than that."[21] The persistent pattern of silence noted in family letters makes one wonder if Ralph resented a consignment to an apprenticeship with an uncle in a distant city that he had not chosen, though it might have been chosen for him by his parents.

At some point in fall 1883, Ralph finally communicated with his sister Ava. Striking a plaintive note, he says,

> Well Sis I see a pretty hard time—I have to get up half past four and open the store and close at ten in the evening. So you see I don't have a very easy time but I get very good wages, my board and washing, and I don't have to pay out anything only for my clothes and I save all I can. I want to go in business for myself when I am twenty one.[22]

Ralph Decides to Study Medicine

A. Studying and Working with His Father

By November 1883, Ralph had rejoined his family and started studying medicine under his father's tutelage. A letter Ralph wrote his sister Ava from Nashville, Arkansas, in the fall of 1883 describes this arrangement:

I will to commence with you by asking you to forgive my not writing before now but the reason is I am traveling with Pa and as we did not know where we would be until now, I would not write. Well dear sis I would like to see you very much and have an old fashioned chat. Well I am getting up cases for Pa. I get one third of every case. I have already got one case of cross eyes and one of club foot and I have only been canvassing for him three days and I have only been out two days.

Well I think I can make enough money this fall and next spring to go to school two years. I believe I can graduate in that amount of time. I am going to study father's profession. I can comprehend the operations in a short time by watching him operate for two seasons.

Well I have got to go with him to operate on a club foot. I will write again soon when I have time.[23]

This undated letter appears to have been written after the Russells moved to southwest Arkansas in October 1883 or as the family was in the process of relocating.

On 3 December 1883, Ava Russell wrote her daughter Ava from Nashville to say that Dr. Russell had left on 27 November with Ralph and Seab for a "Southern trip."[24] By February next, Ava and Eric had joined "the men" as W. J. P., Seaborn, and Ralph did surgery in Mississippi. A 14 February 1884 letter of Mollie Moore to her sister Ava from Cowala, Indian Territory, reports, "Bud Seab says Pa, Ma, Ralph, and E. are on the road to Hazlehurst and want to be there in March."[25] By 17 March, the family had reached Clinton, Louisiana, where W. J. P. wrote his daughter Ava, indicating that Ralph was with him.[26]

Family correspondence indicates that in July 1885 Ralph had gone to Alabama to do medical work on his father's behalf and was planning to go from there to New York to enroll in medical school. In a 2 July letter to his daughter Ava, W. J. P. writes,

Ralph is in the mountains of Alabama 100 miles east of here doing first rate, he averages $500 per month for me. You have no idea how he has improved. He will start for New York the middle of September and will stop and see you. Ma and the boys are in Kosciusko and living at the old place.

I will go home in August and stay a few days only as Seab wishes to keep at work.

We have been striking it rather hard for a month past. In the first place it is the hardest of times about getting money from farmers, just a little of the hardest I have experienced. It must be the people spent all their little savings going to expositions. Then it has been raining all through June and other reasons combined to make June a hard month. But by credit of hard work, selling off horses and pushing we made a very good average. We will go back eastward to Ralph. We are working the mineral region—more money up there than in the Cotton belt.[27]

B. Medical School at Bellevue
and Marriage to Mollie Woodliff

In September 1885, Ralph entered Bellevue Medical College. A letter he sent his sister Ava on 14 September from his residence at 63 Lexington Avenue in New York, four blocks from Bellevue, recounts details of his trip to New York, where he had arrived the day before. He tells Ava that he had visited their aunt Mary and her husband Bryant Strickland in Cartersville, Georgia, en route to Bellevue, and found them as "cold as ice." They had not even offered him hospitality; he stayed at a hotel while visiting them.

From Cartersville, Ralph had traveled to Atlanta, where he stayed with their cousin Octavia, wife of Edward Murphy and daughter of their mother's uncle David Shelton Law. Ralph tells Ava that he found Octavia "one of the most amiable and nicest ladys [*sic*] in existence (our Ma excepted)." From Atlanta, Ralph went by train through Washington, Baltimore, and Philadelphia. He found New York "just grand" and was going to "take the city in" the next day.[28]

Just as Ralph entered Bellevue, Andrew Carnegie had made his first public gift of $50,000 to the school to establish the Carnegie Laboratory, the nation's first laboratory for teaching and investigating bacteria and pathology. Dr. Edward Janeway, later New York City's commissioner of health, was the lab's first director and a distinguished instructor in this field.[29]

There's a dearth of documentation to track Ralph's first year of study. Occupied with his course work, he lapsed into his old habit of sporadic communication with his family. By the end of the spring semester 1886, he appears in the Dallas city directory as a physician and surgeon practicing with his father.[30] Piecing together evidence in family letters, one can infer that after two semesters, Ralph's money had run out, and W. J. P. wanted him to work to earn what he needed to complete his education. Ralph's letter to his sister Ava in the fall of 1883 offering the first hints of his plan to study medicine had stated that he was intending to work for their father to earn enough to go to medical school for two years.

A 28 June 1886 letter Ralph's mother sent her daughter Ava from Dallas states that Ralph was boarding there and had an office on "the principal street."[31] Between that date and August, it seems that Ralph had left Dallas and connected (or reconnected?) with his cousin Mary Belle Law Woodliff, daughter of his mother's sister Lavenia Chester "Chesta" Law Woodliff and her husband Augustin Woodliff in Gadsden, Alabama. On 11 August 1886, Ralph and Mollie married.[32] The wedding announcement in *Atlanta Constitution* states that the couple had never met until the day of their marriage in Flowery Branch, Georgia. They had carried on a romance by correspondence, and neither set of parents approved of the first-cousin union.[33] Ralph did not, in fact, even inform his parents that he was marrying.

On 24 September, Ralph's sister Ava wrote her husband Frank informing him that Ralph had married and that she had learned of this from her cousin Katie Strickland in Cartersville, Georgia, who told her that Ralph and his wife had visited their Strickland relations. Katie had not told Ava whom Ralph had married: Ava states,

> I can't guess who it can be unless it is Mollie Woodliff—Aunt Chesta's daughter. Said they were going to Gadsden to see her mother. I hope he has not gone and played the fool too after condemning early marriages so unjustly. I hope he was only jesting with them and that it will turn out that he is still on the safe side but it is a characteristic of our family to fall in love, get married, settle down, and forget it while others would be getting ready to make up their mind.[34]

The *Constitution*'s report that Ralph and Mollie had not met prior to their marriage in August 1886 is complicated by a certain artifact:

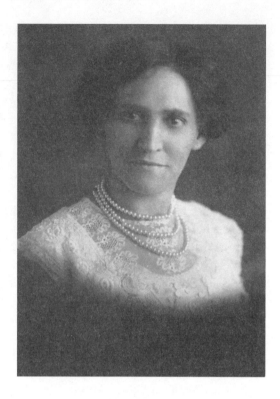

Mollie Woodliff, who married Dr. Ralph Russell on 11 August 1886. *Courtesy of Craig Boden; copy in the Historical Research Center, University of Arkansas for Medical Sciences (UAMS).*

In Gadsden's Forrest Cemetery in which Mollie's parents are buried, there is a grave marker in their family plot that reads, "Infant son of Dr. and Mrs. Ralph M. Russell, 1886." No indication has yet been found of precisely when this child was born and precisely when he died. But if he died in 1886—as the tombstone plainly states—then it is hard to credit the report that Ralph and Mollie first met when they stood before the altar to marry in August 1886.

Ralph's father was "sorely disappointed" in his son's decision to marry his cousin and his failure to inform his parents. On 22 January 1887, W. J. P. wrote his daughter Ava from Wills Point, stating,

> I have heard from a round about source that Ralph has married his cousin. I had promised myself he would have done some good—at least would have finished his medical education before marrying. I am sorely disappointed in him but it is so with all my boys—they bring me nothing but disappointment and trouble. We had one letter from Ralph

last summer wanting money but he said nothing about his having married.

Was ashamed I suppose. I wrote him as he had no one but himself to work for and I had loaned him all I knew he would have to battle his own cause. I could not help him so have had no word from him since. The next news I expect to hear will be a club footed, harelipped, idiotic, deformed child—can't expect anything else from first cousins.[35]

As a man of science, W. J. P. was obviously concerned about possible genetic consequences of such marriages.

Following their marriage, Ralph and Mollie settled in Alabama, where Mollie purchased a lot in Gadsden in April 1887, adjoining where her parents lived.[36] Having married and established a new residence, Ralph made plans to complete his Bellevue studies, and in January 1888, he returned to New York for his final semester. Though he was now married and on his own, he and his father were still professionally linked. As Ralph returned to school, his father wrote the following certificate for him:

Ralph M. Russell has studied medicine under my direction, inclusive of attendance upon lectures from 1st October 1884 to 25 December 1887 being 3 years and 3 months; that he is twenty-one years of age, and of good moral character.[37]

On 10 February 1888, Ralph wrote from New York to his father in Wills Point, Texas. The letter is interesting because of the light it throws on Ralph's troubled yet still-dependent relationship with his father and on his character. Ralph writes,

Dear Father,

Yours of a recent date just received and contents duly noted. I have received no money from Fayetteville. I already received twenty dollars from you which came some three weeks since and in the letter you stated you could send me one hundred dollars by the first of February and owing to all my time being very closely engaged I did not respond simply because I did not deem it necessary. I thought of course you knew my circumstances and knowing I was out of money— would by all means send me the specified amount.

I am now out of money and several weeks behind with my

board and examinations commence two weeks from Monday. Consequently I was all the time reviewing for the examination for you know I came here late and am more than likely to be rejected and if I am of course tis $5,500 thrown away and of course I can't stay here and study situated as I am [*sic*] no money.

You promised to send me money and I should have never come here til next year and if I do not receive the money from you in 10 days I am going to leave New York. I can't stay here in this condition. You know I did not want to come on here. At the time I knew you so well, I told you just how twould be.

I am troubled enough about the examination and now that this has turned out as it has I am just as certain to be rejected as I come up for examination for I am dull in practice anyway. I ought by all means to have studied six months before I came on here. I telegraphed you last night and no answer yet though I have no idea if you called for the message and living off in the country. I do not suppose the operator knows anything about you so I suppose you did not receive it and if you have not sent me the money send it and I will return it in one month after I get back.

I was thinking of a plan to work the prof. Twas this. You see I have a perfect college quiz record and I thought twould be a good idea for you to telegraph me say first of March that 'Mother was dying come home quick' and then you see they would think I was excited and knowing I have a good quiz record would give me an examination hurriedly and let me through. What do you think about it? I am almost certain to fail otherwise.

I am afraid although the prof.—at surgery told me the other day while we were up in the hospital that I need not fret a minute that I would go through perfect. Though I can't help but feel anxious about it.

Excuse short letter am too busy to stop for anything. I am your affectionate son—

R. M. Russell[38]

Worth noting: Ralph's suggestion that his father collude in a charade to allow him to evade a rigorous final exam that he feared he might not pass. 'Telegraph me say first of March that 'Mother was dying come home quick'": this is a *grown married man* requesting his father's help to bend graduation requirements because he was frightened.

Ralph did make it through his final exams and graduated from the prestigious medical college on 12 March 1888.[39] He was one of 144 graduates. He was absent from his graduation ceremony, however, due to a serious injury the day before. Newspaper reports indicate that on 11 March, the number 5 train of the Erie Railroad had jumped the tracks at Scio, New York, killing one passenger and maiming twelve others, of whom four eventually died.[40] *The Saint Paul Globe* reported on the twelfth, Ralph's graduation day, that the injured included Dr. R. M. Russell of Gadsden, Alabama.[41]

Alabama newspapers picked up the story, focusing on the injuries sustained by the local man: On 26 April, *Gadsden Times* reported that Ralph had been crippled in a train wreck in late March or early April at Scio and had been using crutches. The 2 May edition of Birmingham's *Weekly Age* has similar information, adding that Ralph had been compensated $20,000 for injuries.[42] Even more dramatically, *Southern Star* of Newton, Alabama, related the following on 30 May: "Dr. Ralph Russell, of Gadsden, was crippled for life in a railroad wreck at Scio, N. Y., and received $20,000 from the railroad company."[43]

When Ralph had recovered sufficiently, he and Mollie returned to Alabama, where she sold her parents the lot she had bought next to them and bought a new lot in Gadsden on 24 April.[44] As another indicator that the couple was now settling into a new life, Ralph applied and was tested for a medical license in Gadsden on 30 June, using a Dr. Wright, with whom he was in practice, as a local reference.[45]

The following month, he received the license from the Etowah County Board of Medical Examiners. He had scored 79–84 on his exams. In its licensure file for Ralph, Alabama Department of Archives and History has the handwritten original exams Ralph took to obtain his license. In the area of surgery, in which Dr. J. Bevans examined him, he scored particularly high with the exception of a question about the management of gangrene, in which Ralph's answer was barely satisfactory (60%).

Having completed his studies, Ralph resumed work with his father and brother Seaborn, as indicated in a 27 June 1888 letter that W. J. P. wrote his daughter Ava from Cumberland, Mississippi, noting that Seaborn and Ralph were doing surgery in Kosciusko while he toured with Dick. Ralph's application to practice medicine in Gadsden stated that he was in practice with "Dr. Russell" as well as Dr. Wright. On 24 January 1889, *Gadsden Times* reported that Ralph had just returned home with his brother Richard after several months' absence.[46] Apparently, he had spent the latter half of 1888 doing surgical work for his father in Mississippi.

The renewal of a shared practice with his father did not last long. As we noted in discussing W. J. P.'s story, he wrote his daughter Ava from Lake Charles, Louisiana, on 4 June 1890 while she was visiting Ralph and his family in Gadsden, suggesting that, even with the generous financial settlement he had secured from the railroad company, Ralph was still having financial problems and vexing his father with requests for money. W. J. P. was adamant about his intent not to provide Ralph assistance. He wrote:

> Ralph has not shown that Filial regard for either of us since his marriage that calls for any sacrifice on our part. He cares nothing for anybody but self. I have been writing for my Mississippi Licenses for a year and he would not send them. I would have been in the hills of Mississippi now if I could have gotten my licenses in place of being here in the swamps of Louisiana in the heat of summer with gnats, mosquitos, and malaria. I have written to the authorities at Jackson for a duplicate and you tell him he will make himself criminally liable if he loses the original.[47]

The surgical expeditions Russell undertook with his sons required that they produce licenses to practice medicine in at least some of the states they were visiting. As the father had ranged into Louisiana doing surgeries while his sons remained in Mississippi, he needed his Mississippi licenses to return there, and Ralph had not sent them.

Ralph may not, in fact, have been in Mississippi as his father wrote him: The *Directory of Deceased American Physicians* states that he was licensed to practice medicine in Virginia in 1889.[48] Since Ralph and Mollie moved to Birmingham in 1890 or 1891 following the birth of their son Ralph Law Russell on 11 April 1889, Ralph may have been eyeing Virginia as a possible new place of residence as he contemplated leaving Gadsden.

Relocating to Birmingham, Alabama, and Studying at King's College, London

The 1891 volume of *Transactions of the Medical Association of the State of Alabama* states that Ralf [*sic*] Morgan Russell had moved from Gadsden to Birmingham.[49] Also, Ralph filed his license to practice in Jefferson County in 1891, with the document noting that his office was at 404½ 18th Street in Birmingham and that his residence was on 21st Street. An ad in the *Choctaw Herald* (Butler, Alabama) in December 1896 lists Ralph's business address at the corner of 3rd Avenue and 19th Street.[50] Between 1896 and 1900, he and Mollie bought a house at 1315 Huntsville Avenue.[51]

As he established his new practice, Ralph began exploring electromagnetic treatments. This field was becoming popular in American medicine of the period and sometimes featured exaggerated or downright fantastical claims. According to the *Monroe Journal* of Claiborne, Alabama, in October 1896, Ralph invented a device called "the Electro-Medical Apparatus" (he would later call it the Electrozone) in 1891, which he then began using in a medical institute he founded in Birmingham. Noting that it was relying on an article published in a Birmingham paper on 18 September, the *Monroe Journal* offers what is essentially an advertisement, probably written by Ralph himself:

> Dr. R. M. Russell, of the Medico-Surgical Institute, of this city, has demonstrated, beyond a doubt, that the dread disease of consumption can be cured by the use of his Electro-Medical Apparatus, in connection with the X-Rays. This Electro-Medical Apparatus manufactures the same kind of electricity that makes the X-Ray, and this is used to conduct medicines into the diseased tissues of the body. It was originated by Dr. Russell and has been used in his Institution for about five years.
>
> By the aid of the X-Ray machine, equipped with one of the improved tubes of Dr. Russell's own invention, together with the Fluoroscope, he is enabled to locate, exactly, any defective organ of the body and then by the application of proper remedies, by means of Electro-Medication, he is enabled to deal with the worst cases of consumption, having recently effected remarkable cures on more than twenty

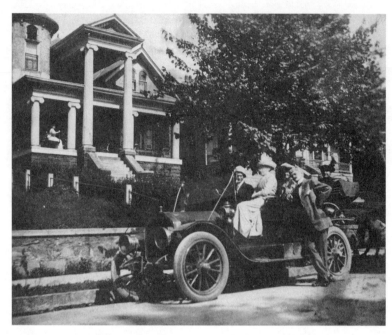

Dr. Ralph Russell leaning on a car in front of his house at 1306 Huntsville Avenue in Birmingham. He lived in the house from about 1904–1908. *Courtesy of Sara Lee Suttle; copy in the Historical Research Center, University of Arkansas for Medical Sciences (UAMS).*

different persons. By the same means the doctor treats all ovarian as well as pulmonary troubles. In the treatment of ovarian troubles and all chronic diseases of women, the doctor has been quite successful. He spent a large portion of last year in Europe, introducing the method of treatment in the hospitals at the great centers. Dr. Russell has persistently refused to let the announcement of his discovery go out to the public until now, for the reason that he wished to thoroughly demonstrate the fact that consumption could be cured. He is an untiring student and worker, and ranks high among the eminent scientists of the world.[52]

As James Harvey Young indicates in a discussion of "device quackery," fascination with the medical application of electricity began in the American medical community and public following

Franz Mesmer's séances in Paris and Ben Franklin's kite experiments in Philadelphia in the latter part of the 1700s.[53] Medical practitioner Elisha Perkins capitalized on the notion that electricity had therapeutic value by inventing "metallic tractors" in this same period. Stating that this device was "gleaned up from the miserable remains of animal magnetism," the Connecticut medical society expelled him from membership due to his claim that his tractors (the first medical device patented under the new US Constitution) cured ailments by drawing off electric "fluid" when passed over the body.[54]

As the nineteenth century proceeded, increasingly fabulous claims were made about electrical devices. Electromagnetic belts were marketed to men concerned about enhancing virility, with frequent claims that they could accomplish even more: As Gerald Carson notes, "A 'voltaic belt' of 1890 could do much more: besides improving health and posture, it could comb the hair, press the clothes, and promote a luxuriant mustache—all in 30 days."[55] Many other electric devices were touted as cure-alls, including wristbands, cravats, anklets, elbow pads, necklaces, headcaps, and corsets, about whose therapeutic value flamboyant avowals were made.[56] As Young observes, "As the utility of electricity became more stunningly apparent to Americans during the ongoing industrial revolution, so too did the utility of electricity increase for quacks."[57] And: "The main currents of device quackery in American history . . . have flowed from electromagnetism and electricity."[58]

As the American Medical Association's *Nostrums and Quackery*, an exposé of unfounded medical claims, stated in 1912 in an article entitled "Mechanical Fakes: The Electropoise—Oxydonor—Oxygenor—Oxygenator—Oxypathor—Oxytonor," "Apparently, there was no disease, known or unknown, that the Electropoise would not cure—according to its exploiter." *Nostrums and Quackery* notes that with his devices such as the Electropoise, Hercules Sanche, who founded an institute in Birmingham called Electrolibration, also sold membership in an organization he named *Fraternitas Duxanimae*, which required patients to take vows and swear an oath of loyalty as a precondition of membership. Along with the devices and fraternity membership came handy donation forms for members to use to send money to Sanche.[59]

About the credulousness of American medical consumers regarding Sanche's claims, the AMA observes,

It might be supposed that an individual who set out to sell, as a panacea for all the ills of the flesh, a piece of brass pipe with one or two wires attached to it, would, commercially speaking, have a hard and rocky road before him. But such a supposition would be incorrect. Not only would the enterprising faker find customers for his gas-pipe, but there would be such a demand for this most inane of 'therapeutic' devices, that two or three imitators would immediately enter the market.[60]

The Electropoise and Oxydonor spawned an imitation invented in 1912 by E. L. Moses of Buffalo, New York, a quack device called the Oxypathor for which the Post Office Department won a criminal fraud case against Moses, the first such case won against a quack device in the US. Because devices were not covered by the 1906 Pure Food and Drugs Law, those seeking to curb medical quackery turned to prosecution by the postal service since such fraudulent devices were sent to gullible customers through the mail.[61]

All of this was in the air when Ralph invented his "Electro-Medical Apparatus" in 1891 as he was setting up his Birmingham practice. By the time that his father died in 1892, Ralph had begun to make a name for himself as an up-and-coming young doctor of Birmingham. He appears in the 1893 city directory as a physician and surgeon with an office at 218½ 21st Street North.[62] A sign that the family had begun to establish itself and put down roots: on 25 November 1894, Mollie joined Birmingham's First Methodist Church.[63]

As his family settled in, Ralph also took a major step: He announced the formation of a Medico-Surgical Institute. The local newspaper *Age-Herald* ran ads for the Institute in February and March 1894.[64] It did not, however, begin operation for several more years; the ads were evidently a trial balloon to test public sentiment—a preliminary to the actual opening of the Institute in 1896.

In the intervening time, Ralph decided to do more study—at King's College in London. On 24 April 1895, he applied for a passport for himself, Mollie, and their son Ralph.[65] The application states that the family would return to the United States within eighteen months. A passport was issued three days later.

As the Russells made their way overseas, their travels were publicized in various newspapers: On 16 May, the *Fort Wayne Weekly Sentinel* reports that Dr. Ralph M. Russell and wife and child of

Birmingham had passed through Fort Wayne the previous day en route to London.[66] A report on 26 May in Montgomery, Alabama's *Advertiser* states that Dr. Ralph M. Russell, son-in-law of Capt. A. L. Woodliff of Gadsden, had sailed with his wife and son for London and would visit Paris, Vienna, Berlin, and other cities.[67] King's College records indicate that Ralph enrolled as an "occasional student" in June 1895, with medical and surgical practice listed as his field of study.[68]

On 14 July, the *Atlanta Constitution* carried the following notice, citing a newspaper in Paris called *Galignani's Messenger*:

> Among the Americans now in Paris are Dr. R. M. Russell, wife and little son, Master Ralph, of Birmingham, Ala. They have just arrived from London, and are domiciled at the grand Hotel Magenta. Dr. Russell is no stranger to the leading medical men of Europe. Being well identified with many of the learned gentlemen of this as well as the American continent for his numerous scientific inventions, original research, and excellent contributions to the medical journals on both sides of the Atlantic. He is esteemed one of the most progressive ophthalmic surgeons of America.[69]

One suspects that Ralph supplied the copy for this article. This was to become something of a pattern, feeding articles that celebrated his accomplishments in glowing terms to newspapers. This penchant for self-advertisement causes one to wonder if the reason he planned a course of study at King's College as he planned his Institute was to enhance his credentials for when he eventually marketed himself—and his electrical devices and, later, his Vi-Be Ni tonic—nationally through the home-treatment book he wrote. It is worth noting that no record has been found of any articles published by Ralph in any medical journals, other than his pamphlet on the treatment of deformities that will be discussed below.

Opening of Russell Medical Institute

In 1896, the Russells returned to Birmingham, and Ralph opened the Russell Medical Institute. The location of the Institute, whose existence is noted in many different documents after Ralph founded it, is something of a mystery: As previously noted, when Ralph applied for his license to practice in Birmingham in 1891, he stated that he had an office at 404½ 18th Street.[70] The city directory for 1900 shows the Institute at this same address and carries an ad suggesting that it had branches in London, Paris, New York, and Chicago:

> Modern and Thoroughly Equipped Institution for the Treatment of Diseases of Women and Children; Chronic and Nervous Diseases; Catarrh; Deformities; Orthopaedic, Plastic and General Surgery, Complete X-Ray Outfit and the Latest European Hospital Methods of Cure.

In addition, the directory indicates that Ralph also had a home office in his residence at 1315 Huntsville Ave. No information found anywhere confirms the existence of branches of the Russell Medical Institute in London, Paris, New York, or Chicago.

As Ralph opened his clinic, *The Marion Times-Standard* of Marion, Alabama, carried a sensational article on 28 May 1896 with the following title: "A MAN WITHOUT FEELING. Subject of a Clinic by Dr. Russell. NOTHING SEEMS TO HURT HIM. He Can Be Stabbed and Shot without Pain and Eats Glass with a Relish—A Wonder."[71] Noting that it is picking up an item published by *The State Herald* on 1 April, the article states that a reporter had attended a clinic at the Russell Medico-Surgical Institute and that he doubted he would be able to sleep for a week afterwards, so great was his wonderment. To a select audience, including Dr. J. C. Dozier, Dr. Jernigan, Dr. Bangston, Rev. R. D. B. Gray of First Baptist Church, Rev. Dr. L. S. Handley of Central Presbyterian Church, Dr. Sol. Palmer of the East Lake Atheneum, Hon. John M. Martin, and Photographer Peddlinghause, Drs. R. M. Russell and E. H. Walker performed various para-medical procedures on a man, Leo Tardo, said to have no feeling.

In the presence of their guests, the doctors pierced Tardo's arm with a scalpel and his tongue with a surgical instrument, penetrated his brachial artery with a rusty instrument, thrust a needle into his cardiac apex, pierced his leg and various nerve chords in different plexuses, ran an electric current through his limbs: The list goes on and on. In front of the audience, Tardo masticated and swallowed a two-ounce bottle "with the ease of a billy goat." Through a tube inserted into his cheek, Tardo drank a cup of gasoline oil, then compressed his lips and lit a flame from the gas produced by this procedure. Tardo invited the journalist to shoot him with a .38 Smith and Wesson pistol, but the reporter declined.

Nothing in the article spells out how the procedures the doctors performed constituted a clinical exhibition or what this exhibition was designed to demonstrate in medical terms—or what it had to do with Ralph's newly opened clinic, except that the clinic was the venue for the performance. Ralph began publishing his *Handbook of Home Medicine*, discussed in detail below, in 1900. Though the book claimed to represent the Russell Medical Institute of Birmingham and speaks as if the Institute occupied an imposing building, there are no photographs of it anywhere in the *Handbook* (or anywhere else for that matter). There is a drawing in Ralph's book, one suggesting that it was an impressive multi-story clinic with a sign on the top story reading, "Dr. Ralph M. Russell's Medico-Surgical Institute," but the text accompanying this drawing locates the building at 406 18th Street, not 404 18th Street, the address given in other sources.[72]

No extant sources have confirmed the existence of a building at either location or anywhere else in Birmingham matching this drawing. It is indubitable that he had an office at 404½ 18th Street. What appears much more dubious is that this office constituted the impressive multi-story "Institute" depicted in the *Handbook of Home Medicine*, which he began marketing nationwide from this Institute in 1900.[73] A number of sources, including Sanborn maps, indicate that a drug company existed at the 18th Street address for a number of years during which Ralph was operating his Institute. It is possible that the Institute was a separate operation within this company and that Ralph rented office space there. The drawing of the Institute appears up to the final edition of Ralph's book in 1911, more than eleven years after the Institute was established.

As noted previously, information about Ralph's new Institute shows up in a 1 October 1896 report in the *Monroe Journal* of Claiborne, Alabama: "Successful Treatment of Consumption by a Birmingham (Ala.) Physician." Several points about this article (transcribed above) deserve attention. First, as with the July 1895 article the *Atlanta Constitution* carried from a Paris newspaper, it appears likely that Ralph supplied the text for this glowing recommendation of his Electro-Medical Apparatus.

Also, the *Monroe Journal* report links the introduction of Ralph's

Appendix.

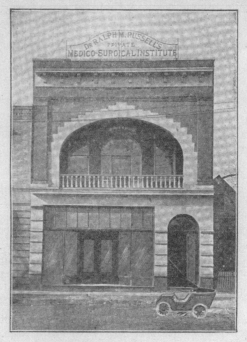

DR. RUSSELL MEDICAL INSTITUTE,
BIRMINGHAM, ALABAMA,
406 Eighteenth Street, Two Blocks North of The Post Office.

A modern and thoroughly equipped institution with a full staff of Specialists for the successful treatment of all manner of nerve, blood, skin, female, chronic diseases and deformities.

Examination by the X-Ray system; latest European hospital methods of cure. Established ten (10) years in Birmingham.

This institution of medicine and surgery is modern in all bearings. We invite the closest scrutiny and seek the widest publicity. Our practice founded on nature and based on common sense, being

Drawing of the Russell Medical Institute appearing in the *Handbook of Home Medicine. A copy of the* Handbook *is in the Historical Research Center, University of Arkansas for Medical Sciences (UAMS).*

electric machine to his new Institute. It explicitly states that Ralph had spent much of the last year in Europe "introducing the method of treatment in the hospitals at the great centers." This strengthens the conclusion that in choosing to do further study at King's College before he founded his Institute, Ralph was following a business plan in which the central features included the Institute's founding, the introduction of electro-therapy machines and his tonic, and the publication of his *Handbook of Home Medicine*. In a different time and place, he was reinventing his father's traveling surgical practice, using new techniques to extend the reach of his practice and secure more income than he could secure through a general medical or surgical practice in Birmingham.

On 30 December 1896, Ralph sent a letter to his sister Ava at Wills Point, using an elegant new letterhead: "Dr. Ralph M. Russell's Private Medico-Surgical Institute, Devoted Special Treatment of Cases of Orthopedic Surgery & General Surgery, Diseases of Women, Chronic and Nervous Diseases, Deformities, Corner Third Avenue and Nineteenth Street, Birmingham, Ala." In the letter, he tells Ava that their mother and Dick had just visited, with Seaborn joining them from Arkansas.

Dick may, in fact, have come to Birmingham to discuss involvement in Ralph's new business ventures. In 1900, he and his family are on the federal census in Birmingham, with his occupation given as chemist. The address of the family's residence is Ralph's office address—404 18th Street.[74] According to Dick's daughter Grace Russell Norton, he moved his family to Birmingham sometime before 1900, so he could work with Ralph to compound and sell a patent medicine, possibly his Vi-Be Ni tonic. The arrangement did not last, and by 1903, the family had returned to Wills Point, where Richard remained the rest of his life working as a stockman and cotton buyer.[75]

In 1896, Ralph registered a trademark for a tonic called Vi-Be Ni, described in its trademark listing as offering "remedies for blood, stomach, nerves, and other diseases."[76] He began marketing the tonic with ads touting the claims of his new clinic to cure a wide range of illnesses from "nervous diseases" to tobacco, alcohol, opium, and morphine addiction. Under a banner reading, "The Dr. Ralph M. Russell Medico-Surgical Institute and Sanatarium, of Birmingham, Ala.," with an engraving of Ralph's face, the *Choctaw Herald* of Butler, Alabama, announced on 17 March and 2 June 1897:

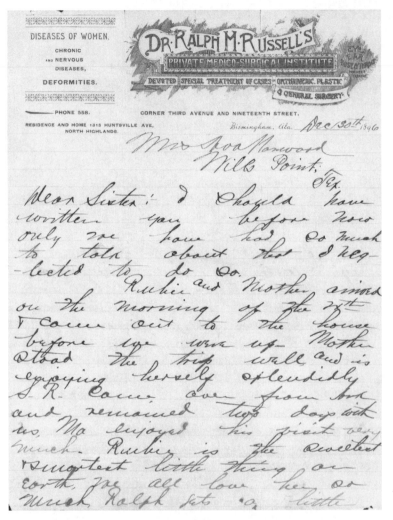

Letterhead used by Dr. Ralph Russell to write a letter to his sister Ava on 30 December 1896. *Original is in the Historical Research Center, University of Arkansas for Medical Sciences (UAMS).*

Successfully treats diseases of women, Chronic and Nervous Diseases, Deformities, Catarrh, Rheumatism, Paralysis, Club, Reel and Crooked Feet, Spinal Curvature, Hip Disease, Hare Lip, Stiff and Crooked Joints, Tumors, Wens, Cross Eyes, Cataract, Blood, Skin, Private and Chronic Diseases generally. Also the Tobacco, Whiskey, Opium and Morphine habit.

We can treat you successfully by mail at your own home, at small cost, and guarantee you a cure.

No Exposure. All Medicine Sent in Plain Package. All Correspondence in Plain Envelopes.

OVER FIVE THOUSAND PATIENTS TREATED SUCCESSFULLY LAST YEAR.

Largest Institution and Best Equipped Sanitarium in the South.

Write for symptom blanks and free catalogues with testimonials of cures effected. Address with stamp the

Dr. R. M. Russell Medico-Surgical Institute
BIRMINGHAM, ALA.
Corner 3d Ave. and 19th St.[77]

The 2 June advertisement carries a voucher stating that "we" (presumably, the *Herald* editors) are "reliably informed" that Dr. Ralph M. Russell is a graduate of "two of the leading Medical Colleges in the world," Bellevue and King's College. He is also author of "many scientific inventions" for which he holds patents, including the world-renowned Cathode Reflector. The voucher recommends that patients seek out his Institute, where they will find relief.[78]

After his return from England, Ralph also published a pamphlet entitled *An Illustrated Lecture on Deformities of the Human Frame, Their Cause, Means of Prevention, and Method of Cure.*[79] It is undated and appears to be an in-house publication, perhaps as a marketing piece for people inquiring about surgeries for cleft lip, strabismus, clubfoot, etc. The pamphlet is lavishly illustrated with drawings replicated in Ralph's *Handbook of Home Medicine,* so it was obviously also used as source material for that text. It can be dated not long after Ralph returned to Birmingham since it mentions his study in England; it also contains testimonial letters from the early 1890s. As a precursor of his *Handbook,* this pamphlet may be an indicator of Ralph's intent to build his Institute and to use it as the basis for a mail-order business. This is the only publication we have found providing a step-by-step description of how Ralph performed cleft-lip surgery—a procedure influenced by his father.

The years 1897 and 1898 were banner ones for Ralph's innovative treatments: In 1897, he received a patent for yet another electric device, the Reflector for Focusing Cathode Rays. The patent file shows

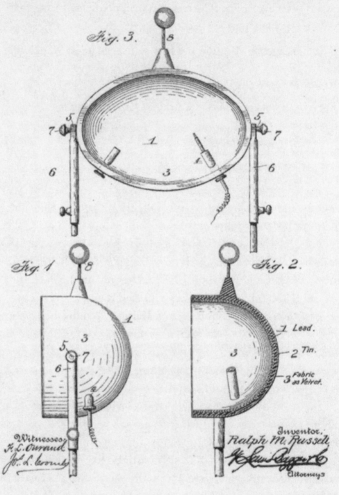

R. M. RUSSELL.
REFLECTOR FOR FOCUSING CATHODE RAYS.

No. 579,808.   Patented Mar. 30, 1897.

Patent diagram for Dr. Ralph Russell's Cathode Ray Reflector. US Letters Patent # 579,808. United States Patent Office, *Official Gazette of the United States Patent Office* (Washington, D.C.: Government Printing Office, 1897), vol. 78, p. 1990. The patent was issued 30 March 1897.

that Ralph applied for a patent on 15 September 1896 and received it on 30 March 1897. The device's description shows that it focuses cathode rays for therapeutic applications; a drawing of the device is appended.[80]

As he developed his Institute and patented his new device, Ralph increased advertising for his medical services. Various newspapers in the late 1890s carried reports about Ralph and his Institute. On 26 March and 9 April 1896, the Birmingham paper *The Weekly Tribune* carried advertisements for Ralph's Institute, listing illnesses it treated and noting that it employed "new European hospital methods of cure," which could be tried in April and May without cost.[81]

Ads Ralph placed in the *Mountain Eagle* in Jasper, Alabama, in December 1896 and August 1897 illustrate that he was not only targeting the urban audience of Birmingham but also smaller communities in the northwest quadrant of the state. The ads tell prospective patients that the Institute is the "best equipped sanitarium for the exclusive treatment of diseases of women and children in the South" and that Ralph's sanitarium could cure opium and morphine addiction with Vi-Be Ni tonic.[82]

On 3 June 1898, an ad in the Centre, Alabama newspaper the *Coosa River News* reported that Dr. Ralph M. Russell, Chief of the Russell Medico-Surgical Institute of Birmingham, "gives *scientific treatment in advance of the age* for the radical cure of Catarrh, Rheumatism, Chronic, Nervous, Blood and Female Diseases, and Deformities, Consumption in its first stages." Chronic sufferers and afflicted persons might consult him in Centre for several days coming.[83]

A few months later, *Montgomery Advertiser* carried an article entitled "Dr. Russell, of London: The Eminent Catarrh Specialist in the City." The article reports that Ralph was at the Mabson Hotel in Montgomery and hoped to establish a branch of his clinic in that city. He was Surgeon-in-Chief of the "famous Russell Medical Institute" in Birmingham, a branch of which was in Chicago. This piece also tells readers that Ralph had graduated from Bellevue and King's College, London. He had acquired "an international reputation" as a catarrh specialist and was distinguished as creator of the "celebrated system of absorption treatment" practiced successfully at his institutes and in Europe.

The *Advertiser* adds,

In a recent lecture delivered at the Academy of Medicine in
Paris, Dr. Russell convinced his distinguished colleagues that
nearly all chronic ailments originate from Tubercular Catarrh
and that such Pathological lesions as rheumatism, blood poi-
son, tumor, nervous prostration, and chronic ailments of the
internal organs could only be relieved by removing the real
cause from the system by absorption.

This theory had been tested at "the great hospitals in Europe" and
found to be "a phenomenal success." The *Advertiser* article then tells
readers that Ralph was the inventor of yet another device called the
Electrozone, "one of the greatest instruments for the relief of nervous
afflictions the country has produced."[84] But he was renowned above all
for his ability to cure and could be consulted at his offices on Dexter
Avenue or the Mabson Hotel.[85]

As this and the *Coosa River News* article suggest, Ralph had torn
a leaf from his father's book and taken his medical show on the road
as he launched an institute and prepared to publish his *Handbook of
Home Medicine*. The ads he placed in these years echo those his father
placed in roughly the same period of his life forty years earlier.

To wit, on 15 December 1898, Ralph placed an ad for his Electrozone
in the *People's Party Advocate* of Ashland, Alabama. "Electrozone"
appears in large bold-face type beside the following text:

> If you are blind, deaf, afflicted with Catarrh, Sexual Debility,
> Painful Menstruation or Lost Manhood, and want to know
> something about Dr. Russell's wonderful discovery, THE
> ELECTROZONE, don't drug and dose yourself to death,
> but write for a free booklet containing full information for
> self-treatment and testimonials of cured. Address RUSSELL
> MEDICAL INSTITUTE, Birmingham, Ala.[86]

Blindness, deafness, catarrh, sexual debility—all this *and* pain-
ful menstruation and "lost manhood" could be cured by this device.
Quite the machine. The following year on 2 June, the Tuscaloosa paper
Tuscaloosa Weekly Times carried an ad covering four columns of the front
page, announcing in boldface, all-caps print, "**HE IS COMING!**"[87]

On 3 November 1899, the *Coosa River News* carried an ad for
Ralph's Vi-Be Ni tonic, making similarly inflated claims for what this
potion could accomplish:

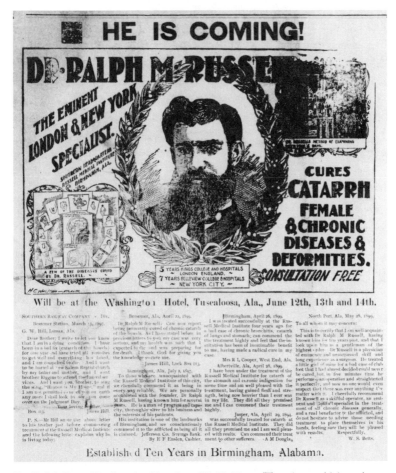

Dr. Ralph Russell's ad in the *Tuscaloosa Weekly Times* (Tuscaloosa, Alabama), 2 June 1899, page 1, columns 1–4.

Vi-Be Ni Malt Tonic, the great liquid food medicine and European hospital remedy for indigestion, loss of appetite, female weakness, chronic and wasting diseases. For sale at the Centre Drug Store.[88]

Again, the interesting touch about "European hospitals" appears. This is clearly part of what Ralph hoped to acquire with his study abroad—the ability to point to the "European" touch as an advertising tool for his clinic, tonic, and electronic devices.

Handbook of Home Medicine

The year 1900 was significant in Ralph's career, as he published his popular and widely circulated self-help book *The Handbook of Home Medicine: Devoted Principally to the Latest and Most Approved Methods of Home Treatment of Diseases Peculiar to the South and West* in that year. It was published by Hammond of Chicago, and eleven editions appeared from 1900 to 1911, when the title then drops from bibliographic sources, including OCLC. A copy held by the Lister Hill Library of the Health Sciences at University of Alabama Birmingham is the eleventh edition and has an inscription by Ralph to Dr. E. T. Fields dated 14 April 1913. This suggests that no further edition had been published two years after the 1911 edition appeared. Only six copies appear to be held by US libraries now, according to OCLC.[89]

Handbook of Home Medicine provides a fascinating glimpse into Ralph's approach to medicine, as well as his business practices. In the 1906 edition, which sold for sixty-five dollars, he introduced a membership certificate, making each family who bought a copy a member of a "Mutual Medical Association" and entitling these families to free medical advice. Editions of the *Handbook* from 1906 onward included a copy of the enrollment form.[90]

Handbook's eleventh edition contains 483 pages, a substantial compendium of information about the most productive ways to treat illnesses at home.[91]

The eleventh edition also contains a description of a training school for nurses founded in 1911. The program is described as a home-training course with "national nurses' text-books" provided for students. Those passing a final examination received a diploma qualifying them as a "Graduate National Nurse." Fees were charged for enrollment, textbooks, instruction, and graduation. The certificate of incorporation showing this nurses' program accredited by the state of Alabama in April 1911 is appended, with Ralph, his son Ralph, and Mollie Russell as incorporating members.[92]

In *Handbook*'s preface, Ralph explains the book's rationale:

> I do not propose to teach the novice how to make a hairsplitting differential diagnosis, nor to make an elaborate chemical analysis of the gastric juice. My object, on the other hand, is to tell the people in simple language how to administer medicine, bind a wound, prepare food for the sick, soothe

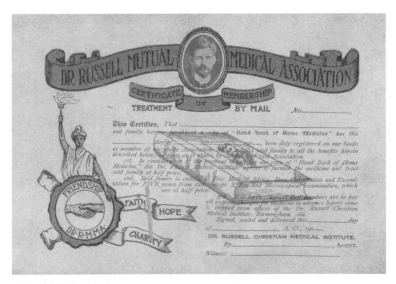

Mutual Medical Association Certificate from the *Handbook of Home Medicine*. Original is in the Historical Research Center, University of Arkansas for Medical Sciences (UAMS).

pain and treat an ordinary complaint in cases of emergency. Trusting that its perusal may contribute somewhat toward extending the popular knowledge of medical subjects, and that it may prove the means of relieving the afflicted in many homes, without further comment I submit the work to the public.[93]

Following the prefatory section, the book presents reproductions of Ralph's diplomas from Bellevue and King's College. An introduction describes the competing schools that have vied for practitioners' and patients' attention, from the allopathic and homeopathic to the eclectic, hydropathic, and electropathic. It also notes that some schools of American medicine endorse divine healing through laying on of hands and "magnetic cure" or through prayer and mental therapy.[94]

This brief survey of the various medical traditions in the United States is designed to introduce the approach of "Russell specialists"—a frankly pragmatic and non-ideological one:

> The Russell specialists discard all schools and select their remedies and methods of treatment from all sources that promise relief to their patients, and it is only by such a course

HANDBOOK

OF

HOME MEDICINE

DEVOTED PRINCIPALLY TO THE

Latest and Most Approved Methods of Home Treatment of Diseases Peculiar to the South and West.

FULLY ILLUSTRATED

With Colored Plates and Wood Engravings, containing a complete description of the wonderful X-Rays, with Radiographs.

WRITTEN IN PLAIN ENGLISH FOR THE PEOPLE

AS A

FAMILY MEDICAL ADVISER

BY

R. M. RUSSELL, M. D.,

Graduate of Bellevue Hospital Medical College, New York City, and Kings College, London, England; Patentee of the Cathode Reflector for Focussing X-Rays; Inventor of the ELECTROZONE; Founder and Chief Consulting Physician to the Russell Medical Institute, etc.

Title page of Dr. Ralph Russell's *Handbook of Home Medicine*. Original is in the Historical Research Center, University of Arkansas for Medical Sciences (UAMS).

that the best interest of the profession and the public can be advanced.[95]

The preface explains that the chapters are designed to teach families how to effectively care for their health and treat illnesses in a pragmatic, results-oriented way at home: "The object of this work (the book) is to teach truths, plain simple truths, no matter from what source, as facts, not fiction, is the crying need of an inquiring public."[96]

The book then launches into a lengthy argument for preventive medicine. This prefatory section notes that the *Handbook* is designed not merely to help families deal with illnesses but also to instruct them about how to safeguard their health so that they will not need medicine and cures. The discussion ends with the following rousing endorsement of preventive medicine that is also a plug for Ralph's book:

> Even our public schools are poorly equipped with plain, simple text-books on hygiene, physiology, physical culture and other health studies.
>
> Unquestionably we are guilty of a most palpable omission here and for this reason *we are certainly behind all* other professions.
>
> The various religious organizations of America publish books and periodicals a plenty for teaching and training their laymen and the same is true for American school teachers and other public organizations. But it seems the vast storehouse of Medical Knowledge has been kept under Latin, lock and key, by we [*sic*] doctors since the days of Aesculapius himself. Is it not time this storehouse was opened wide and the hungry, starving people fed? Surely so![97]

The book proper follows, moving from a presentation of basic anatomy to "hints" about home nursing and diagnosis, and a discussion of 193 diseases patients might encounter. Chapters address diseases of women, men, and the eye. The book also instructs home caregivers in the art of preparing "all kinds of homemade remedies," "palatable prescriptions" and "special prescriptions" to treat illnesses, and food for the sick. Several sections focus specifically on conditions that Ralph, his father, and his brother Seaborn treated, including strabismus, clubfoot, and cleft lip.

Lengthy portions explain the work of the Russell Institute and the therapeutic devices Ralph had introduced, including the Electrozone, the Reflector for Focussing [*sic*][98] Cathode Rays, massage machines, and special braces and supporters devised for use by "Russell specialists" as they treated various illnesses and deformities including clubfoot. A defense of advertising by doctors is followed by an ad for Ralph's cure-all, Vi-Be Ni.

The text is lavishly illustrated with colored plates and wood engravings. These include plates illustrating the anatomy of the head and the male and female torso, as well as a sketch of the Cathode Reflector and a photograph of the Electrozone. The book's eleventh printing replicates prefatory material added when the fifth edition appeared, which states that with this edition, various illustrations had been added, as well as patterns for homemade braces and abdominal supporters.

The final edition also replicates a preface added when the seventh edition was printed, noting that the book had sold several thousand copies and that depictions of an anatomical manikin of the human head and body and a manikin and anatomical chart of a woman had been added. The colored plates are beautifully done and fold out for readers to examine them.

A. *Handbook of Home Medicine*: Long Tradition of American Self-Help Medical Books

Ralph's *Handbook* stands squarely within a long tradition of self-doctoring manuals including Thomson's *New Guide to Health*. With its rallying cry of "Every man his own physician," the Thomsonian system tapped into deep populist veins in Jacksonian America, particularly in frontier areas where access to what passed for professional medicine in the nineteenth century was limited. Thomsonianism eventually coalesced with homeopathy, with its emphasis on providing families "domestic kits" stocked with herbal remedies sold by homeopaths who offered instructions for home doctoring.[99]

All of this—from the encouragement of every family to self-doctor, to the "family rights" sold along with Thomson's book and the enrollment of buyers in a medical fraternity, to the hawking of herbs and tonics as a marketing feature (and an income-generating one) of self-help books: This is all to be found in *Handbook of Home Medicine*,

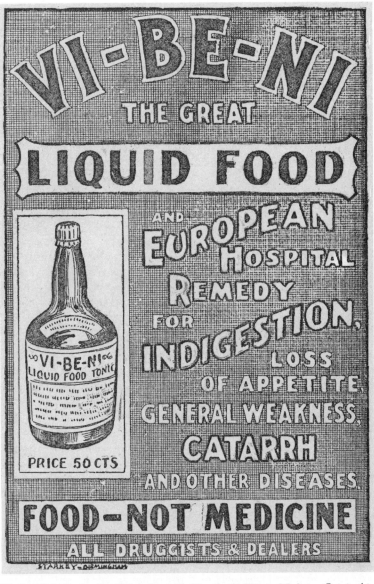

Vi-Be-Ni [*sic*] ad in Dr. Ralph Russell's *Handbook of Home Medicine*. Original is in the Historical Research Center, University of Arkansas for Medical Sciences (UAMS).

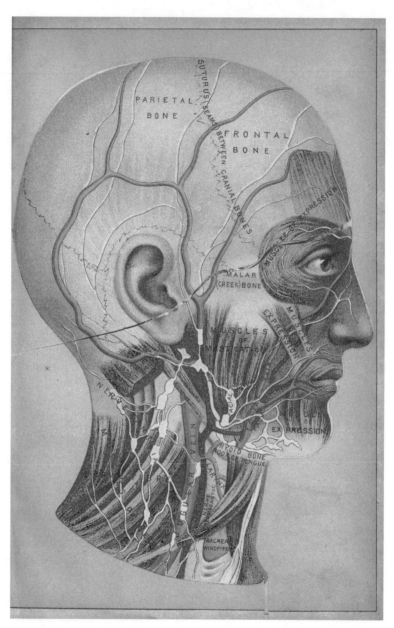

Anatomical plate from Dr. Ralph Russell's *Handbook of Home Medicine*. Original is in the Historical Research Center, University of Arkansas for Medical Sciences (UAMS)

too. It is not in the least accidental that the *Handbook* informs its readers that Ralph's book is designed for use by families living in the South and West, in particular: this is the same market Thomson and others had targeted in the preceding century, a market where trained physicians were scarce and limited to urban areas.

As Michael and Anita Clair Fellman note, even after distrust of medical practitioners began to wane in the final decades of the nineteenth century, Americans continued to have a robust interest in self-help guides.[100] As the medical profession became more established and more Americans sought the assistance of trained doctors, people continued turning to self-help manuals even as they sought professional intervention.[101]

Much of what we find in Ralph's *Handbook* had been built into American medical practice years prior to 1900. As we noted in chapter one, the acclaimed eighteenth-century physician Benjamin Rush, who taught both of William J. Russell's mentors, emphasized the need for practitioners to adopt a pragmatic-democratic approach to diagnosis and treatment. Rush insisted that the practitioner could learn from many different types of people: He instructed students to observe closely how nurses, including elderly women, treated their patients, how they decided what worked and what did not work as they sought a cure. As James Young indicates, from very early on, a "rampant empiricism" was built into the American medical world by formative figures like Rush, resulting in a willingness of American medical consumers to try anything that appeared to cure what ailed them.[102]

Many of the "palatable prescriptions" recommended by *Handbook* echo the emphasis on native pharmacological wisdom bequeathed to American medicine by people like Rush and Thomson. For the treatment of asthma, for instance, Ralph prescribes a mix of the native plant gumweed (*Grindelia robusta*) and orange peel syrup.[103] As he offers readers this and other prescriptions, he notes that some of the prescriptions are original, but others "have been copied from the leading medical authorities of the world," and all are used by "specialists at the Russell Medical Institute."[104] A list of medicinal native plants is appended.[105] It includes Indian tobacco (*Lobelia*), crowfoot, blood root, skunk cabbage, pokeweed, wild carrot, Indian turnip, and liverwort.

As a foundational figure of American medicine, Rush exerted influence on the trajectory of medical practice in the nineteenth century in yet another way, which is also apparent in *Handbook*: This is his willingness to resort to correspondence to carry on his teaching and practice.[106] Ralph's interest in a mail-order practice as exhibited in *Handbook* is not a novel feature of this early twentieth-century work.

Guenter B. Risse notes that published works by practitioners seeking to popularize medical knowledge have existed for centuries.[107] According to Charles Rosenberg, self-help guides were part of American culture from the colonial period forward: Settlers brought not only Bibles and prayer books but also guides to home treatment and midwifery to the colonies. Rosenberg argues that the abundant and richly diverse medical self-help literature found in American culture from very early days has been neglected by scholars and deserves greater attention.[108]

As he notes, prior to the twentieth century, most medical care was provided by individuals who did not think of themselves as physicians. Within this cultural context, the development of medical self-help literature makes eminent sense:

> It is not surprising that prudent families should have assumed the need for a book explaining domestic treatment of the sick, just as they anticipated the need for a cookbook, primer, or Bible. Families provided medical care for every sort of ailment, from acute fevers to chronic ills such as cancer, tuberculosis, and 'dropsy.'[109]

In the post-colonial period, as the settlers of the new nation began moving westward, the need for home medical manuals became even more pronounced, as Christopher Hoolihan points out. Many Americans lived in remote places where doctors were scarce, had little money to hire physicians, and kept doctors at a distance, distrusting their expertise and their "murderous combination of therapies that centered on bloodletting, purging, and drugging with poisonous minerals."[110] To meet the burgeoning market for home therapy instruction in the nineteenth century, hundreds of books on domestic medicine and hygiene appeared in print in North America, along with innumerable pamphlets.[111] Itinerant medical lecturers capitalized on this development by providing a combination of medical education and entertainment in small towns and rural communities, using broadsides and circulars to woo audiences and dramatic exhibits to titillate them.[112]

In particular, as Hoolihan notes, a robust market developed in the

nineteenth century for patent medicines, which were widely advertised with national marketing schemes, though such medicines were
produced in discrete locales. In Hoolihan's view, "Patent medicine
advertising, in fact, created the advertising industry we know today."[113]

American marketers were remarkably creative about devising
endless ways to sell patent medicines: Advertisements were placed in
almanacs, on bookmarks, in calendars, on ink blotters, and in coloring
books and on paper cut-out figures for children to play with. They
appeared in unsolicited form letters mailed out in bulk to American
households and in pamphlets about non-medical themes, including
cooking and etiquette. American families playing parlor games or
opening songbooks, sheet music, or Valentines might expect a medical ad to meet their eyes as they brought out the music or opened the
card.[114] Patent medicine advertisements were, in short, to be found
almost everywhere in nineteenth-century America.[115]

Such advertising was accompanied by a voluminous body of
self-help works published in the nineteenth century for American
(and British and European) audiences. Among the most influential
of these was William Buchan's *Domestic Medicine, or a Treatise on the
Prevention and Cure of Diseases, by Regimen and Simple Medicines:
with An Appendix Containing a Dispensatory for the Use of Private
Practitioners* (London: Strahan, 1803). Buchan's work was, Charles
Rosenberg reports, omnipresent in British and American homes prior
to the Civil War.[116]

Equally popular, especially on the growing edge of the south-
western frontier in the first half of the century, was John C. Gunn's
Domestic Medicine, or, Poor Man's Friend (Knoxville, 1830).[117] As
Rosenberg notes in his introduction to the 1986 facsimile reprint of
this influential self-help book, the volume went through at least nineteen printings from 1830 to 1840. Rosenberg observes, "The manual's
immediate popularity and widespread reprinting in the 'West' indicate
that Gunn, if not precisely a poor man's friend, was able to anticipate
the medical needs of a good many ordinary Americans in the era of
Andrew Jackson."[118]

Buchan and Gunn's books were far from the only self-help man-
uals to be found on the American market in the nineteenth century.
Other widely circulated works published in the US and abroad included
Thomas Johnson's *Every Man His Own Doctor*, published in Salisbury,
North Carolina, in 1798[119]; James Ewell's *The Medical Companion, or*

Family Physician (1807)[120]; Thomas Ewell's *Letters to Ladies, Detailing Important Information, Concerning Themselves and Infants* (1817)[121]; Robert Thomas and David Hosack's *A Treatise on Domestic Medicine* (1820)[122]; Thomas Cooper's *Treatise of Domestic Medicine* (1824)[123]; William Horner's *Home Book of Health and Medicine* (1834)[124]; and William Matthews's *Treatise on Domestic Medicine* (1848).[125]

As a precursor of Russell's *Handbook*, Horner's *Home Book of Health and Medicine* is especially noteworthy. This 1834 volume follows roughly the same trajectory that Ralph's book follows, as it moves from a discussion of anatomy to a focus on hygiene and preventive medicine and then to *materia medica*, analysis of various diseases, and a discussion of pregnancy and parturition, with an appendix about the administering of medicines recommended in the book.

B. *Handbook of Home Medicine*:
Questions about Quackery

As we noted when we told W. J. P. Russell's story, educated practitioners in nineteenth-century America, such as Paul Eve, expended a great deal of energy trying to draw a clear line between genuine medical treatment and quackery in the world of American medicine.[126] The lecture that Eve presented to W. J. P.'s entering class juxtaposes recurring words like "nostrum," "quacks," "empirics," and "charlatans" with "science," "reason" and "education." As Eve noted, from early in its development, American medicine struggled with lax licensing and educational requirements that permitted almost anyone to hang out a shingle and promote remedies accredited physicians knew to be bogus. Eve's lecture singles out "Thomsonian or botanic" doctors for particular critique.

So-called medical authorities making unsubstantiated claims about the curative properties of nostrums had damaged the brand of the medical profession, Eve thought, leaving a gullible public unable to distinguish between authentic and inauthentic treatments. As he wrote,

> The whole system of empiricism is founded upon public credulity, in what is novel, marvelous, or mysterious in treating diseases; and in the popular supposition, that every one can best judge what is good or hurtful to his own system.[127]

As William Helfand indicates in his informative study *Quack, Quack, Quack,* the struggle to distinguish between *bona fide* medicine and quackery has a long history in American culture. "Quack, Quack, Quack," Ben Franklin scribbled in the margin of his copy of a report issued in Paris in 1784 examining the claims of mesmerists.[128] As Helfand notes, the term "quack" probably originates with the Dutch *Quacksalber,* referring to a charlatan, mountebank, empiric, or itinerant seller of medicine. The *Oxford English Dictionary* finds the word in use from the seventeenth century as a designation of "an ignorant pretender to medical skill."[129] As Helfand suggests, the line between quackery and authentic practice was thin to nonexistent in both American and European culture well into the nineteenth century, when accreditation requirements and the formation of professional societies began to draw this line more sharply.[130]

The free-wheeling way in which medicine was practiced in nineteenth- and early-twentieth-century America contributed to the difficulty of distinguishing doctors from quacks. As Helfand notes, the "migratory nature" of the profession strongly stamped American medicine in this period, as "medicine show troupes" traveled throughout the US, making wide use of testimonials, vouchers, advertisements, handbills, broadsides, posters, newspaper ads, books, and pamphlets to market the troupes' purported medical specialties.[131]

Many of these traveling shows offered medical wares with theatrical flair, providing a form of entertainment for small towns and rural communities starved for theatrical performances:

> In their combined aspects of both the healing and the performing arts, these itinerant showmen provided an amalgamation that had later manifestations in the nineteenth-century American medicine show and in twentieth-century television programs.[132]

For those confronted with these shows and their plethora of advertising, it might at one level have seemed easy to distinguish between silver and dross—unlike the doctor, the quack lacked education and especially medical training; the quack promised too much and offered cures that were certain even when all else failed.[133] But at another level, the line between the quack and the trained physician appeared tenuous when, as in the case of the multi-degreed eighteenth-century oculist John "Chevalier" Taylor, the trained doctor functioned to all intents and purposes as a quack.[134] The line between valid medicine and quackery also became difficult to draw when a cure-all touted widely by quacks was, as with Nehemiah Grew and Epsom salts, invented by a trained physician.[135] The reliance on heroic methods also left doctors open to charges of quackery, some of these leveled, in fact, by irregular practitioners.[136]

As Helfand indicates, in the context of nineteenth- and early twentieth-century America, this distinction between doctors and quacks proved all the more difficult due to the confluence of self-help books, many written with the specific purpose of marketing proprietary nostrums and medical devices that could be obtained only from the books' authors and the burgeoning advertising industry. Thomson not only wrote a widely distributed medical-treatment book, but he also linked its distribution to the marketing of herbal cures he had confected.[137] Samuel Solomon's *A Guide to Health*, a British work marketed in the US, which Solomon published to market his cure-all herbal remedy the Cordial Balm of Gilead, went through sixty-six editions in the eighteenth and early nineteenth centuries.[138] With good reason, trained doctors were frequently skeptical about self-help works because of how they popularized and distributed remedies claiming undemonstrated effectiveness.[139]

The widespread use of newspapers to advertise nostrums and quack cures exacerbated the difficulty of drawing a line between genuine medicine and quackery. As Helfand notes, ads for patent medicines and various curative devices—and medical services—proliferated in newspapers from the eighteenth century forward.[140] Advertisements were often accompanied by testimonials whose veracity was not easy to ascertain.[141] In fact, as Helfand points out, "From the earliest days of newspapers, proprietary medicines were among the few brand-name products advertised, most of the space being filled by local merchants and services."[142]

England and the US were outliers in their refusal to apply controls to the hyping of pseudo-medical devices, nostrums, and curatives through newspaper ads and by other means.[143] With its casual belief in the virtue of the free market and advertising, the Anglo-American approach actively encouraged the proliferation of unorthodox practitioners, Helfand suggests:

[T]he unorthodox will be discovered to be those who developed many new marketing, publicity and advertising techniques; fashioned the art of persuasion and salesmanship; created novel distribution systems; pioneered the emphasis on brand-name products; served as an economic link between the hinterland and the urban center; expanded markets; and helped to provide the entrepreneurship necessary for the growth of modern society.[144]

Helfand notes that, up to 1842, only four states—New York, New Jersey, Louisiana, and Georgia—had laws regulating the practice of medicine and seeking to distinguish between authentic and inauthentic practice.[145]

Nor is medical quackery entirely a thing of the past, Helfand thinks. The continuing lack of stringent controls on marketing of para-medical nostrums and devices with dubious claims about their tonic properties and the ability of quacks to evade controls by endless schemes of adaptation permit quackery to thrive today:

> Quackery has shown that it can adapt itself to almost any prevailing political and regulatory system. Practices that many of us would consider unadulterated quackery can be found today in the pages of many newspapers and magazines as well as on the television screen. A visit to any health food store will provide the necessary evidence.[146]

Helfand's historical analysis of quackery in American medicine and of the role of self-help books and aggressive advertising in promoting nostrums and quack medicine is pertinent as we examine Ralph's Institute and his *Handbook*. As noted previously, the AMA sought to alert medical consumers to fraudulent schemes, publishing an extensive two-volume exposé of quackery in 1912 and 1921 entitled *Nostrums and Quackery*.[147] The preface to the first volume states that, beginning in 1905, *Collier's Weekly* had been publishing articles exposing quackery and the peddling of nostrums.[148] The AMA gathered these and printed them in booklet form, and *Nostrums and Quackery* grew out of that project, adding articles printed in the *Journal of the American Medical Association*.[149]

What this AMA exposé tells us about quackery in American medicine in the first decades of the twentieth century raises searching questions about what Ralph was doing at the same time. As we have seen, though his *Handbook* has a drawing of his Institute, in litigation that ensued about his estate following his death, it appears that the multi-story building pictured in this drawing was not, as his *Handbook* implies, entirely occupied by Ralph's Institute. Affidavits in *Hayden v. Russell* (1916) suggest that Ralph occupied several offices in the building and was the sole doctor on the Institute's staff, despite the book's claims that it had multiple specialists. Documents in the case file also indicate that, though Ralph claimed his Institute had a certified pharmacist, most of the compounding of medicine he sold was apparently done by Lucy Hayden and her sons (none of them trained pharmacists, it seems), assisted by Ralph himself, with his brother Richard helping briefly.

A section of *Nostrums and Quackery* entitled "Medical Institutes" provides interesting information about dubious operations that sound similar to Ralph's Institute.[150] As this report indicates, the Reinhardt brothers of Milwaukee operated multiple institutes in the early 1900s, including the "Wisconsin Medical Institute" and "The Master Specialist." These outfits had family ties to the "Heidelberg Institute" in St. Paul, the "Vienna Medical Institute" of Chicago, and the "Copenhagen Institute" of Davenport, Iowa.[151]

The promotional literature of another institute, Boston Medical Institute, printed a picture of its "correspondence" department and claimed that twenty people worked in a 3,000-square-foot space to answer inquiries—but this office and its team of workers were nonexistent.[152] When the clinic was prosecuted, Charles Jessamine, who was compounding medicine for it, testified that not only did he have no training for this work and did it without supervision, but there was also no registered pharmacist working for the clinic.[153] As the AMA study concludes, "Judging from the developments at the trial, it was apparently the custom of the managers of the Boston Medical Institute to employ any one available to do whatever was to be done, regardless of the fitness of the person employed."[154] Among the devices peddled by the clinic was the Boston Electric Belt, which was said to have wide-ranging therapeutic properties, and, in particular, to enhance virility in those wearing it.[155] The clinic's head Edward Hibbard was found guilty of fraud in 1909.

The Epileptic Institute of Cincinnati, run by Otto Kalmus, purported to cure epilepsy.[156] This institute also relied on "symptom blanks" submitted by patients to diagnose illnesses, using a form remarkably similar to the one in Ralph's *Handbook*.[157] When Kalmus's operation received these forms, it then sent out stock letters "diagnosing" the illness along with a set of medicines to treat it, with payment expected on delivery.[158]

As is evident, a primary concern of the AMA in *Nostrums and Quackery* studies is the use of the postal system to defraud medical consumers with claims that illness could be diagnosed and treated by correspondence. As the study notes,

> In his 'Great American Fraud' series Samuel Hopkins Adams calls attention to the absurdity of the proposition put forward by numerous quacks that it is possible to treat diseases by correspondence. As Mr. Adams says, it is 'like mending chimneys by mail.'[159]

A lengthy section of *Nostrums and Quackery* entitled "Mail-Order Medical Concerns" deals with this topic. The Branaman Remedy Company of Kansas City, for instance, advertised cures for deafness, catarrh, asthma, and head noises and secured patients through ads in newspapers and magazines and by correspondence. They were asked to submit "symptom blanks" and return them to Dr. G. M. Branaman for diagnosis. Patients then received a form letter telling them they had either catarrh or deafness, and because their case was too serious to be treated by medicine alone, they needed to purchase Dr. Branaman's "electro-magnetic head-cap."[160]

The Nutriola Company of Chicago, organized in Maine about 1894, elicited critical attention for its use of the mail service to market a preparation called Nu-Tri-Ola Skin Food that was presented as a cure-all for dermatological problems.[161] Likewise, a compound marketed by H. Samuels of Wichita—Professor Samuels' Eye Water—raised eyebrows. Samuels used "symptom blanks" to diagnose patients and claimed that his eye water could cure about any ocular ailment around. This nostrum turned out to be tap water with sugar and table salt added.[162]

As the preface to *Nostrums and Quackery* explains, what set nostrums apart from patent medicines is that the names of nostrums were registered so others could not use them, but their formulas were not revealed. The formulas of patent medicines had to be revealed in a patent application. Because the nostrum formulas were not public, their contents could shift, making it very difficult for trained physicians to track their active properties or assess their effectiveness.[163] As an example, because Ralph's Vi-Be Ni tonic name was registered but the formula not patented, its precise composition is not known and could be changed at any time.

A portion of *Nostrums and Quackery* entitled "Mineral Waters" reminds us that fraudulent claims were made about the healing properties of bottled spring water, including Mountain Valley Water in Arkansas, which was shipped via interstate commerce with labels stating that it was radioactive and cured kidney and bladder ailments, Bright's disease, diabetes, cystitis, and rheumatism. These claims were judged fraudulent, and the company was fined for fraud in 1915.[164] As we noted in our discussion of the story of W. J. P. Russell, part of what motivated his decision to move to Eureka Springs in the early 1880s was his interest in the new water-bottling companies being established in the community as the town began to be marketed as a resort with healing waters.

It is rather difficult to read the AMA's exposé of fraudulent practices in the early twentieth century and not wonder about some aspects of Ralph's Institute and about his *Handbook* as a tool for marketing the Institute. *Did* Ralph's Electro-Mechanical device or the Electrozone really have the miraculous therapeutic effects he claimed it had? A single machine curing blindness, deafness, catarrh, and sexual debility: this stretches belief.

And what about the Vi-Be Ni tonic? Can this cure-all, marketed via the *Handbook*, as were the electrical gadgets, really have accomplished all that Ralph asserted? What sets it apart from nostrums on which the federal government was clamping down in these years? And, again, what to make of the fact that the only picture we can find of Ralph's Institute is a drawing that appears to overstate its physical scope vastly, his claim that the Institute had nonexistent "specialists" on board, or the claim that the Institute had branches in major cities around the world? What to make of the use of "symptom blanks" or the misrepresentation of the clinic's pharmaceutical work as done by a trained pharmacist?

There are some real fissures running through these claims. They point to the possibility—omnipresent in American medicine at all periods—that what was being sold as genuine medical practice was, in key respects, not distant from quackery.

The Final Years

When Ralph Russell published his *Handbook*, he was entering the final full decade of his life, which would be cut short in 1916 by a stroke when he was only forty-nine years old. Ralph's practice appears to have been doing well in 1900, as indicated by the number of land and mortgage transactions for him and wife Mollie in the county deed books.[165]

Birmingham city directories show that the Russells' residence in the 1890s was on 12th Avenue between 20th and 21st streets; in 1900, the family lived at 1315 Huntsville Avenue; and from 1904–1908, it lived at 1306 Huntsville Avenue.[166] Around 1908, the family made one final move to a house at 1320 Huntsville, which remained in the family for ninety years following Ralph's death.[167] A photo of the 1306 Huntsville house is featured in the *Handbook*. Though the family moved from there around 1908, the photo continued to appear in the *Handbook* through its final edition in 1911.

As noted above, Ralph incorporated his nurse training school in 1911. An October 1915 notice in the *Greensboro Watchman* (Greensboro, Alabama) advertises the nursing services of Sim Strong of Newbern, Alabama, who had graduated from "Dr. Russell's Institute at Birmingham." Strong indicates that he was a "colored graduate physician's sick nurse" whose services could be solicited at any time.[168]

As the incorporation of his nurse training program suggests, Ralph continued to seek new opportunities to expand the scope of his business in the final years of his life. The 23 August 1912 edition of the Western North Carolina newspaper *Brevard News* provides a revealing glimpse of efforts Ralph was making at this time to extend his operations: The article reports,

> Dr. R. M. Russell of Birmingham, Ala., has been here several days. His name will be recognized by many here as the author of the medical work handled exclusively by Brevard book men. Dr. Russell has expressed himself very favorably about this country. Some time ago he purchased the lower cottage on North Caldwell from the McMinn-Shipman-Weilt Company.[169]

In 1913, a series of ads appeared in *Brevard News* for Ralph's Vi-Be Ni product, now sold in pill form; these suggest that Ralph was attempting to widen the marketing scope for Vi-Be Ni and perhaps obtain more patients for his Institute. From 24 July through 4 September 1914, an ad appeared in the Brevard paper:

> Recommended for BILIOUSNESS, CONSTIPATION, ALL LIVER AILMENTS. Price 25 cents. 'REMOVE THE CAUSE.'[170]

The ad notes that Vi-Be Ni pills were on sale at several Brevard drugstores, and one could write for a free sample to Doctor Russell Medical Institute, 404 North 18th Street, Birmingham, AL. With the completion of a railroad line to the community in the latter part of the nineteenth century and the building of the luxurious Franklin Hotel in 1900, Brevard was developing a reputation as a cure resort and attracting well-heeled older visitors and new residents seeking its healthy mountain air.[171] Ralph's decision to market here was canny.

On 5 November 1916, Dr. Ralph Morgan Russell died in Birmingham from a cerebral hemorrhage. His death certificate notes that he suffered from hypertension.[172] Ralph's obituary states that notables of Alabama political and professional life, including former US Senator Frank S. White, US District Attorney Robert N. Bell, and Dr. William Gewin, who had organized the Birmingham Infirmary in 1906, served as funeral pallbearers.[173]

Three days after his death, Ralph's wife Mollie filed to probate his estate.[174] The following month, Ralph's former employee Lucy Hayden filed suit to contest the estate.[175] Hayden alleged that she had been Ralph's business partner for a number of years "conducting the business of compounding, manufacturing, advertising, supplying and selling various medicines, from various receipts, prescriptions and appliances for the healing of disease." Her court filing states that the business she shared with Ralph was at 404½ N 18th St. in Birmingham and that her sons assisted her in the pharmaceutical work, though there is no evidence that either she or they had any background in compounding medicine.

When Ralph's heirs Mollie and Ralph Jr. countered Hayden's claims with a filing in January 1917, Hayden responded by filing an amendment to her original complaint, alleging that the will Mollie had presented for probate was not Ralph's last will and that the defendants and their attorney had the last will. It recognized her rights in the estate, she stated, and this is why his heirs were withholding it.

Filings and counter-filings flew back and forth for several years between the parties, with the defendants claiming that Hayden's connection to Ralph had been a business association and not a partnership. The Jefferson County Court ruled in favor of Hayden, only to have the state supreme court overturn the ruling, noting that Hayden had not set forth the terms of any partnership she shared with Ralph in her initial filing. In January 1918, Hayden filed an amendment to her original complaint, stating that the business partnership had been formed in 1911 and had existed continuously up to Ralph's death.

Hayden also alleged that Ralph had received $7,500 from her in 1909–1910, agreeing to invest the money for her benefit. But he had purchased real estate with part of the sum and had used the rest in their business. Hayden also indicated that the two had formed an equal partnership and that all real estate Ralph owned when he died had been bought from her funds.

The case dragged on into the 1920s, with Hayden filing another amendment in May 1920 in which she repeated that she was a legatee of Ralph's last will, which had still not been disclosed. In March 1922, the circuit court ruled in Hayden's favor, affirming that she and Ralph had had a business partnership entitling her to an accounting of the estate. In January 1923, the state supreme court upheld this ruling, and sometime after this date, the case appears to have been settled out of court with no public record of its settlement, leaving a number of questions: Why did Mollie refuse for six years to disclose information to Lucy Hayden about Ralph's business? Why did Lucy continue the case for so long at what was probably considerable expense? What was the final settlement, and what really lay behind this case?

Ralph's widow Mollie died 26 January 1945 in Birmingham and was buried beside her husband in the Elmwood Cemetery. During the course of their life in Birmingham, the couple contributed to a number of local charities, including the Birmingham YMCA and Birmingham College (now Birmingham Southern), a Methodist-affiliated school. From 1920 through 1938, Mollie served as president of the City Mission Board of the Methodist Church's Birmingham District, overseeing the establishment of the Eva Comer Home for Girls and the Bethlehem House for People of Color during her tenure as board president.[176]

CHAPTER 5

Benjamin Franklin Norwood
(1886–1942)
and George Washington Russell
(1915–1989)

The initial pay of an appointee amounts to more than $3,000 a year, which is much better than a young physician is likely to receive when he begins his practice in civil life upon graduation. The known advantages in the way of promotion and certainty of income and final retirement at the age of 64 years or before that time for disability would, it was thought, prove attractive.

—"*Uncle Sam Wants More Army Surgeons,*"
Lafayette County Democrat (Stamps, Arkansas),
1 October 1909[1]

I suspect that, as a surgeon on the battleship the USS Pennsylvania, and having participated in the bloodiest conflicts of the South Pacific campaign where he spent his days trying to save and then care for the severely wounded from the beachheads, he felt his stories were too stern a stuff to share with his two young sons. And so a pattern developed of never talking about the elephant in the room that had affected him so deeply as it has all young men in all past centuries who have been asked to serve and thus seen the unmasked face of war.

—GEORGE SEABORN RUSSELL,
son of George Washington Russell[2]

Two great-grandsons carry the story of the generations of doctors descending from William James Russell to the middle and latter decades of the twentieth century. These are Benjamin Franklin Norwood, son of W. J. P.'s daughter Ava, and George Washington Russell, son of Seaborn. Though Ben and George were first cousins, George was a generation younger because he was Seaborn's last son by his third wife.

Photos of each as they finished medical school—Ben in 1912 and George in 1941—show them looking almost like brothers. The resemblance is remarkable: The same steady regard from underneath their mortarboards, the same firmness of expression, even the same tilt to the head.[3] The gaze of each conveys a certain air, one that bespeaks awareness that they are carrying on a family tradition.

Benjamin Franklin Norwood, Early Life and Education

Benjamin Franklin Norwood was born on 5 January 1886 in Sanford, North Carolina, as his father was conducting business there with wife Ava accompanying him.[4] Since he had his father's name, he was called Ben rather than Frank, to distinguish son from father. Frank and Ava settled initially in Hazlehurst, Mississippi, their home for several years as Frank continued working as a traveling salesman with the Wrought Iron Stove Company. As early as 13 January 1887, when a business associate, G. W. Thompson, wrote Frank from Kennedale, Texas, to encourage him to move to Texas, it appears the Norwoods had begun to consider coming to Wills Point to join Ava's family. Thompson's letter speaks of business Frank needed to do to "wind up" notes that Seaborn had signed.[5]

By 1888, when their last child Ruby Leona Norwood was born, the couple had settled next to Ava's parents in Wills Point, where Ben was raised until the Norwoods moved to Stamps, Arkansas, in the early 1900s to join Frank's family. The 1893–1896 school census of Van Zandt County shows Ben as a pupil, and in March 1899, he appears on a student roster at R. S. Hall Community School #54 near Wills Point.[6]

An invaluable source of information about Ben's life is his naval medical file, which contains information about his and his parents' medical history, illnesses he contracted in service, and his physical examinations.[7] The file indicates that, as a youth, Ben experienced

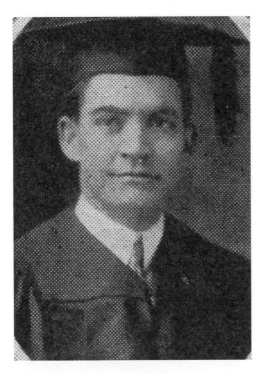

Dr. Ben Norwood's medical school graduation picture from the University of Tennessee yearbook *The Volunteer*, vol. 16, *1912. Courtesy of the Health Sciences Historical Collections, University of Tennessee Health Science Center Library, Memphis.*

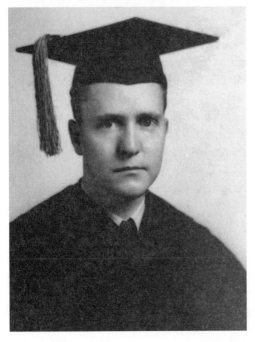

Dr. George Russell's medical school graduation picture from the University of Arkansas for Medical Sciences yearbook *The Arkansas Caduceus 1941. Courtesy of the Historical Research Center, University of Arkansas for Medical Sciences (UAMS).*

a gamut of illnesses common for children of this period, including recurrent malaria, measles at age ten, and a broken collarbone when he was a teen.

The file states that Ben joined the Navy in Fort Worth on 12 January 1904. For the next four years, he served aboard a variety of ships in the Pacific, initially as a painter 3rd class and eventually as a painter 1st class by the time of his discharge,.[8] During this first stint of service, Ben went to the Philippines, Guam, China, and Japan.

His medical file states that Ben contracted gonorrhea in April 1906 and was treated at Cañacao Naval Hospital in the Philippines.[9] In August, he relapsed and required further treatment. As Magnus Unemo and William Shafer note, prior to the discovery of antibiotic treatments in the 1930s, gonorrhea was a challenging illness to cure.[10] Therapies were often gruesome; they included hyperthermia and application of mercury, both taking quite a toll on patients.

Following his honorable discharge on 20 January 1908, Ben returned to Stamps. His military medical records show him suffering xiphoid process injury in the period after he returned home.[11]

In the fall of 1908, Ben went to Memphis to the College of Physicians and Surgeons (later the University of Tennessee).[12] It is interesting to note that he did *not* choose his own state's medical university, the Medical Department of the University of Arkansas. As Ben was entering medical school, Abraham Flexner was writing a ground-breaking evaluation of American medical schools for the American Medical Association. It would be published in 1910, after Ben began school in Memphis.[13]

The Flexner Report was scathing in its assessment of medical education in Arkansas. Noting that the state school was "not even 'affiliated' with the state university whose name it bears" and judging that it was "incredible that the state university should permit its name to shelter" the school, the Flexner Report found its entrance requirements "nominal." Flexner notes that the Arkansas school had no laboratory facilities beyond a dissecting room and an organic chemistry laboratory and that its classrooms had meager equipment and its clinical facilities were "hardly more than nominal."[14]

Flexner's comments about medical education in Tennessee were hardly more flattering, though his appraisal of the College of Physicians and Surgeons in Memphis notes that the school occupied an excellent building with a modern dissecting room and good laboratory. Flexner also gave the school good marks for its clinical education, though the Report looks askance at the practice of having students merely observe obstetrical procedures without actually assisting in them. Regarding the dissecting room and laboratory, the Flexner Report found that instruction in the former was "antiquated" and that lab equipment for pathology, bacteriology, and physiology was insufficient.[15]

Flexner found a plethora of underfunded schools competing with each other in Tennessee. He proposed combining them for better medical education in the state. He also noted (as in Arkansas) the glaring disparity between resources available to majority-culture institutions and those training African American doctors.[16] The only Tennessee school that Flexner praised was Vanderbilt, which he saw as a model for others to emulate.

Since the Flexner Report was published in the year following Ben's matriculation, it cannot have influenced his decision to attend an out-of-state school, though, Ben might have been struck by the quality of the facilities of the Memphis school that Flexner would note the next year. What may have weighed more than anything in Ben's choice was that a Norwood cousin had gone to the Memphis college, and a friend from Stamps, Herschell Kitchens, entered at the same time Ben did.

A newspaper clipping Ben's mother preserved in her scrapbook allows us to infer that he was esteemed by his classmates. Under the heading "Freshman Class Organized," this notice from an unidentified newspaper states that Ben was elected president of his freshman class.[17] His graduating yearbook shows him as captain of the school's football team in 1909 and a member of Chi Zeta Chi fraternity.[18]

Ben graduated as an MD from the University of Tennessee in the spring of 1912, ranking near the top of his class, a point emphasized by a 10 May 1912 article in his hometown *Lafayette County Democrat*.[19] After having been interviewed by the state board, he was licensed to practice in Tennessee.[20] Shortly before Ben's graduation, the College of Physicians and Surgeons had merged with two other schools to form University of Tennessee Medical School. As a result, documents identify his alma mater as the University of Tennessee.

On 26 April, the Stamps paper published a report indicating that

Ben had come home the previous week to visit family and had then gone east to take a "lucrative position in New York."[21] This evidently refers to his internship at St. Mary's Hospital in Hoboken, New Jersey. By 1914, Ben had completed the internship and launched his practice in Memphis, where he appears in the city directory with a downtown office.

City directories show Ben living in Memphis from 1909–1917.[22] But as articles from Ben's hometown paper suggest, he continued to maintain close ties to the medical community of Arkansas, and his family and friends back home followed his budding career with interest. The statewide *Arkansas Gazette* carried an article on 6 May 1917 noting that Dr. Ben F. Norwood of Memphis had been in Stamps to lecture on hygiene and sanitation for "Baby Welfare Week," and then on 10 May, the *Gazette* reported that Ben had been brought from Memphis to Stamps by Mrs. T. A. Brown, president of the town's Woman's Study Club, to work with local physicians and a nurse to examine children as part of a welfare campaign.[23]

Naval Medical Career Begins

Following his five years of practice in Memphis, Ben launched a distinguished career as a naval medical officer on 30 May 1917, when he accepted his oath of office in the Naval Medical Corps. On 23 July he was assigned to the Sault St. Marie Naval Station in Michigan.[24]

In accordance with the National Defense Act of 1916, President Woodrow Wilson confirmed Ben's nomination as an officer on 1 August. Those nominated under the act were either members of the Officer Reserve Corps or honor graduates of universities. As a medical school honor graduate, Ben was appointed assistant surgeon in the Navy the following day.[25] He entered active duty in the Navy Medical Corps with the rank of lieutenant junior grade on 26 September 1917. At the time he was commissioned, Ben was one of only four Arkansas physicians in the naval service.[26]

Military service was an honored tradition in the Russell family network. Ben and George had a cousin, Colonel Beverly Wyly Dunn of Clinton, Louisiana, who was an 1883 graduate of West Point and an artillery officer. In 1906, Dunn had invented the ammonium picrate-based explosive known as "Dunnite," the first explosive used in aerial

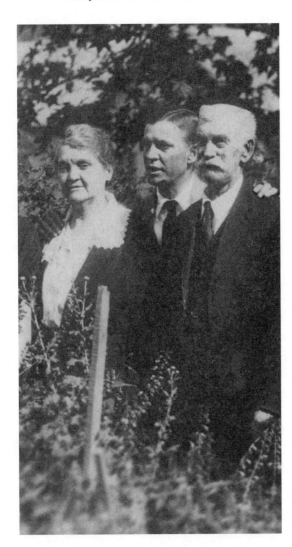

Dr. Ben Norwood
with his parents,
Ava and Frank
Norwood, in
Stamps, Arkansas,
circa 1920. *Courtesy
of Sara Lee Suttle;
original is in the
Historical Research
Center, University of
Arkansas for Medical
Sciences (UAMS).*

bombing operations (performed by Italian pilots against Libya) in 1911 and later used by the Allied forces during World War I. Dunn wrote a book entitled *Development of Power in the Modern Military Rifle* in 1913, and his two sons were the first brothers to graduate in the same class at West Point in 1910 and at the Army War College in 1928.[27]

Ben initially spent a few months at the Naval Medical School in Washington, D.C., before reporting to the Naval Operating Base in Hampton Roads on 17 January 1918 for a two-year assignment.[28]

While at Hampton Roads, Ben was commissioned a full lieutenant of the Naval Medical Corps.[29] His medical file indicates that, during the time he was assigned to Hampton Roads, Ben also shipped out with a Marine contingent on 25 November 1919 to Guantanamo Bay and then Nicaragua, aboard the USS *Ingram*.

From the beginning of 1920 into 1922, Ben did shore duty with the American Legation's Marine Detachment in Nicaragua. By March 1921, he had been assigned to assist in establishing a military hospital at the fort in Campo de Marte.[30] During this period, he published the first of several articles based on his work as a naval doctor. The article, in the *United States Naval Medical Bulletin* in April 1921, was entitled "The Application of the Schick Reaction to 2,911 Naval Recruits and the Immunization of Susceptibles to Diphtheria with Toxin-Antitoxin."[31] Based on Ben's clinical experience with recruits, the article argues that "a systematic application of the Schick reaction to the personnel of the Navy, including all officers and men below the age of fifty, with particular attention to the recruit, and the administration of proper doses of toxin-antitoxin, would practically eliminate diphtheria from the Navy."[32] Ben's medical records show that as he was stationed in Nicaragua and studying the Schick reaction, he was dealing with a case of tapeworm that he appears to have contracted in Central America.

Ben followed this clinical study with another in October 1921, also in the *United States Naval Medical Bulletin*, entitled "A Case of Poisoning by Oil of Chenopodium."[33] This focuses on the use of the oil of *Chenopodium ambrosioides*, wormseed, which grows wild in the southern US, to deal with intestinal nematodes. Noting that the treatment had become popular in recent years, Ben maintains that "more prominent workers" had not allowed wormseed to supersede thymol as the treatment of choice for nematode infection.[34]

In a small number of infections, however, he and other naval doctors using both drugs had found a greater percentage of egg-free stools when they treated with *Chenopodium* rather than thymol, though they also found that whipworm seemed especially resistant to *Chenopodium*. The article describes the dangers of *Chenopodium* treatment and symptoms of *Chenopodium* poisoning.[35] It reports on a case in which a Marine sergeant had reported to sick bay in Managua on 12 July 1920, presenting with symptoms of amebic dysentery. Testing confirmed motile *Entameba histolytica*. The patient was dosed with *Chenopodium* and, by the fourth day, was exhibiting signs of severe poisoning with cardiac and respiratory failure. The prognosis became grave by the seventh day. As a concerted effort was made to control the effects of the poisoning, the patient began regaining consciousness on the ninth day and returned to full consciousness on the tenth day, though mental confusion persisted. The patient gradually recovered and after ten months showed no signs of infection.[36]

After his Latin American stint, in November 1922, Ben was assigned to the Naval Recruiting Station in San Francisco, where he worked at the naval hospitals in San Francisco and Mare Island.[37] During this period, his father died of epithelioma of the lip in Stamps on 5 February 1924.

In April 1925, Ben was promoted to the rank of lieutenant commander and ordered to medical duty aboard the USS *Nitro* and the USS *Cincinnati*, an assignment that continued to January 1928, with a brief period in September 1925 at the US Naval Hospital in New York City.[38] In July 1926, he published another article in the *United States Naval Medical Bulletin*, this one reporting on an outbreak of food poisoning aboard the *Cincinnati*.[39] The article chronicles what happened when corned-beef hash had been allowed to incubate in a warm copper for ten hours before it was cooked and served: numerous sailors became sick, with a stool and urine sample of one of the sickest showing gram positive coccus and gram positive spore-bearing bacillus, *B. coli communis*.

In January 1928, Ben sailed on the USS *Chaumont* to Shanghai, returning to San Francisco on 25 February. The *Chaumont* was a transport ship for moving Marines and supplies that made at least one yearly voyage to Shanghai from 1925 to 1937 to support units deployed to the international settlement there to protect US nationals and business interests.[40] After his return from Shanghai, Ben shipped out on the USS *Cincinnati*.

Marriage and Final Years

Following his assignments to the West Coast and aboard the *Chaumont* and *Cincinnati*, Ben was ordered to Boston in March 1929 for several months' training at Massachusetts General, after which he was assigned to the position of chief of surgery at the Naval Hospital in D.C. and then to the Marine Barracks at Quantico.[41] In September 1930, he returned to Massachusetts General for additional training and was then assigned (after a brief intervening period of service in 1931 aboard the USS *Nitro* as it voyaged to Cuba) to the US Naval Hospital at League Island on 5 October 1932. During this assignment, he performed two months of temporary duty studying medicine at University of Pennsylvania Graduate School of Medicine. While in Philadelphia, Ben met Anne Parker Robinson, daughter of John Albert and Margaret Brown Robinson, whom he married in Philadelphia's First Presbyterian Church on 18 October 1933.[42] Anne was twelve years Ben's junior.

A month before marriage, Ben was assigned to the US Naval Hospital at Charleston, where he remained until June 1935, when he was made chief medical officer aboard the USS *Nevada* and promoted to commander.[43] During the Charleston assignment, his mother Ava died of heart failure on 12 February 1935 in Stamps. Ben's naval medical history file meticulously documents the dates, places, and causes of his parents' deaths, as well as his own health challenges, showing that he had persistent dental problems, having had six teeth extracted by 1924, and was a heavy smoker, smoking fifteen to twenty-five cigarettes a day through his adult life.

From June 1935 to June 1937, Ben served as senior medical officer on the USS *Nevada* and then the USS *California* and USS *Arizona*, after which he was ordered to serve as commanding officer in charge of the Navy Dispensary at Long Beach, California, where he remained until April 1940, when he was reassigned to the USS *California*.[44] The 1940 federal census for Los Angeles shows Ben serving as a councilman for the city's 15th District.[45] His medical records show he contracted mumps while in California.

In March 1941, Ben was stationed briefly at the naval yard in Puget Sound, and in July, he was promoted to the rank of captain and ordered to the Naval War College in Newport, Rhode Island.[46] Ten days after his graduation on 2 December 1941, he received his last assignment, to the US Navy Medical Supply Depot in Brooklyn. He and wife Anne spent a month living at the Towers Hotel there before moving to an apartment at London Terrace on West 23rd Street in New York City on 12 January 1942, the day Ben died.

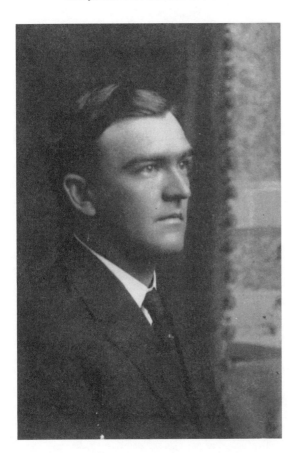

Dr. Ben Norwood,
circa 1933. *Courtesy
of Sara Lee Suttle;
copy is in the
Historical Research
Center, University of
Arkansas for Medical
Sciences (UAMS).*

As his obituary in Brooklyn's *Daily Eagle* reports,[47] Ben Norwood's death was attributed to coronary thrombosis, though following his sudden death at age fifty-six, his widow Anne filed suit against two insurance companies to contest the cause of death. Newspaper coverage indicates that Great American Indemnity and Prudential Insurance Company had sought to attribute the death to heart trouble due to high blood pressure. Anne's counsel successfully showed that Ben died as the result of a head injury he sustained when he slipped on a bar of soap and fell in the shower. The trial resulted in a large settlement for Anne.[48]

Ben's medical file contains extensive documentation of Anne's appeal to the Board of Veterans' Appeals, contesting the initial determination of the cause of death by a naval doctor. A detailed statement Anne provided to the board describes the circumstances of Ben's death:

> Captain Norwood never had a heart condition. He had never been treated for a heart condition. He was on active duty, and had never lost time. He had passed his annual physicals every year; had never failed these physicals, and he was promoted to Captain in July of 1941. That was the last physical that he had, because we went to the War College and then he died, January 12, 1942. The cause of his death in my estimation, and I have never changed my opinion about this, was the fall in the bath tub on a piece of soap.
>
> We had moved from the Towers Hotel in Brooklyn, January 12, 1942. Captain Norwood died the same day.
>
> Captain Norwood had been ordered to Washington. Then War was declared, and he was ordered to the Navy Supply Depot at Brooklyn. We lived in the Towers Hotel in Brooklyn from December 12, 1941 to January 12, 1942. On that day we moved to the London Terrace Apartments, 435 W. 23rd Street, New York, City. We moved 6 o'clock in the evening.
>
> The Captain was on duty until 5 o'clock. He came home to the Towers Hotel in Brooklyn. The Navy took all our baggage to New York City. We arrived at the London Terrace around a quarter after six, and we got ready to go to dinner. We had dinner at the Bouvert, taking a taxi from and to the London Terrace. We came home about nine o'clock, and I took a bath and the Captain read the evening paper while I was bathing. Then he took a bath and I heard the shower turned off. I was in the adjoining room, and in just a minute, I heard a thud. (This was around ten o'clock).
>
> I opened the door to the bathroom; he was just getting out of the tub and he handed me a small piece of soap saying, 'I was trying to end my life on a piece of soap.' He had no impairment of speech. He came out in a few minutes and sat down, smoking a cigarette. While he smoked a cigarette he rubbed the back of his head, and said that he had struck his head on a vital spot. In a few minutes we went to bed. I went to sleep. The light from the Court was shining in the window, and I happened to get awake. The light was also shining on

the Captain, but I noticed he was not sleeping, and asked him why. He retorted that he did not feel very well, and could not get to sleep. (This was about 10:30 P.M.). I immediately asked him if he thought it was the result of the fall. He said he thought it was, and reiterated in the next few minutes that he had struck his head; that his head did hurt him.

I wanted to call the house doctor and he said, I was talking to a doctor. In a few minutes he decided to smoke another cigarette. He made himself comfortable, putting a pillow behind him, and we chatted while he smoked. He was pale and very apprehensive.

I was very much concerned and urged him to call a doctor, and as he was putting the cigarette out he said he felt that his heart was missing a beat. Again I urged him to contact a physician and he said 'No—just turn over and go to sleep, I will be all right.' I watched him pull the bed clothing over his shoulders, and in just a second he turned over and gasped. He was dead before I could step from my bed to his.

The house doctor, whom I had called and had arrived within ten minutes, said he had been dead at least fifteen minutes; that he died about eleven o' clock. . . . He asked me if Captain Norwood had ever been ill. I said 'No.' I told him he had had a fall. He stated that he could not say whether the Captain had had a heart condition, or died from the fall; that either could have caused his death. Then I called Admiral Melhorn; he was my husband's Commanding Officer, and he, of course, notified the Navy Department. He came to the apartment with Mrs. Melhorn about one o'clock in the morning. In the meantime, the manager of the hotel had been there, and he had notified the Brooklyn Naval Hospital, where post mortems are performed and bodies prepared for burial. The undertaker came with a Dr. Chasserot, who was a Junior Grade Lieutenant in the Naval Reserve, and I gave him the facts concerning Captain Norwood's death, but they were enlarged upon later on.

He at no time told me that he had a pain in his heart. . . . [T]he original death certificate shows Hypertensive Heart Disease, which is the principal cause of death, and on the final death certificate, the principal cause of death is Edema of Brain, which was decided by the court.[49]

Ben F. Norwood was buried at Arlington National Cemetery. His distinguished career included service during both world wars. Among the medals he earned were the Philippine Campaign medal, the Marine Corps Expeditionary medal (Nicaragua, 1920–1922), with a second award of the same medal in 1927, the Yangtze Service medal for 1927, the American Defense Service medal, the World War I Victory medal, and the World War II Victory medal.

Ben's widow Anne did not remarry and died 7 September 1987 at the age of eighty-eight at her home in Philadelphia. As her *Philadelphia Inquirer* obituary notes, she became one of the first women to work in a brokerage house (Hopper Soliday) in Philadelphia following Ben's death. Anne is buried beside her husband.[50] The couple had no children.

George W. Russell, Early Life and Education

We have already met George Washington Russell in his father's diary: "old George W. Russell," about whom Seaborn wrote on George's seventh birthday, 22 February 1922, "God bless his dear good manly soul. He is great company for me now."[51]

Given the closeness of father and son and the tradition of sons following in fathers' footsteps as doctors in this family, it is perhaps not surprising that George Russell chose to become a doctor, representing the fourth generation in the line of doctors descending directly, father to son, from William James Russell. Seaborn's aspirations for George are subtextually patent in his diary: the beloved son, the son hand-picked to represent the rest of Seaborn's family on visits to cherished relatives and to church, the last-born son whom Seaborn often took with him to his office and on visits to patients.

But as we have also noted, all was not rosy in this household: From the beginning, Seaborn and Lounetta's marriage appears to have been tempestuous with frequent separations in which Lounetta provided for the children while Seaborn lived elsewhere. It is George who tells us in a letter to his cousin that, while Seaborn was "a highly perceptive, highly intelligent man who was devoted to helping people," he was "totally impractical" when it came to money. George concludes his reminiscences in the 1976 letter by stating plaintively,

During the times my mother and father were separated my
mother would have to rent out rooms in order to have food
and to live because he either had no money or wouldn't send
her any or at most only a few dollars.[52]

George's frankness hints at more than a little ambivalence in his
relationship with his father, understandable when one considers the
anguish a child feels at seeing his mother abandoned for periods of
time and left to fend for herself and her children with no financial
support. It is noteworthy that the line of Russell doctors ended with
George himself. George's sons George and Paul and their sister Ann
indicate that their father discouraged them from becoming doctors.[53]
Given the strong impetus within the family for generations for sons
to succeed their fathers as doctors, one has to wonder if George's
decision to discourage his children from medical practice had much
to do with ambivalence he felt about his own father and perhaps with
the economic difficulties he witnessed in his father's professional life.

Seaborn's diary documents key events in the life of this final son,
including his birth on 22 February 1915, when the Russell family was
living in southwest Little Rock. George's birth certificate confirms
that he was born at home and that his father delivered him.[54]

George graduated from Little Rock's Senior High School in 1935
and then joined the Civilian Conservation Corps program, where he
worked as a mechanic to help pay for his college education.[55] In the
same year, George enrolled in Little Rock Junior College, the precursor of the University of Arkansas at Little Rock, graduating in 1937.
He was vice-president of the Science Seminar and a member of Phi
Theta Kappa honor society.[56]

George then enrolled in the University of Arkansas, from which
he graduated in 1939 with a Bachelor of Science degree with a specialty
in medicine. The 1940 federal census shows him living at home with
his mother Lounetta and sister Martha, and Frank Strong, the former
husband of George's half-sister Mabel. The census lists George and
Frank as mechanics in a garage.[57]

It appears that the garage work was a way for George to continue
earning money while he was pursuing medical studies. He graduated
from the University of Arkansas School of Medicine on 10 June 1941.
The 1941 UAMS yearbook tells us George was a member of Phi Chi

medical fraternity and intended to go to the US Naval Hospital in San Diego after graduation.[58]

Naval Service

Immediately following graduation, George entered naval service. On 19 June, he accepted a commission for the Navy Medical Corps as an acting assistant surgeon with the rank of lieutenant and was assigned to the Naval Hospital at San Diego for basic medical officer orientation.[59] On 3 July George was ordered to the Naval Hospital in Washington, D.C., where he served as a medical intern. In March 1942, the hospital was relocated to Bethesda, Maryland, where George continued his internship until July 1942. During this period, he met President Franklin D. Roosevelt while the president was receiving medical care there.[60] Two days after Roosevelt died, George wrote his wife-to-be Jeanette Roberts from the US Naval Hospital in Memphis where he was stationed:

> The news of our great President's death stunned me. It may sound silly and emotional but tears actually came to my eyes for a moment. He always seemed so benevolent and fatherly that I actually must have had some personal feeling for him. Then, too, I had the privilege in 1941 of seeing him and being near him when he came out to the medical center for x-rays. I was overwhelmed by his dynamic personality. I only hope his death will not affect the future of our country too much.[61]

On 3 July 1942, George completed his internship and was nominated on 23 September as a naval assistant surgeon with the rank of lieutenant junior grade.[62] In November, George received orders to proceed to the Pacific as an assistant surgeon aboard the battleship *Pennsylvania*. The USS *Pennsylvania* was conducting training operations off the coast of California and was then dispatched to the Aleutians, where it was involved in three bombardment missions against the Japanese, resulting in the liberation of Attu and Kiska—a campaign in which, though George was unaware of it at the time, Army Lieutenant William L. Russell, son of George's half-brother James Wilson Russell, was also involved.[63] William L. Russell, who ended the war with eight purple hearts, received the first of these for his actions in the Aleutian campaign.[64]

Following the Aleutian operations, during which George received a promotion on 1 May 1943 to the position of assistant surgeon with rank of full lieutenant, the USS *Pennsylvania* sailed for the South Pacific for bombardment operations against the Japanese forces on the Gilbert and Marianna Islands.[65] For this period of George's service, a valuable collection of documents exists: a set of letters that George and his wife-to-be Jeanette Roberts exchanged from the end of 1943 to June 1945, when the couple married. George's son George S. Russell, who now owns these letters, has transcribed them in an unpublished manuscript entitled *Letters from the War.*

As George's son George explains in an overview of the collection of letters,

> This book is a true love story written in the words of the two lovers who found each other in a world torn apart by war. It begins in the middle of the Second World War with a Victory Christmas card written to the mother of an old family friend by a lonely Lieutenant Commander in the Navy serving aboard a battleship in the South Pacific. He hopes that by sending the card to the mother of his best friend in high school, he can get someone, anyone to respond and send him news of home. The youngest sister of his old friend, ten years younger than him, begins to write to him. She was just a young teenage girl when he last saw her. Now he is twenty eight years old and living with 5,000 other young men aboard the largest battleship in the Navy, the USS *Pennsylvania*, and he knows she is now eighteen and living on her own attending junior college in Washington, DC. Desperate for normal conversation outside of the horrors of war, where his days are spent as a surgeon trying to save the most badly injured from the beachheads and taking a launch at day's end to bury at sea those he couldn't save, he writes back. She is anxious to finish her secretarial training at junior college and will get a government job as a clerk/typist like so many thousands of other young girls who came to Washington to help with the war effort and to see the world outside their hometowns.[66]

George's correspondence with Jeanette began on 12 December 1943 when he sent a Christmas card to her mother to which Jeanette, who was by this point studying and working in Washington, D.C., unexpectedly replied.[67] A letter George sent her on Christmas Day, with a return address of USS *Pennsylvania*, c/o fleet postmaster in San Francisco, responds to Jeanette's reply, telling her that the *Pennsylvania* had just returned from the battle zone.[68]

By March 1944, George and Jeanette had become regular correspondents when he wrote her on the fourth and twelfth to say that, due to censorship regulations, he could not disclose information about where he was or what he was doing. The 4 March letter tells Jeanette he is sending her a necklace but cannot say where he purchased it—only that "it is characteristic of the place from which it comes."

On the twelfth, George added, "As far as news is concerned, you can read more in the newspapers than I can tell you—you know, censorship regulations." This letter contains an interesting aside in which George tells Jeanette that he has heard via "ye old grapevine" that his request to do postgraduate work had been approved, and if things worked out well, this might mean that he would be able to see Jeanette when she returned to her family in Little Rock for spring vacation.[69] George had made a request to be transferred from the *Pennsylvania* to the Naval Hospital in Philadelphia, where he hoped to study neuropsychiatry—a request granted on 7 February, though George had not received word of this yet.[70]

By 20 March, confirmation reached George of approval of his request to study psychiatry. In a letter with that date, George states,

> As I understand it, eventually I will be at the University of Penn Medical School most of the time and most of the lectures will be delivered by Dr. Edward Strecker—certainly the foremost neuropsychiatrist in the United States and probably in the world today. I have read several of his text books—he has written 8 or 10 which are considered standard. Of course, I will not be detached until another doctor relieves me—he is on his way out now!

In addition, George had been granted twenty days of leave with five additional travel days. He expected to be in Little Rock in late April or early May and proposed that Jeanette arrange her vacation so they could rendezvous. If so, he would drive Jeanette to Conway, where she had studied at Hendrix College for a year, and introduce her to his aunt. George ends this letter full of excitement about the new assignment: since the train ride from Philadelphia to D.C. was only two-and-a-half hours, he expected he'd "be up about every weekend," and he could think of nothing better than being assigned to a D.C. position when he finished his studies.

George appends some specific instructions about how Jeanette should reply, given the uncertainty about his location as he headed back to the States:

> Using a typewriter (or a pen as you wish) make three copies of your answer, (2) mail one to me in care of general delivery, San Francisco, California; (3) mail one to me on the ship (USS Pennsylvania) just in case I'm still aboard at the time; and (4) mail one copy in a plain envelope (sealed and placed within another envelope) addressed as follows: Dr. Norman East, Intern's Cottages, Queen's Hospital, Honolulu, T.H.[71]

In April, George began studies under Edward A. Strecker at the Naval Hospital in Philadelphia. The Navy was eager to train him in the fields of psychiatry and neurology due to the anticipated volume of service members who would be suffering from what is now termed post-traumatic stress disorder. Strecker was a leading figure in psychiatry with over ten books to his credit, along with numerous papers; his books included standard textbooks used in psychiatry. In 1943, he had been president of the American Psychiatric Association. Having served in the army during both world wars, he had conducted research on battle fatigue.[72]

The letters George wrote Jeanette from Philadelphia show him growing increasingly enamored of her. Several times in July and again in September, he wrote to share school gossip and news of parties he'd attended and to tell her he was thinking of her and wishing to see her.[73]

In September, having completed his work under Strecker, George received a new assignment—to the psychiatric staff of the Naval Hospital in Millington, Tennessee, near Memphis, where he would soon direct a new electroencephalographic laboratory.[74] The new assignment began a period of vexation for the young couple who, though they were both in the US, were separated by many miles. George's letters from this time until the couple married in June 1945 speak repeatedly of his unsuccessful attempts to obtain a new assignment closer to her, preferably in D.C. or, failing that, New York.

George began his new assignment in early October. On the eighth, he wrote Jeanette from Memphis to say that he had driven down from Philadelphia in his "old gas buggy," having stopped in Roanoke to buy a new radiator. The following day, he'd be leaving for Fort Worth to take some patients to the hospital there. Then he adds, "You know we have to take neuropsychiatric patients all over the U.S. and one of the main places is Bethesda, MD (Washington, DC). I'm going to get the next draft of patients going up there so I can see you."[75]

In a letter of the twenty-sixth, George again expresses his hope to be sent with patients to Bethesda, something he had not been able to accomplish since only officers were sent there and the Memphis hospital had no officers in his care.[76] A 7 December letter again bemoans his inability to get to Bethesda, and then on 20 December, George writes,

> Baby, I am pulling strings in Washington to get a transfer and have contacted a friend at the Naval Hospital at St Albans, Long Island, New York to try to get duty there. I am also considering to try to get Bethesda, Md. there in Washington. Either of these would be good places and I could be near you. I haven't heard anything yet but am hoping and keeping my fingers crossed. You do the same, Sweet.[77]

A 31 October letter to Jeanette explains why—in addition to his desire to be closer to her—there was a sense of urgency about George's attempt to be reassigned. Things were in a state of flux in Memphis, with three medical officers having been shipped out for foreign duty the previous day and several others given similar orders. Because of the tremendous need for doctors in the Philippines, he anticipated that he might be reassigned for foreign duty. The one bit of good news he had to share was, however, that he had just been named officer of the day.[78]

On 2 February 1945, George had big news of an entirely different sort to share:

> Part of the hospital burned up last night, but we had no casualties. However, I did miss a lot of good sleep. I ran down without any hat, socks or tie on. I was afraid it might be in the orthopedic ward where the boys are in casts and couldn't get out but luckily it was in the auditorium and ship service store. One whole wing was lost and we almost lost the entire hospital—as it was only one wing was lost. What a mess—we

evacuated patients outside—many of them very sick and it was very cold. The fire engine caught fire and we had to put that out.

This letter also conveys news that the hospital was getting an electroencephalograph machine and hiring a technician for it. The commander had instructed the doctors in its use, and because George had given a lecture about electroencephalography, he was assigned to work with the Kennedy General expert in this field, Dr. Stephenson, a well-regarded electroencephalographist who had trained at Harford Hospital, which specialized in this diagnostic procedure. George tells Jeanette,

> I am very enthusiastic as there are only a few doctors in the U.S. that know anything about E.E.G.s. But to get to where you and I come in—I think that after I have worked a couple of weeks with Dr. Stephenson I will put in a request for post graduate work in this field and will probably be sent to either Washington, DC (St Elizabeth Hospital & Naval Center) or Leahy Clinic in Boston. I sure hope this goes through and that we can be together again.

George added that he'd been saving cigarettes from his two-packs-a-day allotment and would send them to Jeanette as a Valentine's present.[79] Both were heavy smokers throughout their adult lives, according to their children.

The 2 February letter is one for which Jeanette's reply is extant: She replied on the seventh that the news of the fire interested her because her Barton Hall residence at West Potomac Park in D.C. had also had a fire, caused by a woman who went to sleep with a cigarette in her hand. Jeanette's letter also indicated that she was excited at the news of George's possible reassignment and happy to hear about the cigarettes he had saved for her. Just that day, she had waited in a line that went halfway down the block to buy cigarettes, and when she got to the counter, only "spuds" were left.[80]

George wrote Jeanette on the twenty-second, concerned that he had not heard from her. It is in this letter that he notes it was his birthday and that he had spent his birthday the previous year aboard the *Pennsylvania* working with casualties all day and then taking those who died out to sea for burial at the end of the day.[81]

George and Jeanette continued corresponding throughout March and April, sharing inconsequential news of their daily lives, with Jeanette acknowledging on 3 April roses George had sent her.[82] On 9 April, Jeanette sent news about her new apartment on R Street. She was sharing it with a roommate and trying to learn to cook but was failing at this. She had wanted to fry southern-style chicken, but the butcher told her that he had not seen chicken for months.[83]

On 6 June 1945, George W. Russell married Jeanette Laverne Roberts, daughter of William and Annie Gardner Roberts, in Elkton, Maryland.[84] On the tenth and thirteenth, Jeanette wrote George in Memphis to ask him to send clippings about their wedding.[85] A letter George sent on the fourteenth contains the surprising information that he had not told his mother that he was marrying Jeanette but had called her after the marriage, and she had seemed pleased. He also says that the EEG machine was ready to be installed.[86]

On 10 July, George entered the Naval Hospital in Memphis for treatment of smoke inhalation damage he had suffered in the fire in February.[87] He remained at the Memphis hospital until 13 September, when he was transferred to the Naval Hospital in Sampson, New York, for further diagnosis and treatment. While there, George was promoted on 3 October to the rank of surgeon lieutenant commander.[88] He also received the Navy Unit Commendation award on 15 January 1946 for his battle service aboard the *Pennsylvania*.[89]

On 28 January 1946, while he was at Sampson, George was ordered to report to the Naval Board of Medical Examiners to determine his physical fitness to perform his duties. On 8 March, the board found evidence of a tubercular infection that was no longer active. But there was evidence of lung damage compromising his ability to continue performing his naval duties. On the thirteenth, the board found him unfit for service and ordered him to appear before the Naval Retirement Board.[90]

George ended his stay at Sampson on 26 April and then took a driving trip home to Little Rock from 29 April to 2 May to visit his family.[91] In June, George was separated from active duty with 100% disability. He had earned the Navy Unit Citation, the World War II Victory medal, the Asiatic-Pacific Campaign medal with three stars, and the American Defense Service medal with a Fleet Clasp. A 15 June separation and commendation letter to him from Secretary of the Navy James Forrestal states,

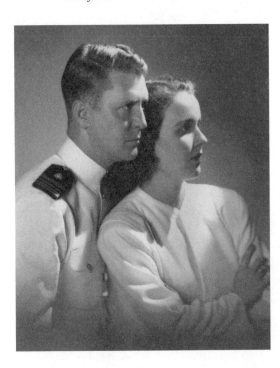

Dr. George Russell
and wife Jeanette
Roberts Russell,
circa 1945. *Courtesy
of George S. Russell;
copy is in the Historical
Research Center,
University of Arkansas
for Medical Sciences
(UAMS).*

I want the Navy's pride in you, which it is my privilege to express, to reach into your civil life and to remain with you always. You have served in the greatest Navy in the world. It crushed two enemy fleets at once. . . . It brought our land-based airpower within bombing range of the enemy, and set our ground armies on the beachheads of final victory. . . . No other Navy at any time has done so much. For your part in these achievements you deserve to be proud as long as you live. The Nation which you served at a time of crisis will remember you with gratitude.[92]

On 1 November, George was placed on inactive status.[93]

Post-Naval Psychiatric Practice in Pennsylvania

In anticipation of his retirement, George began a psychiatry residency at Friends Hospital in Philadelphia on 1 May.[94] During his residency, Jeanette had their first child, Ann Roberts Russell, on 31 October 1946. George completed the residency on 7 September 1947 and continued a teaching fellowship in psychiatry at Women's Medical College of Pennsylvania that he had begun while in residency.[95]

On 11 March 1948, two days before his next child, George Seaborn Russell, was born, George was licensed by the Pennsylvania state medical board to practice.[96] The following June, he earned a certificate of proficiency in neurology and psychiatry from the University of Pennsylvania Graduate School.[97] During this period and into 1951, George was also serving as psychiatric consultant and director of the electroencephalographic laboratory at Lakeland Hospital in Blackwood, New Jersey.[98]

On 15 November 1949, George and Jeanette's last child, Paul Hoobler Russell, was born, and the couple began to make plans to buy a house near Philadelphia. In 1952, they purchased a comfortable three-story house built in 1875 in Wyncote some five miles north of Philadelphia's city center. In the same year, *Who's Important in Medicine* published a biographical notice about George, outlining his considerable accomplishments, including his membership in the American Medical Association, the Pennsylvania Medical Association, the Medical Club of Philadelphia, the Pennsylvania Psychiatric Society, the American Psychiatric Association, the World Federation of Mental Health, and the American Board of Psychiatry and Neurology.[99]

In the decade 1952–1962, as the family settled into its new residence, George served as assistant professor of psychiatry at Temple University and assistant director of the university's child psychiatric clinic. His Temple chair and mentor was noted psychotherapist O. Spurgeon English, nationally recognized as one of the first psychotherapists to document the connection between mental and physical health, with numerous books and textbooks to his credit.[100] According to George's children, George and English became close friends.

In the final period of his employment at Temple, George also served (1959–1962) as co-supervisor of residency training at Eastern Pennsylvania Psychiatric Institute.[101] Early in 1960, he moved into a new non-academic venue that would occupy his attention for the first half of the decade and where he would make important contributions: he accepted an appointment as director of the Bucks County Mental Health Guidance Center, established in 1958 in Doylestown.[102]

At his new post, George quickly began laying a foundation for the center to expand community outreach and therapeutic services

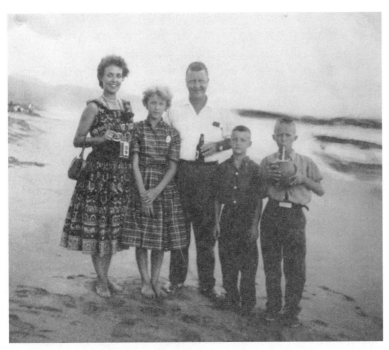

Family vacation in Mexico, 1958. Jeanette Roberts Russell and Dr. George Russell with their children Ann Roberts Russell, Paul Hoobler Russell, and George Seaborn Russell. *Courtesy of George S. Russell; copy is in the Historical Research Center, University of Arkansas for Medical Sciences (UAMS).*

through educational initiatives, implementation of an "after-care" program, and the addition of a psychiatric social worker.[103] These initiatives led to robust growth in the program: On 20 June 1960, the *Daily Intelligencer* reported that the Doylestown center had just approved a new annual budget of $96,000. Two years later, the center was handling 10,000 visits a year. By August of the following year, annual visits had increased to 11,500, with the center having set a new record for the number of patients served when its June 1963 quarter ended.[104]

The Final Years

In 1964, George leveraged his conspicuous success at directing the Bucks County mental health center by starting his own clinic. The last twenty-five years of his medical practice were spent directing his Russell Psychiatric Clinic at Allentown.[105] As he made this move,

George and Jeanette also began preparations to re-settle their family in an eighteenth-century farmhouse sited on an eighty-six-acre working farm they bought in 1961 in the Blue Mountain Valley of the Poconos near Saylorsburg. The Russells moved in 1966, allowing George to reconnect to a mountain landscape similar to that of his youth in Arkansas, and giving Jeanette, who was an antiques collector, access to numerous outbuildings to house her finds.[106]

In the 1970s, while still operating his clinic, George branched out of medicine by founding G. W. Russell & Associates, Ltd., an enterprise offering a variety of wholesale trade-durable products, including sheepskin vests and boots from Afghanistan, inflatable tire jacks utilizing air from exhaust pipes, and a Mowtron automatic lawn mower guided by wires buried in the ground. The most successful product his business provided was Spiky ice cleats, a German product that could easily be affixed to footwear to prevent slippage on ice and snow. In a good year, this product alone grossed as much as $400,000 for George's business.[107] He also went into partnership with his son George to create the Pocono Abstract Agency, incorporated on 10 March 1981. It focused on real estate developments and purchases in Allentown, including the Maple Leaf Mobile Home Park and an apartment complex at Grant and 5th Street.[108]

In interviews with their distant cousin William L. Russell Jr., George's children described their father as cerebral, independent, and fair-minded, always encouraging them to pursue their goals without caring what others thought of them or their choices. Though he remembered his naval years with great fondness and liked to wear his dress white uniform to events at the officers' club, he refused to discuss his war experiences, experiences that may in part, his children think, have accounted for his unwillingness to encourage them to pursue medical careers.

George's children remember him as quiet and thoughtful and reserved in the presence of visitors he did not know until he had consumed a few drinks. From his naval years, George developed the habit of binge drinking at times of stress, a habit that continued in his adult life as a way, they suspect, of dealing with the unacknowledged trauma of what he witnessed as a naval surgeon in the war.

His children also noted their father's diffidence about organized religion, a diffidence he shared with his favorite philosopher Bertrand Russell. He did not attend church and did not want his children to do

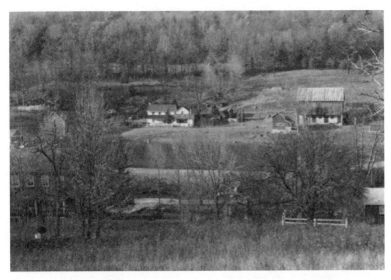

Dr. George Russell family farm in the Blue Mountain Valley of Pennsylvania near Saylorsburg. *Courtesy of George S. Russell; copy is in the Historical Research Center, University of Arkansas for Medical Sciences (UAMS).*

so until they reached the "age of reason," which he interpreted as about thirteen or fourteen. They remember George praying only on one occasion, on the day that President John F. Kennedy was assassinated, when he uttered a brief prayer at the dinner table. The prayer stands out in their memory because of its uniqueness. George described his father Seaborn to them as "a religious nut," and they have concluded, on the basis of what he told them, that his reluctance to encourage them to adopt any kind of religious practice had much to do with what he remembered of his father.

In the late 1980s, George was diagnosed with metastatic lung cancer, with tumors in his brain, liver, abdomen, and adrenal system. On 9 February 1989, he was admitted to Palmerton Hospital in Palmerton, Pennsylvania, where he died on 21 February 1989 at the age of seventy-three. Like his cousin Ben, George was buried in Arlington National Cemetery. Jeanette continued living on the Blue Mountain Valley farm, where she died on 4 March 2003. She is buried beside her husband at Arlington.

The death of George W. Russell closes this saga of the dynasty of doctors descended from William James Russell—a story spanning almost two centuries and multiple locations in a period in which

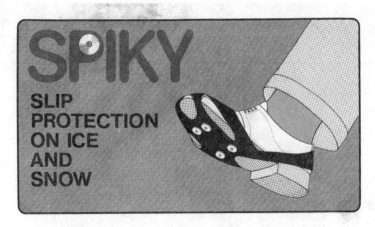
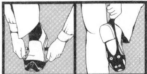
Print advertisement for Spiky shoe attachments, one of Dr. George Russell's non-medical businesses, circa 1980. *Courtesy of George S. Russell; original is in the Historical Research Center, University of Arkansas for Medical Sciences (UAMS).*

American medicine changed in ways the generation of George's great-grandfather could not have imagined. In addition to the ties of blood and geography linking these doctors, one motif binds their stories together: their shared commitment to "the only profession that labors incessantly to destroy the reason for its own existence."[109]

AFTERWORD

I have often wondered about the winds of war. As a young child growing up without any extended family within thousands of miles, I wondered why we, the children of George Washington Russell, were living near Philadelphia, which played such a large role in the American Revolution, and yet all of our extended family were in the South, particularly in Texas and Arkansas. I came to realize that it was because my father, who was born and raised in Little Rock, had come up to Philadelphia after stopping on his way to be part of the medical team for President Franklin Delano Roosevelt and had, like a leaf in the wind, been blown there.

He had served as an assistant surgeon on the USS *Pennsylvania* in the Second World War. After participating in the Aleutian campaign, he then headed to the South Pacific and Kwajalein, where he worked hard after bloody battles to save the Marines from the beachheads and then, at the end of the day, buried at sea those not fortunate enough to survive. As the war was drawing toward a successful close, he was ordered back to Philadelphia to be re-trained as a psychiatrist to help as many of the millions of bloodied soldiers returning and suffering from battle fatigue—the World War II name for PTSD—as he could. Having made good friends while he was studying this new field and possibly because he had seen enough blood in the battle zone, he decided to return to Philadelphia after his final assignment at the Memphis Naval Hospital, where he helped returning veterans in their readjustment to civilian life. As a result of this decision, my parents, both of whom were from Little Rock, saw their aunts, uncles, cousins, nieces, and nephews only rarely over the next forty years.

As I have wondered about the winds of war that blew my father and his family to Philadelphia, it has occurred to me that this was not the first time that they had breathed their dragon breath on the Russell family. When the first of my Russell ancestors, James and a Robert Russell many researchers think is his father, came over to Pennsylvania in the mid-1700s, the Scots Irish were unhappy with their treatment by the English and by their Anglo-Irish landlords in Ulster, who were effectively confiscating their land at the end of ninety-nine-year leases.

This discontent and the eventual American Revolution were building when these forebears arrived in the colonies, and that conflict continued to have generational impacts on the Russell family as James's son William died at an early age and William's son William James then set out on the course of his life from infancy as an orphan. He became a champion of other orphans and established a wonderful medical practice and also built up a large agricultural plantation business near Atlanta. Family stories recount that Sherman's troops decided not to burn his plantation as they passed in their March to the Sea because, after they had hanged him up above a fire to coerce him to tell where he might have hidden his money and valuables, he told them that whatever little he had left was for his children and that they should do their worst. With respect, they packed up and passed him by.

But the winds of war breathed their dragon breath once again, and William James's son William James Park was forced to flee to Northwest Arkansas near Indian Territory as he feared for his life because he had been a spy for the Union during the Civil War conflict. His reasons, I am sure, were complex, but having served as an American soldier during the Mexican War, he must have felt a strong bond to the Union. As a result of the choices he made during the Civil War, his life as a doctor and traveling surgeon was difficult, as was true for so many people in the South in the aftermath of the Civil War. The struggles W. J. P. endured seem to have strongly affected his son Seaborn, who apprenticed with him to follow in his father's footsteps as a doctor and spent his time traveling with his father drumming up business for the traveling surgical practice. This traveling lifestyle seemed to affect Seaborn for his entire life—he apparently had a case of the wandering spirit—as he moved around frequently and had trouble keeping connected with just one family.

This brings us back to my father again, with whom we started this afterword. In a family diary written by his father in 1922, we have seen a glimpse of my father George W. Russell as a young six-year-old living with his elderly father Seaborn. George was thirteen years old when his father died with little or no estate, and he needed to muster the Russell character to be able to struggle along and continue the family tradition of becoming a doctor in a much more complicated and regulated world. He succeeded in doing so during the largest military conflict that this world has ever known. And then the winds of war and their dragon breath blew him to another part of the world like many generations of Russells before him.

Fortunately, modern travel has made the world a smaller place, and because of that, there are fewer and fewer isolated branches of families like the Pennsylvania branch of the Russell family in which I grew up. Due to technology today, we have increasing opportunities to find ways, if we wish, to unite far-flung branches of families in the tranquility and warm breezes of familial love and respect. And future generations of all our families can look forward to the day when the dragon finds his eternal rest and breathes his winds of war no more.

GEORGE S. RUSSELL

ILLUSTRATIONS AND PHOTOGRAPHS

Chapter 1

John Chester Buttre engraving of Dr. William James Russell of Gwinnett County, Georgia, circa 1855.

Portrait of Dr. William James Russell, circa 1830.

Portrait of Sophia Park Russell, wife of Dr. William James Russell, circa 1830.

Photograph of Lawrenceville, Georgia, including the home of Dr. William James Russell, circa 1907.

Photograph of Iantha Missenia Huff Russell, wife of Dr. William James Russell, circa 1855.

Chapter 2

Image of a photographic portrait of Dr. William James Park Russell, circa 1855.

Photograph of Ava Octavia Dunn Law Russell, wife of Dr. W. J. P. Russell, circa 1850.

Dr. W. J. P. Russell's ad in the *Tuskegee Republican* (Tuskegee, Alabama), 10 June 1858.

Cane Hill, Arkansas, looking northwest, circa 1895.

Dr. W. J. P. Russell's business card when practicing in Dallas, Texas, circa 1885.

Dr. W. J. P. Russell, circa 1888.

Family photo taken 25 December 1905 in Birmingham, Alabama. Seated left to right are sisters Sallie Law Parker, Ava O. D. Law Russell, and Chesta Law Woodliff. Standing left to right are Ava Russell Norwood, Dr. Ralph Morgan Russell, his wife Mollie Woodliff Russell, and her sister Ollie Woodliff.

Chapter 3

Photograph of Dr. Seaborn Rentz Russell, circa 1880.

Photograph of Seaborn Rentz Russell, age eighteen, photo taken in Fayetteville, Arkansas, circa 1878.

Photograph of Dr. Seaborn Russell's first wife Alcie Daisy Bachelor, circa 1880.

Photograph of Dr. Seaborn Russell's second spouse (no marriage record found) Emma Sear holding youngest daughter Mamie Russell, circa 1898.

Letterhead used by Dr. W. S. R. (Seaborn) Russell when he was practicing in Lorado, Arkansas, in 1897.

Photograph of Dr. Seaborn Russell's third wife Mary Lounetta Hoobler Smith Russell with stepdaughters Mabel and Mamie Russell, circa 1902.

Photograph of Dr. Seaborn Russell in his Little Rock medical office with his brother, Richard D. Russell (left), circa 1926.

Chapter 4

Photograph of Dr. Ralph Morgan Russell, circa 1886.

Photograph of Dr. Ralph Russell's wife, Mollie Woodliff, circa 1900.

Photograph of Dr. Ralph Russell leaning on a car in front of his house at 1306 Huntsville Avenue in Birmingham.

Drawing of the Russell Medical Institute appearing in the *Handbook of Home Medicine*.

Letterhead used by Dr. Ralph Russell to write a letter to his sister Ava Russell Norwood on 30 December 1896.

Patent diagram for Dr. Ralph Russell's Cathode Ray Reflector.

Dr. Ralph Russell's ad in the *Tuscaloosa Weekly Times* (Tuscaloosa, Alabama), 2 June 1899.

Reproduction of the Mutual Medical Association Certificate from the *Handbook of Home Medicine*.

Reproduction of the title page of Dr. Ralph Russell's *Handbook of Home Medicine*.

Vi-Be-Ni [*sic*] ad in Dr. Ralph Russell's *Handbook of Home Medicine*.

Anatomical plate from Dr. Ralph Russell's *Handbook of Home Medicine*.

Chapter 5

Dr. Ben Norwood's medical school graduation picture from the University of Tennessee yearbook *The Volunteer*, v. 16, *1912*.

Dr. George Russell's medical school graduation picture from the University of Arkansas for Medical Sciences yearbook *The Arkansas Caduceus 1941*.

Photograph of Dr. Ben Norwood with his parents, Ava and Frank Norwood, in Stamps, Arkansas, circa 1920.

Photograph of Dr. Ben Norwood, circa 1933.

Photograph of Dr. George Russell and his wife Jeanette Roberts Russell, circa 1945.

Photograph of Jeanette Roberts Russell and Dr. George W. Russell with their children Ann Roberts Russell, Paul Hoobler Russell, and George Seaborn Russell on a family vacation in Mexico, 1958.

Photograph of Dr. George Russell's family farm in the Blue Mountain Valley near Saylorsburg, Pennsylvania.

Print advertisement for Spiky shoe attachments, one of Dr. George Russell's non-medical businesses, circa 1980.

NOTES

Introduction

1. In its historiographical approach giving a prominent place to family history, this book walks through the door opened by Peter Laslett in his *The World We Have Lost: England Before the Industrial Age* (London: Methuen, 1965). Laslett argues that the denigration of genealogy as an historiographical tool and the characterization of this historiographical approach as "glorified gene-alogy" are short-sighted. The door Laslett opened has yielded such important works as Arkansas historian Carolyn Earle Billingsley's *Communities of Kinship: Antebellum Families and the Settlement of the Cotton Frontier* (Athens: Univ. of Georgia Press, 2004), Ricky Lee Sherrod and Annette Pierce Sherrod's *Plain Folk, Planters, and the Complexities of Southern Society* (Nacogdoches: Stephen F. Austin Univ. Press, 2014), David J. Russo's *Families and Communities: A New View of American History* (Nashville: American Assoc. for State and Local History, 1977), and Joseph A. Amato's *Jacob's Well: A Case for Rethinking Family History* (St. Paul: Minnesota Historical Soc., 2008).

2. William D. Lindsey, ed., *Fiat Flux: The Writings of Wilson R. Bachelor, Nineteenth-Century Country Doctor and Philosopher* (Fayetteville: Univ. of Arkansas Press, 2013).

Chapter 1

1. John Livingston, "William J. Russell, M.D., of Lawrenceville, Gwinnett County, Georgia," *Portraits of Eminent Americans Now Living: With Biographical and Historical Memoirs of Their Lives and Actions*, vol. 3 (New York: R. Craighead, 1854), p. 281. Livingston reports information provided by Russell himself.

2. Livingston, *Portraits of Eminent Americans*, p. 281..

3. Livingston, *Portraits of Eminent Americans*, p. 282.

4. Annie Mae Kent and Edith Huff Green, "Dr. William James Russell," in *Gwinnett County, Georgia, Families, 1818–1968*, ed. Alice Smythe McCabe (Atlanta: Cherokee, 1980), pp. 431–32.

5. Cabarrus Co., NC, Court of Pleas and Quarter Sessions, Minutes, Bk. 1, 1797–1805, 23 July 1801, 21 October 1801, 19 October 1803, and 3 April 1804.

6. Cabarrus Co., NC, Court of Pleas and Quarter Sessions, Minutes, Bk. 1, 1797–1805, 23 April 1801 and 19 October 1802.

7. Cabarrus Co., NC, Court of Pleas and Quarter Sessions, Minutes, Bk. 1, 1797–1805, 17 October 1804.

8. See Kent and Green, "Dr. William James Russell," pp. 431–32; Bobby Gilmer Moss, *The Patriots at the Cowpens* (Blacksburg, SC: Moss, 1985), p. 4; Mary Lou Stewart Garrett, *History of Fairview Presbyterian Church of Greenville*

County, South Carolina (Fountain Inn, SC: Fairview Presbyterian Church Session, 1986), pp. 5, 9, 63. Alexander's obituary notes his Revolutionary War service at King's Mountain and Cowpens, where he commanded a troop: see *The Athenian* (Athens, GA), 14 May 1830, p. 3, col. 3–4. Alexander's tombstone in Fairview Presbyterian Cemetery in Lawrenceville, GA, describes him as a patriot, soldier, and Christian. Alexander represented Spartanburg County in the state legislature before moving his family to Georgia in the early 1820s.

9. Livingston, "William J. Russell," p. 282.

10. Clarence F. Blume and Mabel Rumple Blume, *Historic Rocky River Church Buildings and Burying Grounds: Cabarrus County, Concord, North Carolina, 1751–1958* (n.p.: Rocky River Historical Foundation, 1958), p. 40. The couple's original marriage bond, 16 August 1797, in Cabarrus Co., NC, gives Sarah's maiden name as McCree, though various published sources give it as McRee. Russell's tombstone in Rocky River Cemetery, which dates from the time of his death, also states that he married Sarah McCree.

11. "Death of Dr. W. J. Russell," *Gwinnett Herald* (Lawrenceville, GA), 9 October 1872, p. 3, col. 2.

12. On Thomas Williamson Alexander, see Joseph Gaston Baillie Bulloch, *A History and Genealogy of the Habersham Family* (Columbia, SC: R.L. Bryan Co., 1901), p. 95.

13. William Chapman Herbert, *A Brief History of Medicine in the Spartanburg Region and the Spartanburg County Medical Society, 1700–1990* (Spartanburg: Spartanburg Medical Society, 1992), p. 13.

14. See Herbert, *Brief History of Medicine*, p. 13. See also Tom Moore Craig, ed., *Upcountry South Carolina Goes to War: Letters of the Anderson, Brockman, and Moore Families, 1853–1865* (Columbia: Univ. of South Carolina Press, 2009), p. xxx; and J. B. O. Landrum, *History of Spartanburg County* (Atlanta: Franklin, 1900), pp. 50, 192.

15. On Charles Moore's education, see a 15 March 1899 letter from Thomas J. Moore to J. B. O. Landrum transcribed in Landrum, *History of Spartanburg County*, p. 49. A pamphlet compiled by Spartanburg Historical Society (2016) regarding Walnut Grove states that Rocky Spring was established in 1770 with Charles Moore as first schoolmaster until Nazareth Presbyterian Church took over the school.

16. See Herbert, *Brief History of Medicine*, p. 13.

17. See Herbert, *Brief History of Medicine*, p. 13.

18. See Herbert, *Brief History of Medicine*, p. 14.

19. See Herbert, *Brief History of Medicine*, p. 14.

20. Livingston, "William J. Russell," p. 282.

21. William S. Harris, *Historical Sketch of Poplar Tent Church, Cabarrus County, North Carolina* (Concord, NC: Times Book and Jobs Press, 1924), p. 21.

22. William Frederick Norwood, *Medical Education in the United States Before the Civil War* (Philadelphia: Univ. of Pennsylvania Press, 1944), p. 32. On the preceptorship method in the colonial and post-Revolutionary period, see pp. 32–41. See also Norwood, "Medical Education and the Rise of Hospitals: II: The Nineteenth Century," *JAMA* 186, no. 11 (Dec. 1963), p. 134.

23. Norwood, *Medical Education*, pp. 32–33.

24. Martin Kaufman, "American Medical Education," in *The Education of American Physicians: Historical Essays*, ed. Ronald L. Numbers (Berkeley: Univ. of California Press, 1980), p. 7.

25. Norwood, *Medical Education*, pp. 34–35, citing Stephen Wickes, *History of Medicine in New Jersey and of Its Medical Men, from the Settlement of the Province to A. D. 1800* (Newark: Martin R. Dennis, 1879), pp. 100–1. Norwood reproduces an apprenticeship contract between William Clark of Monmouth County, New Jersey, and Jacob Hubbard of Gravesend, New York, dated August 1760.

26. Norwood, *Medical Education*, p. 35.

27. Norwood, *Medical Education*, p. 35.

28. Norwood, *Medical Education*, p. 38.

29. John Duffy, "The Changing Image of the American Physician," in *Sickness and Health in America: Readings in the History of Medicine and Public Health*, ed. Judith Walzer Leavitt and Ronald L. Numbers (Madison: Univ. of Wisconsin Press, 1978), p. 131.

30. Duffy, in *Sickness and Health in America*, p. 131.

31. Duffy, in *Sickness and Health in America*, p. 131.

32. Duffy, in *Sickness and Health in America*, p. 135.

33. See Frederick C. Waite, "The Professional Education of Pioneer Ohio Physicians," *Ohio State Archaeological and Historical Society* 48 (1939), pp. 189–97.

34. A. D. Griesemer, W. D. Widmann, K. A. Forde, and M. A. Hardy, "John Jones, M.D.: Pioneer, Patriot, and Founder of American Surgery," *World Journal of Surgery* 34, no. 4 (April 2010), pp. 605–9.

35. Gert H. Brieger, "Surgery," in *Education of American Physicians*, ed. Ronald Numbers, (Berkeley: Univ. of California Press, 1980), p. 178, citing John Morgan, *A Discourse upon the Institution of Medical Schools in America* (Philadelphia, 1765; repr. Baltimore: Johns Hopkins Press, 1937), p. xv.

36. Brieger, "Surgery," pp. 182–83. See also Griesemer, Widmannn, Forde, and Hardy, "John Jones"; and Blair O. Rogers, "Surgery in the Revolutionary War, Contributions of John Jones, M.D. (1729–1791)," *Plastic and Reconstructive Surgery* 49, no. 1 (January 1972), pp. 1–13.

37. Brieger, "Surgery," pp. 179–80.

38. Brieger, "Surgery," p. 184, citing Frank H. Hamilton, *Introductory Lecture before the Surgical Class of Geneva Medical College* (Geneva: Merrel, 1840), p. 7.

39. Brieger, "Surgery," pp. 197–98, citing Samuel D. Gross, *A System of Surgery*, (Philadelphia: Blanchard and Lea, 1862), p. 36.

40. Brieger, "Surgery," pp. 188–89, citing Edward D. Churchill, ed., *To Work in the Vineyard of Surgery: The Reminiscences of J. Collins Warren (1842–1927)* (Cambridge: Harvard Univ. Press, 1958), p. 30.

41. Brieger, "Surgery," p. 190, citing Stephen Smith, "Union of Didactic and Clinical Instruction," *American Medical Times* 9 (1864), p. 121.

42. Brieger, "Surgery," p. 188.

43. Brieger, "Surgery," p. 190. See also A. D. Bevan, "The Study and Teaching and the Practice of Surgery," *Annals of Surgery* 98 (1933), p. 486.

44. Kemp Plummer Battle, *History of the University of North Carolina*, vol. 1, *From its Beginning to the Death of President Swain, 1789–1868* (Raleigh, N.C

Edwards & Broughton, 1907), p. 66. Noting that Harris taught primarily by preceptorship, William M. McLendon challenges Battle's claim: "Edenborough Medical College: North Carolina's First Chartered School of Medicine," in Dorothy Long, ed., *Medicine in North Carolina: Essays in the History of Medical Science and Medical Service, 1524–1960*, vol. 2, *Medical Education and Medical Service in North Carolina* (Raleigh: North Carolina Med. Soc., 1972), p. 353. See also George T. Blackburn, "Harris, Charles Wilson," in *Dictionary of North Carolina Biography*, vol. 3, *H–K*, ed. William S. Powell (Chapel Hill: Univ. of North Carolina Press, 1988), p. 51; and Guide to Charles Wilson Harris Papers, collection 315, Southern Historical Collection at the Louis Round Wilson Library, Univ. of North Carolina, online at http://finding-aids.lib.unc.edu/00315/ (accessed November 2016).

 45. Daniel Augustus Tompkins, *History of Mecklenburg County and the City of Charlotte: From 1740 to 1903*, vol. 1 (Charlotte: Observer, 1903), pp. 82–83.

 46. See John Hill Wheeler, *Historical Sketches of North Carolina: From 1584 to 1851* (Philadelphia: Lippincott, 1851), p. 68; and C. L. Hunter, *Sketches of Western North Carolina Illustrating Principally the Revolutionary Period of Mecklenburg, Rowan, Lincoln and Adjoining Counties* (Raleigh, 1877), pp. 97, 162.

 47. D. M. Furches, "Judge Harris, of Iredell," *North Carolina Journal of Law* 2, no. 6 (June 1905), p. 267.

 48. Wheeler, *Historical Sketches*, p. 68. As Wheeler notes, Harris's tombstone states, "Dr. Harris was engaged in the practice of medicine and surgery forty years; eminent in the former, in the latter preeminent."

 49. Wheeler, *Historical Sketches*, p. 59, transcribing a letter of Charles Wilson Harris to Robert Wilson Harris dated 78 [*sic*] February 1799.

 50. Wheeler, *Historical Sketches*, p. 60, n. 2.

 51. Harris, *Historical Sketch of Poplar Tent*, p. 21. William S. Harris was a son of Dr. Charles W. Harris. Charles's brother Samuel was for many years presiding elder of this church.

 52. Lucie Miller Johnson, "John Robinson," *Dictionary of North Carolina Biography*, vol. 5, *P–S* (Chapel Hill: Univ. of North Carolina Press, 1994), pp. 236–37. See also Harriet Sutton Rankin, *History of First Presbyterian Church, Fayetteville, North Carolina: From Old Manuscripts and Addresses* (Fayetteville, NC: First Presbyterian Church, 1928), reproducing A. L. Phillips, *An Historical Sketch of the Presbyterian Church of Fayetteville, North Carolina* (Fayetteville, NC: J.E. Garrett, 1889), which reproduces a portrait of Rev. Robinson dated 1800 (p. 12).

 53. William Henry Foote, *Sketches of North Carolina: Historical and Biographical, Illustrative of the Principles of a Portion of Her Early Settlers* (New York: Robert Carter, 1846), pp. 441–42, 446. P. 445f is a biography of John Robinson.

 54. Robert H. Morrison, "John Robinson," in *Annals of the American Pulpit*, vol. 4, *Presbyterian*, ed. William B. Sprague (New York: Robert Carter & Brothers, 1859), p. 113, citing a 24 August 1848 letter by Rev. Robert H. Morrison, Cottage Home, North Carolina.

 55. Harris, *Historical Sketch of Poplar Tent*, p. 21.

 56. Dorothy Long, ed., *Medicine in North Carolina*, vol. 1, *Development of*

Medical Science, Medical Administrative Agencies, and Medical Service Facilities in North Carolina (Raleigh: North Carolina Med. Soc., 1972), pp. 58–59. Long does not provide a specific citation for the *Raleigh Register* reference.

57. Both the Harrises and Russells had Ulster Scots Presbyterian background. Many of the earliest schools in the Carolina backcountry were established by Presbyterians who brought to the colonies strong interest in education, reflecting uncommonly high literacy rates in post-Reformation Scotland, where the ability of lay believers to read the Bible was prized: see James C. Leyburn, *The Scotch-Irish: A Social History* (Chapel Hill: Univ. of North Carolina Press, 1962), pp. 212–13; David Hackett Fischer, *Albion's Seed* (New York: Oxford Univ. Press, 1989), pp. 645–46; Arthur Herman, *The Scottish Enlightenment: The Scots' Invention of the Modern World* (New York: Random House, 2001); William R. Hoyt, "Presbyterianism," in *Encyclopedia of Religion in the South*, ed. Samuel S. Hill (Macon: Mercer Univ. Press, 1984), pp. 607–11; and Charles Reagan Wilson, "Religion and Education," in *Encyclopedia of Southern Culture*, ed. Charles Reagan Wilson and William Ferris (Chapel Hill: Univ. of North Carolina Press, 1989), p. 262.

Of early doctors in Arkansas with college degrees, two were Pennsylvania-educated—Matthew Cunningham and James A. Dibbrell Sr., both educated at University of Pennsylvania School of Medicine: see W. David Baird, *Medical Education in Arkansas 1879–1978* (Memphis: Memphis State Univ. Press, 1979), p. 3. Baird notes wide variations in training of early Arkansas practitioners, with the majority "reading medicine" rather than having formal medical education (p. 2).

58. Salem College File Card Register of Students, 1840 and 1842, transcribed by Lelia Graham Marsh, alumnae secretary, in a letter 2 March 1959 to Mrs. W. L. (Ruby Norwood) Kitchens, a granddaughter of William. Original is in the William James Park Russell Family Letters, 1878–1928, Small Manuscript Collection S4082, University of Arkansas for Medical Sciences Library, Historical Research Center, Little Rock, AR.

59. Norwood, "Medical Education and Rise of Hospitals," p. 134.

60. Carl Binger, *Revolutionary Doctor, Benjamin Rush, 1746–1813* (New York: W. W. Norton & Company, 1966), p. 184.

61. Binger, *Revolutionary Doctor*, p. 184

62. Binger, *Revolutionary Doctor*, p. 184

63. Dagobert D. Runes, "Preface," in *The Selected Writings of Benjamin Rush*, ed. Runes (New York: Philosophical Library, 1947), p. vii.

64. Ibid.; and Norwood, *Medical Education*, p. 35.

65. Runes, "Preface," p. vii.

66. See Benjamin Rush, *The Autobiography of Benjamin Rush: His "Travels Through Life" Together with His Commonplace Book for 1789–1813*, ed. George W. Corner (Princeton: Princeton Univ. Press, 1948), pp. 93-94.

67. Norwood, "Medical Education and Rise of Hospitals," p. 135.

68. Thomas H. Broman, "The Medical Sciences," in *The Cambridge History of Science*, vol. 4, *Eighteenth-Century Science*, ed. Roy Porter (Cambridge: Cambridge Univ. Press, 2003), p. 484.

69. Norwood, "Medical Education and Rise of Hospitals," p. 135.

70. Norwood, "Medical Education and Rise of Hospitals," p. 135, citing Richard Harrison Shryock, *American Medical Research Past and Present* (New York: Commonwealth Fund, 1947), p. 21.

71. Alex Berman, "The Heroic Approach in 19th-Century Therapeutics," in *Sickness and Health in America*, p. 77.

72. David Dary, *Frontier Medicine* (New York: Knopf, 2008), p. 172. See also Binger, *Revolutionary Doctor*, p. 180.

73. Duffy, "Changing Image," p. 133.

74. Fielding H. Garrison, *An Introduction to the History of Medicine*, 4th ed. (Philadelphia: W. B. Saunders Company, 1929), p. 379.

75. See Myrl Ebert, "The Rise and Development of the American Medical Periodical, 1797–1850," *Bulletin of the Medical Library Association* 40 (1952), pp. 248–49.

76. Runes, "Preface," p. viii.

77. Binger, *Revolutionary Doctor*, pp. 181–82. Binger does not provide a citation for the lecture he is citing.

78. On Rush's favorable view of "natural" remedies, see Binger, *Revolutionary Doctor*, p. 182.

79. Binger, *Revolutionary Doctor*, p. 185.

80. Garrison, *Introduction to History of Medicine*, p. 310.

81. Norwood, "Medical Education and Rise of Hospitals," p. 134.

82. Garrison, *Introduction to History of Medicine*, p. 405.

83. Norwood, "Medical Education and Rise of Hospitals," p. 134.

84. Norwood, "Medical Education and Rise of Hospitals," p. 134; and Garrison, *Introduction to History of Medicine*, p. 393.

85. Norwood, "Medical Education and Rise of Hospitals," p. 135.

86. Ebert, "Rise and Development of American Medical Periodical," pp. 245–46.

87. Ebert, "Rise and Development of American Medical Periodical," pp. 248–49, 253, 259.

88. The term "sects" is from Ronald L. Numbers, "Do-It-Yourself the Sectarian Way," in *Sickness and Health in America*, p. 87.

89. Numbers, "Do-It-Yourself the Sectarian Way," p. 87.

90. Ebert, "Rise and Development of American Medical Periodical," p. 257.

91. Numbers, "Do-It-Yourself the Sectarian Way," p. 87.

92. Numbers, "Do-It-Yourself the Sectarian Way," pp. 87–88; and Ebert, "Rise and Development of American Medical Periodical," p. 257.

93. Numbers, "Do-It-Yourself the Sectarian Way, pp. 87–88; Ebert, "Rise and Development of American Medical Periodical," p. 257; and Baird, *Medical Education in Arkansas*, p. 4.

94. Numbers, "Do-It-Yourself the Sectarian Way," p. 88, citing Samuel Thomson, *New Guide to Health, or Botanic Family Physician* (Boston: House, 1825), part 1, p. 10.

95. Numbers, "Do-It-Yourself the Sectarian Way," pp. 89–90.

96. See *supra*, n. 48.

97. Livingston, "William J. Russell," pp. 282–83.

98. Edward Baptist, *The Half Has Never Been Told: Slavery and the Making of American Capitalism* (New York: Basic Books, 2014), pp. 18–19.

99. Baptist, *The Half Has Never Been Told*, and p. 186.

100. Albert M. Hillhouse, *A History of Burke County, Georgia, 1777–1950* (Swainsboro, GA: Magnolia, 1985), p. 63.

101. The South Carolina upcountry had experienced drought and hunger immediately before 1820, as economic depression also affected various other areas of the nation: see John R. Finger, *Tennessee Frontiers: Three Regions in Transition* (Bloomington: Indiana Univ. Press, 2001), pp. 255–56, on the ways in which this depression spurred westward movement at this period.

On migration of kinship networks to the frontier of the old Southwest in the early 1800s, see Billingsley, *Communities of Kinship*. On such migration from Eastern North Carolina to Georgia shortly before 1800, see Sherrod and Sherrod, *Plain Folk, Planters, and the Complexities of Southern Society*, p. 27, citing Mary Alice Jordan, *Cotton to Kaolin: A History of Washington County, Georgia* (Milledgeville: Boyd, 1989), pp. 9, 152–53, 181. On the extension of the cotton kingdom from Virginia and the Carolinas into Georgia, Mississippi, Alabama, and Tennessee, see Malcolm J. Rohrbough, *The Trans-Appalachian Frontier: People, Societies, and Institutions 1775–1850* (New York: Oxford Univ. Press, 1978), pp. 196–97.

102. Livingston, "William J. Russell," p. 283.

103. Livingston, "William J. Russell," p. 283.

104. On Gwinnett's formation from Jackson County after Georgia acquired the Wofford purchase from the Cherokee Nation in 1804, see Frary Elrod, *Historical Notes on Jackson County, Georgia* (Jefferson, GA: n.p., 1967), pp. 34–36. On Winn's role in laying off Lawrenceville, see James C. Flanigan, *History of Gwinnett County, Georgia*, vol. 1, *1818–1943* (Hapeville, GA: Tyler, 1943), pp. 15, 27; and Gwinnett County Historical Society, *Gwinnett County: It All Started Here* (Dacula, GA: Dacula Rapid Press, 1978), p. 4.

105. Flanigan, *History of Gwinnett*, vol. 1, pp. 27–28, 82; and Gwinnett County Historical Society, *Gwinnett County*, p. 5.

106. See James C. Flanigan, *History of Gwinnett County, Georgia*, vol. 2, *1818–1960* (Hapeville, GA: Tyler, 1943), p. 152.

107. On the demographics of Gwinnett County in 1820, citing the 1820 federal census for the county, see Flanigan, *History of Gwinnett*, vol. 1, p. 32f.

108. Norwood, *Medical Education*, p. 276

109. James H. Cassedy, "Why Self-Help? Americans Alone with Their Diseases 1800–1840," in *Medicine Without Doctors: Home Health Care in American History*, ed. Guenter B. Risse, Ronald L. Numbers, and Judith Walzer Leavitt (New York: Science History Publications, 1977), p. 38.

110. Cassedy, "Why Self-Help?," pp. 36–37.

111. Cassedy, "Why Self-Help?," p. 38.

112. On the quick growth and prosperity of Gwinnett (in particular, its elite class), see Flanigan, *History of Gwinnett*, vol. 1, p. 97f. As Flanigan notes, Gwinnett's initial small farms gradually "went into the hands of large landowners and the plantation replaced the farm. These plantations were cultivated by slaves and there was developed a landed aristocracy that grew in power, wealth and influence until it was destroyed by the Civil War."

113. On the role of Elisha Winn in early Lawrenceville, see an unpublished 26 November 1885 manuscript of his son Richard Dickson Winn, transcribed

by Frederick Ware Huff, *Four Families, Winn, Thomas, Ware, Garrett of the Southern United States from 1600s to 1993* (Kennesaw, GA: priv. publ., 1993), pp. 130–31, 133–36. Huff does not provide information about the current owner or repository of the unpublished manuscript. This document is also cited in C. L. Pentecost and Aldyne Maltbie, "William Maltbie," in *Gwinnett County, Georgia, Families*, pp. 319–21. Frederick Ware Huff has sent us his typed transcription of the manuscript. See also Flanigan, *History of Gwinnett*, vol. 1, pp. 92–94, 321, on the founding of Lawrenceville Academy.

    114. Flanigan, *History of Gwinnett*, vol. 1, pp. 95–96.

    115. See 23 December 1837 act of the Georgia legislature: *Acts and Resolutions of the General Assembly of the State of Georgia Passed in Milledgeville at an Annual Session in November and December 1837* (Milledgeville: P. L. Robinson, 1838), pp. 18–19.

    116. Livingston, "William J. Russell," p. 283.

    117. Livingston, "William J. Russell," p. 283.

    118. Greene Co., GA, Marriage Bk. 1829–1849, p. 241; Morgan Co., GA, Marriage Bk. 1855–1854, p. 56; Greene Co., GA, Will Bk. 4, p. 90. James Daniel Park was a prosperous planter of Greene County; on 23 March 1788, he acquired 862½ acres on the east side of Oconee from Abraham Sanders (Greene Co., GA, Deed Bk. 1, pp. 349–50). By his death, he had 1137½ acres that were divided in 1826 between his wife Phebe and 14 children (Greene Co., GA, Superior Court Minutes, Bk. 6, pp. 44, 507–8).

    On the Park family, see Lucian Lamar Knight, *Georgia's Bi-Centennial Memoirs and Memories: A Tale of Two Centuries, Reviewing the State's Marvelous Story of Achievement, Since Oglethorpe's Landing in 1733*, vol. 1 (Atlanta: priv. publ., 1931), pp. 141–44; Alfred J. Morrison, "Militia Officers, Prince Edward County, 1777–1781," *Virginia Magazine of History and Biography* 21 (1913), pp. 201–2; and J. T. McAllister, *Virginia Militia in the Revolutionary War* (Hot Springs, VA: McAllister, 1913), p. 225.

    The marriage to Sophia Park connected William J. Russell to the kinship network of Lawrenceville's founder Elisha Winn, whose daughter Martha Ann had married Clark Howell; after Martha's death, Howell married Sophia's sister Effiah Jane. In 1827, two years after William J. Russell and Sophia Park married, an announcement in *The Athenian* (Athens, GA), 14 December 1827, p. 1, shows Russell acting as guardian for Sophia's minor sister Rebecca as their father James Park's estate was settled.

    119. In "An Old Land Mark Is Being Removed," *Gwinnett News-Herald* (Lawrenceville, GA) reports 7 February 1910 (no author is given) that the house had been "rolled back from Perry Street to face Oak Street" to make room for the Ware family's house. According to Bob Wynn, "Ramshackle House Holds Slice of History," *Gwinnett Daily News* (Lawrenceville, GA), 6 November 1986, p. C-1, after Russell's death in 1872, when his wife Iantha married his business partner Dr. Andrew J. Shaffer, she and Shaffer lived in the house.

    120. The date and place of birth and death of W. J. P., Wallace, and Richard Russell are recorded in the Bible of W. J. P.'s wife Ava Law Russell. The Bible, published in 1843, passed from Ava to her son Eric, to Eric's daughter Mary Russell Hurley, and then to Mary's son Lloyd Hurley. Its present location is

unknown. William L. Russell of Maumelle, AR, has seen the original and made photocopies of the Bible register. Sarah's dates of birth and death are on her tombstone at Fairview Presbyterian Cemetery in Lawrenceville, and Mary Catherine's are on her tombstone in Shadowlawn Cemetery, Lawrenceville. See also Kent and Green, "Dr. William James Russell," p. 431. Bryant Strickland's sister Harriet Emeline married Dr. John Winn Maltbie, son of William Maltbie and Philadelphia Winn, in 1848.

121. Fairview Session Minutes, 1823–1835, 11 February 1826, p. 29.

122. Fairview Session Minutes, 1823–1835, 25 August 1826.

123. See Jackson Co., GA, Superior Ct. Minutes, 1801–1803, unpaginated, 29 June 1804, for a case in which Elisha Winn and his father-in-law James Cochran testified about James Smith assaulting Asa Hearn at Winn's house, with Hearn losing his ear in the fight. Though the record book is labeled 1801–1803, it contains minutes for sessions in 1804. Cochran himself was repeatedly charged with assault: see Jackson Co., GA, Superior Court Minutes, 1814–1822, unpaginated, 24 March, 28 September, 30 September 1818, and 29 Sept. 1819; Jackson Co., GA, Superior Ct. Minutes, 1822–31, unpaginated, 14–15 September 1824, 12 September 1825. In his unpublished family history cited *supra*, n. 113, Richard Dickson Winn notes the volatility of Cochran's temperament and his tendency to drink, which exacerbated the volatility.

124. Flanigan, *History of Gwinnett*, vol. 1, p. 131.

125. See "Fairview Presbyterian Church History," compiled by Fairview Presbyterian Church, online at its website at http://www.fairviewpres.org/ historyfull.html.

126. Dickson D. Bruce Jr., "Frontier, Influence of," in *Encyclopedia of Religion in the South*, ed. Samuel S. Hill, p. 274. See also Gregory A. Wills, *Democratic Religion: Freedom, Authority, and Church Discipline in the Baptist South, 1785–1900* (New York: Oxford Univ. Press, 1997), p. 9, noting the function of churches as "moral courts of the frontier." In the voluminous body of literature discussing the role of religion on the frontier, William Warren Sweet's documentary histories of various churches stand out: see *Religion on the American Frontier*, vol. 1, *The Baptists, 1783–1830* (New York: Henry Holt, 1931); *Religion on the American Frontier*, vol. 2, *The Presbyterians, 1783–1840* (New York: Cooper Square, 1964); *Religion on the American Frontier*, vol. 4, *The Methodists, 1783–1840* (New York: Cooper Square, 1964). See also David T. Bailey, "Frontier Religion," in *Encyclopedia of Southern Culture*, ed. Wilson and Ferris, pp. 1286–88.

127. Marian Silveus, "Churches and Social Control on the Western Pennsylvania Frontier," *Western Pennsylvania Historical Magazine* 19 (1936), p. 128. On the function of Presbyterian sessions, see p. 127. See also Martin Marty, "North America," in *The Oxford Illustrated History of Christianity*, ed. John McManners (New York: Oxford Univ. Press, 1990), p. 397, on the role of Presbyterian churches in bringing social control to frontier settlements.

128. On the Southern penchant for violence, particularly when honor is involved, see Bertram Wyatt-Brown, *Honor and Violence in the Old South* (New York: Oxford Univ. Press, 1986); Raymond D. Gastil, "Violence, Crime, and Punishment," in *Encyclopedia of Southern Culture*, ed. Wilson and Ferris, pp. 1473–76; and Edward L. Ayers, "Honor," in ibid., pp. 1483–84. See J. H. Elliott,

Spain, Europe and the Wider World, 1500–1800 (New Haven: Yale Univ. Press, 2009), p. 119, on how Puritan divines constrained westward migration from New England due to fear that the church would lose social control.

129. Fairview Session Minutes, 1823–1835, 8 March 1828, p. 87. Sophia's case is discussed in the online history of Fairview Church cited *supra*, n. 125.

130. Fairview Session Minutes, 1823–1835, pp. 121–35. Noting that he had been a ruling elder for forty years, had been born in Ireland, and had served in the Revolution, Fairview minutes state that Russell's stepfather John Alexander died on 9 May 1830 (p. 102).

131. Livingston, "William J. Russell," pp. 283–84.

132. See Flanigan, *History of Gwinnett*, vol. 2, p. 45.

133. "Proceedings of the Anti-Van Buren Convention," *Southern Recorder* (Milledgeville, GA), 10 May 1836, p. 2, col. 4. The article is dated 2 May 1836, which is when the convention occurred.

134. *Columbus Enquirer* (Columbus, GA), 13 May 1836, p. 3, col. 3; Livingston, "William J. Russell," p. 282.

135. "Obituary [of Mrs. Sophia P. Russell]," *Southern Recorder* (Milledgeville, GA), 9 April 1844, p. 3, col. 6–7.

136. Edith Huff Green and Mildred Huff Breedlove, "John Huff," in *Gwinnett County, Georgia, Families*, p. 247; Kent and Green, "Dr. William James Russell," p. 432; Gwinnett Co., GA, Marriage Bk. 4, 1843–1864, p. 31; and *Southern Recorder* (Milledgeville, GA), 6 May 1845, p. 3, col. 6.

137. Kent and Green, "Dr. William James Russell," p. 431.

138. *Catalogue of the Classes and Graduates of the Philadelphia College of Medicine for 1849–50, and 1850* (Philadelphia: Hughes & Gaskill, 1850), p. 7. This is the notice of William J. P. Russell's matriculation at the Philadelphia College of Medicine in March 1850; p. 8 states that he graduated at the end of term, with commencement in July 1850.

139. See "Medical Intelligence," in *The Southern Medical and Surgical Journal* 1, no. 4 (1845), p. 224, listing graduates of the institution in March 1845. Lowe's dissertation was a study of dysentery.

140. 1850 federal census, Gwinnett Co., GA; roll M432_71, p. 235A, image 473; and 1860 federal census, Gwinnett Co., GA, District 407; roll M653_125, p. 613, image 163. Shaffer continues in William J. Russell's household on the 1870 federal census: 1870 federal census, Gwinnett Co., GA; roll M593_154, p. 92B, image 300449.

141. See B. Y. Martin, *Reports of Cases in Law and Equity, Argued and Determined in the Supreme Court of the State of Georgia from November Term, 1859, at Milledgeville, to June Term, 1860, at Macon, Inclusive*, vol. 30 (Atlanta: Franklin, 1862), pp. 400–12.

142. See Flanigan, *History of Gwinnett*, vol. 2, which notes that Lucretia Douglas gave her diary to her nephew K. H. Walker in 1893, and he then published it with the title *Grace for Every Trial*.

143. Letter of William J. Russell to Governor Joseph E. Brown, in Governor Joseph Emerson Brown correspondence file, 1861–1865, Georgia Archives, Series 245, Governors Subject Correspondence, 3335–16, unit 93–1219A.

144. The biographical sketch is transcribed in Flanigan, *History of Gwinnett*, vol. 1, pp. 382–85.

145. See Phyllis Hughes and Marvin Hughes, "National Register Narrative, Isaac Adair House, c. 1827," National Register of Historic Places Registration Form, 20 October 2000; online at National Park Service website at https://focus.nps.gov/GetAsset?assetID=4c81ecfc-55ae-48e8-ac3a-f36443df5180 (accessed January 2017).

146. James M. Gordon, "A Remarkable Case of Volvulus and Strangulation of the Intestines Within the Abdomen," *Southern Medical and Surgical Journal* 1, no. 8, new series (August 1845), pp. 444–47. The case account is also in *Boston Medical and Surgical Journal* 33, no. 2 (August 1845), pp. 39–41.

147. Gordon, "Remarkable Case," p. 445.

148. See *supra*, n. 140.

149. James M. Gordon, "Contributions to Practical Midwifery, with Cases Occurring in Obstetrical Practice," *Southern Medical and Surgical Journal* 3, no. 12 (December 1847), pp. 703–17.

150. James M. Gordon, "Observations on Ranula: with Cases, Treatment and Cure," *Southern Medical and Surgical Journal* 5, no. 2 (February 1849), pp. 65–69.

151. Gordon, "Contributions to Practical Midwifery," p. 708.

152. Gordon, "Contributions to Practical Midwifery," p. 709. It is interesting to note that the cases Gordon records in this article describe patients variously as "of nervous bilious temperament" or "of nervous sanguine temperament."

153. James M. Gordon, "Letter," *Southern Medical and Surgical Journal* 5, no. 2 (February 1849), pp. 120–21.

154. Stanley Finger, *Origins of Neuroscience: A History of Explorations into Brain Function* (Oxford: Oxford Univ. Press, 2001), p. 161.

155. See Frank Kells Boland, *The First Anesthetic: The Story of Crawford Long* (Athens: Univ. of Georgia Press, 1950).

156. Richard D. Winn, "Dr. James M. Gordon," in Flanigan, *History of Gwinnett*, vol. 1, pp. 383.

157. *Gwinnett Herald* (Lawrenceville, GA), 19 March 1873, p. 3.

158. A death notice is in *Southern Recorder* (Milledgeville, GA), 9 March 1847, p. 3, col. 6.

159. See "Frozen to Death," *Concord Weekly Gazette* (Concord, NC), 31 January 1857, p. 2.

160. "The Yellow Fever," *Baltimore Sun* (Baltimore, MD), 12 September 1854, p. 2, col. 1.

161. "The Yellow Fever," *Richmond Dispatch* (Richmond, VA), 15 September 1854, p. 2, col. 2.

162. "List of Persons Adjudged Insane and Ordered to Be Committed to the Insane Asylum at Milledgeville from the *Atlanta Constitution* Newspaper 1870–1914," online at the website of the Baldwin Co., GA, GenWeb page, maintained by Eileen Babb McAdams, at http://theusgenweb.org/ga/baldwin/cshinmates.html (accessed August 2018). See also "Roundabout in Georgia,"

Atlanta Constitution (Atlanta, GA), 29 June 1877, p. 3, col. 4, noting that Dr. Jesse Lowe had been committed to the state insane asylum.

163. Fairview Presbyterian Church (Lawrenceville, GA) Session Minutes and Register, 1835–1880, held by Columbia Theological Seminary, p. 75.

164. Fairview Presbyterian Church Session Minutes and Register, 1835–1880, pp. 202–3.

165. See *supra*, n. 140.

166. *Southern Banner* (Athens, GA), 24 April 1851, p. 4, col. 2.

167. *Acts Passed by the General Assembly of the State of Georgia, Passed in Milledgeville, at a Biennial Session in November, December, and January, 1851–2* (Macon: Samuel J. Ray, 1852), pp. 208–9.

168. "A Letter from the Great Western Canal Survey," *Atlanta Constitution* (Atlanta, GA), 8 February 1872, p. 1, col. 2.

169. The article notes that Dr. A. J. Shaffer led this discussion and that Tyler Macon Peeples, editor of the *Gwinnett Herald*, was part of the meeting.

170. "Death of Dr. W. J. Russell."

171. See, e.g., William E. Lass, *A History of Steamboating on the Upper Missouri River* (Lincoln: Univ. of Nebraska Press, 1962), p. 58, noting that in 1865, Charles A. Maurice, the founder of Maurice and Company, and Joab Lawrence formed the firm of Joab Lawrence & Co., which was both engaging in cotton factoring business and extending railway systems west.

172. Gwinnett Co., GA, Will Bk. D, pp. 70–75.

173. "Death of Dr. W. J. Russell."

174. Baptist, *Half Has Never Been Told*, pp. 90–95. Notes of William L. Russell, Maumelle, AR (2016), state, "The Gwinnett county records show no fewer than twelve recordings of guardianships, sureties, executorships, and sheriff sale actions from 1827–1857."

175. Gwinnett Co., GA Deed Bk. N, pp. 228–31.

176. Gwinnett Co., GA, Tax Digest, 1864, p. 67.

177. On the 1860 and 1870 census, see *supra*, n. 140.

178. *Gwinnett Herald* (Lawrenceville, GA), 2 October 1872.

179. "Death of Dr. W. J. Russell," noting that he died two days previously, on Sunday, at noon.

180. "Death of Dr. W. J. Russell." For Iantha' probate of the will on 7 April 1873, see Gwinnett Co., GA, Will Bk. D, pp. 74–75.

181. 1860 federal census, Bidwell, Butte Co., CA, post office Bidwell's Bar; roll M653_56, p. 725.

182. See his CSA service papers, Co. I, GA 55th Infantry, which show him enlisting at Lawrenceville on 6 May 1862, being made sergeant the following day, and then raised to the rank of lieutenant on 7 December 1862. The service papers also record his date and place of capture and information about his imprisonment at Johnson's Island: see Carded Records Showing Military Service of Soldiers Who Fought in Confederate Organizations, Compiled 1903–1927, Documenting the Period 1861–1865, M266, roll 532, RG 109 NARA.

183. The letters are in the Mary M. Sneed Owen Papers, Williamson Co., TN, Archives, Franklin, TN.

184. Gwinnett Co., GA, Marriage Bk. 4, #2, 1871–1882, p. 182.

185. "Death of Dr. Shaffer," *Atlanta Constitution* (Atlanta, GA), 27 May 1887, p. 3, col. 4.

Chapter 2

1. *Tuskegee Republican* (Tuskegee, AL), 3 June 1858, p. 2, col. 6.

2. William J. P. Russell to Major General William S. Rosecrans, 17 August 1863 in Union Citizens' File, Union Provost Marshals' File of Papers Relating to Individual Civilians, 1861–1867, file 22632, M345, RG 109, NARA.

3. The date is recorded in the Bible of his mother Ava. In a 10 January 1889 affidavit in Van Zandt Co., Texas, as he filed for a Mexican War pension, W. J. P. Russell states the same date and place of birth (Mexican War pension application 21053, certificate 18030).

4. Fairview Session Minutes, 1823–1835, p. 101: "Infant of Dr. Wm J Russell was baptized named William James Park Russell."

5. Flanigan, *History of Gwinnett*, vol. 1, pp. 122, 143–44, transcribing 26 November 1885 manuscript of Richard Dickson Winn on the history of the Winn family. Flanigan transcribes minutes from a meeting of Gwinnett citizens in early 1837, at which a resolution was made to erect a monument honoring the county's men killed at Goliad. See also Huff, *Four Families*, pp. 133–36; Flanigan, *History of Gwinnett*, vol. 2, pp. 624–25; George W. Clower, "Thomas Winn (c. 1741–1797) and His Remarkable Connection with Atlanta Through His Descendants," *Atlanta Historical Bulletin* 12, no. 4 (1967), p. 41; and Mabel Ward Cameron, *The Biographical Cyclopedia of American Women*, vol. 2, *American Biographical Notes* (New York: Halvord, 1924), p. 433.

6. See Army Register of Enlistments, January 1847–June 1849, p. 213; MIUSA1798_102882, roll 23, RG 94, NARA. Russell's enlistment papers have the same physical description: see Mexican War Enlistment Papers, 1st Series, 1798–1894, box 675, Entry 91, NARA. See also pension application cited *supra*, n. 3.

7. Medical College of Georgia, Register of Students 1832–1861, Students of the Session of 1848–1849, pp. 92–93; Students of the Session of 1849–1850, pp. 110–11. On requirements for entering medical colleges in the 1840s, see Glenna R. Schroeder-Lein, *Confederate Hospitals on the Move: Samuel H. Stout and the Army of Tennessee* (Columbia: Univ. of South Carolina Press, 1994), p. 28: "To enter a medical school in the 1840s, a prospective student needed to be a white male who could read and write. He did not need to know Greek and Latin, nor did he need to have a college degree. . . ."

8. Paul D. Eve, *The Present Position of the Medical Profession in Society: An Introductory Lecture Delivered in the Medical College of Georgia, November 5, 1849* (Augusta: James McCafferty, 1849), p. 3.

9. Eve, *The Present Position of the Medical Profession in Society*, pp. 5–6.

10. Eve, *The Present Position of the Medical Profession in Society*, pp. 8–9.

11. Eve, *The Present Position of the Medical Profession in Society*, p. 9.

12. Eve, *The Present Position of the Medical Profession in Society*, p. 11.

13. Eve, *The Present Position of the Medical Profession in Society*, p. 11.

14. Eve, *The Present Position of the Medical Profession in Society*, p. 15. On

the emphasis of physicians of the period on science as a counter to quackery, see Steven M. Stowe, *Doctoring the South: Southern Physicians and Everyday Medicine in the Mid-Nineteenth Century* (Chapel Hill: Univ. of North Carolina Press, 2004), p. 2. See also Baird, *Medical Education in Arkansas,* on concern about quackery in nineteenth-century medicine (pp. 8–9).

15. Eve, *Present Position of the Medical Profession,* p. 19.

16. Eve, *The Present Position of the Medical Profession in Society,* p. 20.

17. See Minutes of the Medical College of Georgia Board of Trustees Meetings, 1829–1892, p. 140 (20 March 1849); original at Medical College of Georgia, online at Augusta University's Open Repository at http://augusta. openrepository.com/augusta/handle/10675.2/965 (accessed February 2017). P. 182 provides a list of thesis topics of each graduate of the class. According to the college's archivist, the school did not retain copies of theses at this period but returned them to students.

18. Minutes of the Medical College of Georgia Board of Trustees Meetings, 1829–1892, p. 184 (March 1850 minutes—the day is blurred and is perhaps 2nd). Pp. 185–86 present a list of the year's graduates with thesis subjects.

19. Record Book 1 of the Faculty of the Medical College of Georgia, October 1833–November 1852, 1–2 March 1850. The handwritten minutes are in the archives at Medical College of Georgia's Robert B. Greenblatt Library; scans are online at Augusta University's Open Repository at http://augusta. openrepository.com/augusta/handle/10675.2/966. The Greenblatt Library also has a typed transcript; the 1–2 March 1850 faculty meetings are recorded on pp. 140–41.

20. Emailed communication, Sarah Braswell, historical research coordinator, Office of Medical Historian in Residence, Augusta University, to Mary Ryan, Little Rock, AR, July 2017.

21. *Twenty-Fifth Annual Announcement of the Medical College of Georgia* (Augusta: Medical College of Georgia, 1850), online at Augusta University's Open Repository website at http://augusta.openrepository.com/augusta/ handle/10675.2/319890 (accessed February 2017). The 1848 catalog, *Seventeenth Annual Announcement of the Medical College of Georgia* (Augusta: Jas. McCafferty, 1848), is also extant.

22. *Twenty-Fifth Annual Announcement of the Medical College of Georgia,* p. 12. On the history of Medical College of Georgia, see Norwood, *Medical Education,* pp. 276–79.

23. Stowe, *Doctoring the South,* p. 23.

24. *Catalogue of the Classes and Graduates of the Philadelphia College of Medicine for 1849–'50, and 1850,* p. 7. See also Harold J. Abrahams, "Extinct Medical Schools of Nineteenth Century Philadelphia: (II) The Philadelphia College of Medicine," *Transactions and Studies of the College of Physicians of Philadelphia* 30 (1963), p. 176, noting Russell's matriculation in March 1850. In her Bible, Ava Russell recorded that W. J. P. graduated from Philadelphia College of Medicine on 3 March 1850, but the school's catalog states that this was the matriculation date and that he graduated on 19 July.

25. Abrahams, "Extinct Medical Schools," p. 163.

26. Abrahams, "Extinct Medical Schools," p. 164. See pp. 166–69 for a list of the school's faculty from 1847–1858.

27. Abrahams, "Extinct Medical Schools," p. 165.

28. Norwood, *Medical Education*, p. 99. On debates in this period about how many terms were needed to achieve an M.D., with most educators emphasizing two consecutive terms, see Stowe, *Doctoring the South*, p. 24.

29. *Catalogue of the Classes and Graduates of Philadelphia College of Medicine*, p. 8, noting that commencement was 19 July 1850.

30. W. David Baird, *Medical Education in Arkansas*, pp. 2–3. See also Stowe, *Doctoring the South*, pp. 19–20, noting that before 1830, relatively few American men with interest in medicine attended medical school and learning by apprenticeship was the norm. Stowe provides a detailed sketch of the preceptorship method on pp. 27–31.

31. Stowe, *Doctoring the South*, pp. 16–19.

32. Stowe, *Doctoring the South*, p. 15.

33. Hall Co., GA, Marriage Bk. A, 1819–1870, p. 184. The date is also recorded in Ava's Bible, which also gives her birthdate (11 October 1832), as well as the names and birthdates of both sets of parents. The date of marriage is also stated in Russell's Mexican War pension affidavit (see *supra*, n. 3). Following Russell's death, Ava filed a widow's pension application on 14 April 1892, stating the same date and place for their marriage. The application also includes a transcript of the marriage record from Hall Co., GA, showing that license was granted 14 November 1850: see Mexican War pension widow's application 10579, certificate 9137.

34. Hall Co., GA, Will Bk. A, p. 64.

35. On coverture, its roots in English law and application in the American colonies and states, see, Merril D. Smith, *Women's Roles in Eighteenth-Century America* (Santa Barbara, CA: Greenwood, 2010), p. 9; Angela Robbins, "Alice Morgan Person: 'My Life Has Been Out of the Ordinary Run of Woman's Life,'" in *North Carolina Women: Their Lives and Times*, ed. Michele Gillespie and Sally G. McMillen (Athens: Univ. of Georgia Press, 2014), p. 157; and Thomas E. Buckley, "Placed in the Power of Violence: The Divorce Petition of Evelina Gregory Roane, 1824," *Virginia Magazine of History and Biography* 110, no. 1 (January 1992), p. 32.

36. Hall Co., GA, Deed Bk. G, p. 360.

37. Hall Co., GA, Deed Bk. G, p. 419.

38. Hall Co., GA, Deed Bk. I, p. 587.

39. Polk Co., GA, Deed Bk. A, p. 91.

40. The names and birthdates for both sons are recorded in Ava's Bible in her hand. Places of birth appear to have been added later by someone else.

41. Also buying lots in Calhoun in 1853 was Dr. George William Young, who was roughly Russell's age. One of the first purchasers of lots was also Ava's uncle David Shelton Law, a founding trustee of the academy established in Calhoun in 1852: see Lulie Pitts, *History of Gordon County, Georgia* (Calhoun, GA: Calhoun Times Press, 1933), pp. 311–12, 327.

42. The date and place of birth are in Ava's Bible.

43. Ava's Bible.

44. See *supra*, n. 1.

45. Goodspeed's *Reminiscent History of the Ozark Region* (Chicago: Goodspeed, 1894), pp. 408–9. Pierce was a native of Ava's home county, Hall. By 1860, federal census records place his family in Dawson County in north central Georgia: see 1860 federal census, Dawson Co., GA; roll M653_119, p. 69, image 69.

46. The date and place of birth are in Ava's Bible. See also Diary of Seaborn Rentz Russell, 7 September 1922, original in possession of George S. Russell, Saylorsburg, PA. A transcription is in the William James Park Russell Family Letters.

47. See N. J. Hammond, *Reports of Cases in Law and Equity, Argued and Determined in the Supreme Court of the State of Georgia, at Milledgeville, June Term 1867, and Part of December Term 1867*, vol. 36 (Macon: J. W. Burke, 1868), pp. 494–98.

48. *Southern Banner* (Athens, GA), 23 September 1858, p. 3, col. 2.

49. Polk Co., GA, Deed Bk. A, pp. 96–97. On Boring's marriage to Nancy Wardlaw, see Paulding Co., GA, Marriage Bk.1, p. 185; see also 1880 federal census, Sumter Co., GA, roll 186, p. 184A, ED 73, listing him as a physician; and "Methodist Minister Dies: Dr. J. J. Boring Passes Away After a Long Illness at Americus," *Atlanta Constitution* (Atlanta, GA), 11 December 1897, p. 3, col. 3. An ad for Boring's medical services is in *Atlanta Constitution* (Atlanta, GA), 1 July 1868, p. 1.

50. On Seaborn's diary entry, see *supra*, n. 46.

51. *Southern Banner* (Athens, GA), 1 July 1858, p. 3, col. 2.

52. See *supra*, n. 1. On the use of cards to advertise doctors' services, see William H. Helfand, "Advertising Health to the People: The Early Illustrated Posters," in *Right Living: An Anglo-American Tradition of Self-Help Medicine and Hygiene*, ed. Charles E. Rosenberg (Baltimore: Johns Hopkins, 2003), pp. 173–74.

53. *Tuskegee Republican* (Tuskegee, AL), 10 June 1858, p. 2, col. 6. Note that the terms "hare lip" and "hair lip" (both will be encountered in documents cited in this historical study) are now considered offensive. "Cleft lip" is now the preferred term. Because this is an historical study, we have been careful always to replicate terms as we find them in historical documents, as we cite these documents as direct quotes or report about them in indirect quotes.

54. *Hinds County Gazette* (Raymond, MS), 23 March 1853, p. 3.

55. *Arkansas Gazette* (Little Rock, AR), 3 April 1878, p. 6. In February 1880, the *Gazette* announced that surgeons from Indianapolis's Central Surgical Infirmary would be in Little Rock at Capitol Hotel and in Hot Springs for consultation and surgery for "any disease of the Eye or Ear": ibid., 5 February 1880, p. 1. For similar announcements in other Southern communities, see *The Times* (Shreveport, LA), 11 March 1884, p. 4; *Times-Picayune* (New Orleans, LA), 28 April 1884, p. 2; and *Richland Beacon* (Rayville, LA), 4 May 1889, p. 3.

56. See, e.g., *Semi-Weekly Mississippian* (Jackson, MS), 11 September 1860, p. 1; *Arkansas Gazette* (Little Rock, AR), 22 February 1870, p. 2; *Times-Picayune* (New Orleans, LA), 3 February 1872, p. 2; *Dallas Daily Herald* (Dallas, TX), 4 January 1876, p. 3; *The South-Western* (Shreveport, LA), 17 November 1889, p.

3; and *The Meridional* (Abbeville, LA), 14 May 1892, p. 1. The practice of offering vouchers from fellow physicians was standard procedure in this period: for instance, the *Times-Picayune* (New Orleans, LA), 17 December 1884, p. 4, prints a voucher for Dr. A. J. Miller, apparently of Alexandria, by Dr. A. Cockerille, regarding Dr. Miller's ability to cure strabismus with surgery.

57. *Arkansas Gazette* (Little Rock, AR), 8 July 1871, p. 4.

58. As Charles Rosenberg notes, "Until the last decades of the nineteenth century, voluntary surgery represented only a small part of medical practice"— hence the good market for itinerant surgeons, like the Russell doctors, who offered surgical treatment in communities where it was otherwise not available (see Charles E. Rosenberg, "Health in the Home: A Tradition of Print and Practice," in *Right Living*, p. 4).

59. Again, note that the male pronoun is used here to reflect historical reality: with one or two rare exceptions, there simply were not female doctors practicing in American communities during this time.

60. Abrahams, "Extinct Medical Schools of Nineteenth Century Philadelphia," p. 170, citing Robert Druitt's *The Principles and Practice of Modern Surgery* (Philadelphia: Lea and Blanchard, 1844); Robert Liston, *Practical Surgery, with Notes and Additional Illustrations by George W. Norris* (Philadelphia: James Crissey, 1838), and *Elements of Surgery* (Philadelphia: Ed. Barrington & Geo. D. Hasswell, 1842); William Gibson, *Institutes and Practice of Surgery: Being Outlines of a Course of Lectures* (Philadelphia: Edward Parker, 1824); George McClellan, *Principles and Practice of Surgery* (Philadelphia: Grigg & Elliott, 1848); and Alfred Velpeau, *New Elements of Operative Surgery* (New York: Henry G. Langley, 1845–1847).

61. 1860 federal census, Bosqueville, McLennan Co., TX; roll M653_1300; p. 405.

62. 1860 federal census, District 569, Hall Co., GA; roll M653_126, p. 32.

63. "Last Roll: L. A. Whatley," *Confederate Veteran* 19, no. 10 (October 1911), p. 488. Burwell Wilson Ornan Whatley is perhaps the W. O. Whatley who enlisted in Co. K, 1st Regiment Texas Heavy Artillery, CSA, in Marlin, Texas, on 8 February 1863. Lucius Adolphus Whatley served in the Texas state legislature, and his legislative biography notes that his family came to Texas in 1858: see Lewis E. Daniell, *Personnel of the Texas State Government: With Sketches of Distinguished Texans, Embracing the Executive and Staff, Heads of the Departments, United States Senators and Representatives, Members of the XXth Legislature* (Austin: City Printing, 1887), pp. 191–92.

64. Bosqueville was just being laid out in 1858, so it is possible that Russell was exploring the community, in a region with rich, alluvial soil suitable for cotton, as the venue of a newly founded practice. On the town's early history, see Dayton Kelley, *The Handbook of Waco and McLennan County, Texas* (Waco: Texian, 1972); Vivian Elizabeth Smyrl, "Bosqueville, Texas" in *The Handbook of Texas Online* at the website of the Texas State Historical Association at https://tshaonline.org/handbook/online/articles/hnb63 (accessed January 2017); and Nancy Roberts Detlefsen, "Bosqueville," in *Historic McLennan County: An Illustrated History*, ed. Sharon Bracken (San Antonio: Lammert, 2010), p. 19.

65. See Ava Law Russell's Bible.

66. *Times-Picayune* (New Orleans, LA), 21 December 1860, p. 4.

67. See Russell's Mexican War pension affidavit, 26 March 1889, cited *supra*, n. 3. The affidavit appears to have been given in Caddo Parish, LA, but states that he lived in Van Zandt Co., TX.

68. Undated affidavit of Ava Law Russell in ibid.

69. Peter Cozzens, *The Darkest Days of the War: The Battles of Iuka and Corinth* (Chapel Hill: Univ. of North Carolina Press, 1997), pp. 31–32.

70. See "Case of Elisha H. Forsyth, Citizen, Tried in September 1863," Records of the Office of the Judge Advocate General, Army Court Martial Case Files, 1809–1894, box 2025, file 778, RG 153, NARA. The trial was held in Nashville. Russell testified 22–24 September 1863 and Emmel on 1 October. Russell testified that he collaborated with Eugene Shine, St. Louis treasurer of Maurice & Co., as Union Cotton Co. was formed to bring members of the previous firm in Mississippi to carry on business "as we did in Mississippi." Emmel testified that Shine joined Union Cotton after Russell went to St. Louis to purchase supplies for the army and asked Shine to come to Tennessee. Maurice & Co. had extensive railroad interests, and in the late 1850s and early 1860s, the firm undertook to build the Texas and New Orleans Railroad line connecting Houston and New Orleans: see Fay Hempstead, *Historical Review of Arkansas: Its Commerce, Industry and Modern Affairs*, vol. 3 (Chicago: Lewis, 1911), pp. 1186–88. Directors of this project included Truesdail, who had worked for a number of railroad firms prior to his connection to Rosecrans: see John Fitch, *Annals of the Army of the Cumberland* (Philadelphia: J. B. Lippincott, 1863), pp. 346–48; and "Telegraphic Intelligence," *The Daily Delta* (New Orleans, LA), 8 August 1860, p. 2, col. 1, noting that Truesdail was arriving in New Orleans for an organizational meeting of the Texas and New Orleans Railroad Company, of which he was a director.

By summer 1860, Maurice & Co. was operating railroad stores at Beaumont, Liberty, and Gentry: see *Beaumont Banner* (Beaumont, TX), 8 January 1861, p. 3, publishing ads from July and September 1860. It was Corinth's importance as a town in which two rail systems converged that caused the Union-Confederate struggle for its control: see Timothy B. Smith, "A Siege from the Start: The Spring 1862 Campaign against Corinth, Mississippi," *Journal of Mississippi History* 66, no. 4 (2004), pp. 403–24.

71. The ledger is entitled "List of Mail Scouts and Police Vouchers cashed by Col. Taylor Chief Quarter Master Department of the Cumberland from Nov. 1st 1862 to May 1st 1863," Records of the Provost Marshal General's Bureau, entry 41, "Correspondence, Reports and Other Records Relating to Policemen," RG 110, NARA.

72. William Feis, professor of history, Buena Vista Univ., Storm Lake, IA, email communication to William L. Russell, Maumelle, AR, 8 August 2017.

73. See "Contingent Expenses of the War Department, &c." in *Third Session, Forty-First Congress, Executive Documents Printed by Order of the House of Representatives 1870–'1* (United States Congressional Serial Set 1453) (Washington, D.C.: Government Printing Office, 1871), p. 24. There are two separate payments to W. J. P. Russell dated 10 August–10 September and 10 September–10 October, for $98.64 and $92.07, respectively.

74. William B. Feis, *Grant's Secret Service* (Lincoln: Univ. of Nebraska Press, 2002), pp. 127–28, citing Dodge to Rawlins, 5 May 1863, entry 6159, RG 393, NARA.

75. Feis, *Grant's Secret Service*, p. 128.

76. Feis, *Grant's Secret Service*, p. 129.

77. Feis, *Grant's Secret Service*, p. 129.

78. Feis, *Grant's Secret Service*, p. 89.

79. Feis, *Grant's Secret Service*, pp. 109–12.

80. Feis, *Grant's Secret Service*, p. 178.

81. Young's letter is transcribed in *The Papers of Andrew Johnson*, vol. 6, *1862–1864*, ed. Leroy P. Graf and Ralph W. Haskins (Knoxville: Univ. of Tennessee Press, 1983), pp. 87–88. Young ended up imprisoned on charges of double-dealing as a spy: see the *Gallipolis Journal* (Gallipolis, OH), 3 September 1863, p. 3, which reports that the "gasconading rebel" Young had been sent to Nashville from Akron, where he had been confined for nine months, to be tried by a military commission on charges of spying. Graf and Haskins identify the Dr. Russell on whom Young reported as W. J. P. Russell: *Papers of Andrew Johnson*, vol. 6, *1862–1864*, p. 88, n. 2. The note cites Fitch, *Annals of the Army of the Cumberland*, pp. 499–50; and "Proceedings of the Military Commission in the Case of Elisha H. Forsyth," RG 153, NARA. On Fitch's accolades for Truesdail and his police work, see William B. Feis, "'There Is a Bad Enemy in This City': Colonel William Truesdail's Army Police and the Occupation of Nashville, 1862–1863," *North and South* 8, no. 2 (March 2005), p. 43.

82. As George Worthington Adams notes, doctors in both armies were civilians working under contract: see *Doctors in Blue: The Medical History of the Union Army in the Civil War* (Baton Rouge: Louisiana State Univ. Press, 1952), p. 9.

83. See *supra*, n. 47.

84. On Stones River as the point after which Russell ceased working as Assistant Chief of Police, see his pension affidavit, 26 March 1889, cited *supra*, n. 3. On Truesdail's ledger showing his payments to Russell, see *supra*, n. 71. A 10 February 1863 telegram of Provost Marshall William Wiles to Brigadier General Boyle of Louisville, Kentucky, confirms that Russell was no longer serving as Assistant Police Chief by that date. Wiles had telegraphed Truesdail from Murfreesboro on 9 February to ask if he had sent Russell to Louisville and, if so, on what business. Truesdail replied that Russell was no longer working for him, and when Wiles telegraphed Boyle the following day, he stated that Russell had been sent to Louisville on unknown business but was no longer working for Truesdail: see "Provost Marshal, Letters and Telegrams Sent 1863," Department of the Cumberland, entry 1091, p. 17, #50, p. 18, #56, RG 393, pt. 1, NARA. Truesdail resigned due to ill health in October 1863, and his operations then definitively ceased: see Feis, "'There Is a Bad Enemy in This City,'" p. 43.

85. See "Dr. J. R. Hudson, Smuggling and Other Offences," Files of Union Provost Marshal 4275 (Nashville, 1863), held by Tennessee State Library and Archives and online at http://share.tn.gov/tsla/UnionProvostPDFs/4275. pdf (accessed February 2017). "Dr. J. R. Hudson, List of Military Prisoners," Files of Union Provost Marshal 4348 (Jackson, 1863) shows Hudson and his

wife imprisoned and sent south for helping Confederate prisoners escape before the end of March 1863. The file is online at http://share.tn.gov/tsla/UnionProvostPDFs/4348.pdf) (accessed February 2017). On 15 April 1863, *Nashville Daily Union* reports ("Local and Commercial, Further Arrests," p. 3, col. 1) that Hudson and his wife were among "secessionists" arrested on 14 April 1863. Union Provost Marshal File 4789, "Dr. Hudson and Wife," has a letter dated 25 May 1863 from Truesdail to General James D. Morgan stating that the Hudsons had sought to facilitate illicit prisoner exchanges. See also Stanley F. Horn, "Dr. John Rolfe Hudson and the Confederate Underground in Nashville," *Tennessee Historical Quarterly* 22, no. 1 (March 1963), pp. 38–52; and Fitch, *Annals of the Army of the Cumberland*, p. 511. Biographical information about Araminta Hudson is in "Last Roll: Mrs. Araminta Claiborne Hudson," *Confederate Veteran* 12, no. 4 (1904), p. 194, noting that the Hudsons' house Cliff Cottage was behind the penitentiary in which Confederate prisoners were kept and that the family shielded escapees.

86. "Case of Elisha H. Forsyth." As a 15 May 1863 communication that Truesdail sent Wiles's office from Murfreesboro indicates, Russell was by then under investigation for possible involvement in cotton running: the note provides information about "a certain cotton transaction of Dr. W. J. P. Russell" and others, the cotton having been purchased from slaves belonging to a Mr. Hall— see "Provost Marshal, Register of Letters Received, January 1863–December 1864," Department of the Cumberland, pt. 1, entry 1095, #47, RG 393, NARA. It is clear that Truesdail sent the communication as Army officials were gathering information about cotton running in preparation for a hearing. Two weeks after Truesdail sent this communication, Wiles telegraphed Temple Clark (care of Truesdail) at Nashville to tell him that Truesdail was closing up shop with his police operation and that Clark was to consult with General Morgan about the continuation of the police force: see "Provost Marshal, Letters and Telegrams Sent 1863," Department of the Cumberland, entry 1091, #358, RG 393, pt. 1, NARA.

87. Union Citizens' File, Union Provost Marshals' File of Papers Relating to Individual Civilians, 1861–1867, file 22632, NARA, contains a statement dated 2 September 1863 from the arresting officer Major James J. Scarritt to Wiles stating that, per orders, he arrested Russell on suspicion of cotton running on 15 July. On 4 September, Scarritt sent a clarification to Wiles indicating that he had been in error in stating previously that Russell belonged to Forsyth & Co. as he gathered cotton.

88. "Latest News," *Nashville Daily Union* (Nashville, TN), 15 August 1863, p. 3, col. 2.

89. "Case of Elisha H. Forsyth."

90. See *supra*, n. 2. Calvin Goddard's 17 August 1863 note that Russell had been arrested and tried twice is in the same file.

91. Feis, "'There Is a Bad Enemy in This City,'" p. 42. As David G. Moore states, the conflict between Johnson and Rosecrans had to do with the relationship between military versus civilian authority in Middle Tennessee: see *William S. Rosecrans and the Union Victory: A Civil War Biography* (Jefferson, NC: McFarland, 2014), p. 76.

92. Paul H. Bergeron, *Andrew Johnson's Civil War and Reconstruction* (Knoxville: Univ. of Tennessee Press, 2011), pp. 28–29; and Hans L. Trefousse, *Andrew Johnson: A Biography* (New York: W. W. Norton, 1989), p. 163. On Johnson's animosity to Truesdail, see also Feis, "'There Is a Bad Enemy in This City,'" pp. 42–43.

93. See Stephen E. Towne, *Surveillance and Spies in the Civil War: Exposing Confederate Conspiracies in America's Heartland* (Athens, OH: Ohio Univ. Press, 2014), p. 66.

94. Feis, "'There Is a Bad Enemy in This City,'" pp. 37, 41.

95. Feis, "'There Is a Bad Enemy in This City,'" p. 37, citing Truesdail to Rosecrans, 15 January 1863, Records of the United States Army Continental Command, part I, entry 925, box 20, RG 393, NARA. On Nashville as "the great centre to which thronged all the hordes of smugglers, spies, and secret plotters of treason, whom a love of treachery or of gain had drawn to the rebel cause," see Fitch, *Annals of the Army of the Cumberland*, p. 457, as cited, Horn, "Dr. John Rolfe Hudson and the Confederate Underground in Nashville," p. 39.

96. "Fall of Rosecrans," *Washington Chronicle* (Washington, D.C.), 24 October 1863, p. 1. The article was picked up by other newspapers, including the *Shelby Volunteer* (Shelbyville, IN), which ran it on 5 November 1863, p. 1, col. 3–5. The *Chronicle* states that it published its piece to refute positive treatment of Rosecrans by Fitch's *Annals of the Army of the Cumberland*, which was published in fall 1863.

For a countervailing assessment of Rosecrans's and Truesdail's activities, see John S. C. Abbott, *Comprising a Full and Impartial Account of the Origin and Progress of the Rebellion, of the Various Naval and Military Engagements, of the Heroic Deeds Performed by Armies and Individuals, and of Touching Scenes in the Field, the Camp, the Hospital, and the Cabin*, vol. 2 (New York: Henry Hill, 1866), p. 361, which claims that Truesdail's police work reduced smuggling, profiteering, and spying in Nashville; and the pro-Rosecrans *Nashville Daily Union's* (Nashville, TN) 8 April 1863 article "A Trip to Murfreesboro," applauding the "iron will and untiring energy" of Rosecrans (p. 3, col. 1).

97. See "Case of Elisha H. Forsyth." On 2 October, Forsyth was found guilty of obtaining money under fraudulent pretenses and conspiring to bribe government officials. He was fined $6,000 and sentenced to a month of imprisonment at hard labor. A 23 August 1864 note from Major General Lovell Rousseau in Forsyth's case file remits the prison sentence.

98. Robert Wiles was in Corinth in late summer 1862: see "List of Arrivals," *Corinth War Eagle* (Corinth, MS), 7 August 1862, p. 2, col. 2, listing guests at Corinth House Hotel; see also 24 September 1863 testimony of W. J. P. Russell in "Case of Elisha H. Forsyth"; and Towne, *Surveillance and Spies*, p. 66. In their annotated edition of Johnson's papers, Graf and Haskins explain that Forsyth and Robert Wiles had been in the cotton business together: *Papers of Andrew Johnson*, vol. 6, *1862–1864*, p. 350, n. 2, and p. 351, n. 4, citing "Case of Elisha H. Forsyth." In a 12 September 1863 article entitled "Cotton Speculators—Singular Reports," *Nashville Daily Union* (Nashville, TN) reports (p. 1, col. 7) that Forsyth and Wiles had been arrested for confiscating cotton from Confederates and buying cotton from Unionists while falsely representing themselves as

US agents. The article states that Russell had been named but not charged in the case.

99. Russell's apprehensions were well founded. See the chain of communications from Wiles to General Morgan in July–August 1863 in M345 Union Provost Marshals' File of Papers Relating to Individual Citizens, roll 236, NARA: Wiles to General Morgan, 30 July, "Letters and Telegrams Sent 1863," entry 1091, p. 144, #530 and p. 145, #533; Wiles to Captain Goodwin, 31 July, ibid., entry 1091, p. 148, #546, stating that in Wiles's view, Russell was "acting rascally"; and a 3 August telegram from Wiles called for Russell to be arrested, ibid., entry 1091, #568. Wiles telegrammed Morgan on the fourth, instructing him to send Russell to Rosecrans's Winchester headquarters on the fifth: See ibid., entry 1091, p. 175, #639. On the fourteenth, Stanley sent Wiles's office a communication stating that Russell and George Telan would be important witnesses before the commission investigating cotton speculation, which had convened on the thirteenth at Murfreesboro: See ibid., entry 1095, #145. In preparation for this, Russell had provided a statement on the tenth: See ibid., entry 1095, #56. On the sixteenth, Wiles wrote Stanley telling him that Russell and others were at Winchester under guard at Stanley's request: see ibid., entry 1091, p. 177, #652.

100. M345 Union Provost Marshals' File of Papers Relating to Individual Citizens, roll 236, NARA. Since the letter was written in haste and Russell was agitated, some words are unclear. We have indicated words we cannot read with bracketed question marks. The letter is accompanied by a summary on 21 August stating that Russell was leaving Nashville: "Starts for home today address for next ten days will be Jonesboro Illinois—is afraid of being arrested & put out of the way by Taylor Wiles & others &c." The following day, Wiles telegraphed General Granger to tell him that Russell, "Cotton Speculator with others," had been paroled and it had been reported to Wiles that he was being permitted to go beyond the limits of the Department of the Cumberland. Wiles was telegraphing to ask if this information was correct and, if so, by whose authority this was done: See Letters and Telegrams Sent 1863," entry 1091, p. 182, #670. On the twenty-third, Wiles telegraphed Granger's assistant to notify him that Forsyth, Russell, and others, "Cotton men" who had been paroled, were to remain at Nashville by command of the Provost Marshal and were to take the train next day to Stevenson, Alabama, where Stanley's commission would reassemble on 24 August: see ibid., entry 1091, #685.

See also Wiles's 1 September letters to Andrew Johnson and Stanley's assistant William Henry Sinclair, telling Johnson that he was preparing a statement about Russell's involvement in cotton speculation and responding to Stanley's query about Russell's 15 July arrest: Union Provost Marshals' File of Papers Relating to Individual Citizens, roll 236, M345, NARA; Union Citizens' File, Union Provost Marshals' File of Papers Relating to Individual Civilians, 1861–1867, file 22632, NARA; and "Letters and Telegrams Sent 1863," entry 1091, p. 202, #739.

101. Union Co., IL, Deed Bk. 19, pp. 496–97.

102. Union Co., IL, Collection Book, List of Taxable Real Estate, 1864, pp. 201–2; ibid., 1865, pp. 168–69.

103. The date and place of birth are in Ava's Bible.

104. *The War of the Rebellion: A Compilation of the Official Records of the Union*

and Confederate Armies, series 2, vol. 5, serial 118: *Correspondence, Orders, etc.,*
Relating to Prisoners of War and State, Dec. 1, 1862–June 10, 1863 (Washington:
Government Printing Office, 1899), pp. 521–22.

105. "From the West: The Cotton Business," *New York Times* (New York,
NY), 4 December 1864, p. 3, col. 6. See also "The Cotton Crop in Illinois," *Alton
Telegraph* (Alton, IL), 24 November 1865, p. 6, col. 4, stating that the fall crop
was the largest ever raised in Illinois; and "Cotton in Union County," *Ottawa
Free Trader* (Ottawa, IL), 3 February 1866, p. 2, col. 1, reporting that 4,000 bales
of the 1865 crop had been shipped from Union County with bales averaging 400
pounds each, for a net of $640,000 for local planters.

106. The death date is in Ava's Bible with a statement that William is buried
in Jonesboro.

107. Union Co., IL, Deed Bk. 21, pp. 446–47. There are actually two deeds for
this sale. The first shows W. J. P. and Ava as grantors (Union Co., IL, Deed Bk.
21, p. 28). The second (pp. 446–47) has Ava as grantor, which is in line with her
deed of purchase. The land description and acreage are the same in both deeds,
but the dates, grantees, and price of the land are different: On 25 May 1865,
W. J. P. and Ava sold 280 acres to E. Mackindsee for $1,100. On 25 October 1865,
Ava sold the same 280 acres to Alex Cruse for $3,000.

The family's move to Alexandria after they left Illinois is mentioned
later in letters exchanged by W. J. P. and Ava's daughter Ava Leona to
Benjamin Franklin Norwood, who became connected to her father in business
ventures as early as 1880 and later married Ava Leona.

108. John D. Winters, *The Civil War in Louisiana* (Baton Rouge: Louisiana
State Univ. Press, 1963), pp. 331–32.

109. The date and place of death are in Ava's Bible.

110. See John Spurgeon, "Trail of Tears National Historic Trail," in
Encyclopedia of Arkansas History and Culture, online at website of Butler Center
for Arkansas Studies at http://www.encyclopediaofarkansas.net/encyclopedia/
entry-detail.aspx?search=1&entryID=4887 (accessed November 2017).

111. Goodspeed's *History of Benton, Washington, Carroll, Madison, Crawford,
Franklin, and Sebastian Counties, Arkansas* (Chicago: Goodspeed, 1889), p. 268.

112. Frank Norwood, Hope, AR, 10 November 1881 letter to Ava Leona
Russell in Eureka Springs, AR, William James Park Russell Family Letters.

113. Ava Leona Russell, Boonsboro, AR, to Frank Norwood, [Alexandria,
LA?], 24 April 1881, in ibid.

114. W. J. P. Russell, Eureka Springs, AR, to Frank Norwood [Alexandria,
LA?], 27 December 1881, in ibid. Several other family letters mention the livestock business.

115. Baird, *Medical Education in Arkansas*, p. 10.

116. Stowe, *Doctoring in the South*, p. 8.

117. Baird, *Medical Education in Arkansas*, p. 12.

118. Baird, *Medical Education in Arkansas*, pp. 13–14.

119. Baird, *Medical Education in Arkansas*, p. 14.

120. *Van Buren Press* (Van Buren, AR), 7 September 1866, p. 2, col. 4.

121. See Jacob Barker, *The Rebellion: Its Consequences, and the Congressional
Committee, Denominated the Reconstruction Committee, with Their Action* (New
Orleans: Commercial Print, 1866), pp. 221–22; and Gregg Andrews, "The Racial

Politics in Ralls County, 1865–1870," in *The Other Missouri History: Populists, Prostitutes, and Regular Folk*, ed. Thomas Morris Spencer (Columbia: Univ. of Missouri Press, 2004), p. 15.

122. Washington Co., AR, Deed Bk. R, p. 310.

123. Goodspeed's *History of Benton, Washington, Carroll, Madison, Crawford, Franklin, and Sebastian Counties, Arkansas*, p. 305.

124. See Ava's Bible.

125. Washington Co., AR, Marriage Bk. C, p. 349. Wallace and Julia divorced, and he then married Martha Gray on 8 January 1879: Crawford Co., AR, Marriage Bk. A, p. 191.

126. *Arkansas Gazette* (Little Rock, AR), 13 October 1868, p. 3, col. 5.

127. *Arkansas Gazette* (Little Rock, AR), 15–16 October 1868, p. 2.

128. *Arkansas Gazette* (Little Rock, AR), 20 October 1868, p. 2.

129. *Arkansas Gazette* (Little Rock, AR), 21 October 1868, p. 3.

130. *Arkansas Gazette* (Little Rock, AR), 13 November 1868, p. 3.

131. See Julanne S. Allison, "Cane Hill (Washington County)," in *Encyclopedia of Arkansas History and Culture*, online at website of Butler Center for Arkansas Studies at http://www.encyclopediaofarkansas.net/encyclopedia/entry-detail.aspx?entryID=2705# (accessed February 2017).

132. Ava's Bible records both Lilly's and Dick's dates and places of birth. It states that Dick was born near "Bethesday Camp Ground."

133. Albert Burton Moore, *History of Alabama and Her People*, vol. 2 (Chicago: American Historical Society, 1927), pp. 528–29.

134. Washington Co., AR, Real Estate Tax Record, 1878, p. 201, delinquent taxes, August 1878, noting that Russell had not paid taxes on land in Section 12, Range 33 West since 1875. He forfeited ten acres, the southeast corner of the southeast corner of Section 14, Township 14, Range 33 West.

135. Washington Co., AR Personal Property Tax, 1870, p. 67, Vineyard Township.

136. See *supra*, n. 73.

137. The birthdate and place of birth are recorded in Ava's Bible in her hand.

138. On the collection entitled William James Park Russell Family Letters, see *supra*, n. 46.

139. Ava Law Russell, Boonsboro, AR, to Mary Bedell, 14 April 1878, William James Park Russell Family Letters.

140. Rohrbough, *Trans-Appalachian Frontier*, pp. 285–88.

141. Sarah M. Fountain, "Introduction," in *Sisters, Seeds and Cedars: Rediscovering Nineteenth-Century Life Through Correspondence from Rural Arkansas and Alabama*, ed. Fountain (Conway, AR: Univ. of Central Arkansas Press, 1995), pp. xiii-xvi.

142. Bethany May, "Eureka Springs," in *Encyclopedia of Arkansas History and Culture*, online at website of Butler Center for Arkansas Studies at http://www.encyclopediaofarkansas.net/encyclopedia/entry-detail.aspx?entryID=843 (accessed March 2017).

143. The original handwritten ledger of the Fayetteville attorney is held by the Fayetteville Public Library—see "Dr. Russell's Account," p. 104.

144. Ava Leona Russell, Eureka Springs, AR, to Frank Norwood, 12 July 1881, William James Park Russell Family Letters.

145. W. J. P. Russell, Eureka Springs, AR, to Frank Norwood, 27 December 1881, in ibid.

146. Ava Russell, Boonsboro, AR, to Ava Norwood, 18 June 1883, in ibid. The letter also speaks of Ava Norwood's former music teacher, "Mrs James Jr. Jones," whose husband had been elected to Congress and who was in D.C. with him. Musical education for daughters was a preoccupation of families of the class to which the Russells belonged in the American South. The musical accomplishments of the Russell women are mentioned frequently in family correspondence. In a 20 August 1973 oral interview, Lavetta Russell Pack, a daughter of Seaborn Russell, described her grandmother Ava to William L. Russell as "an accomplished musician." In a 4 January 1974 conversation with William L. Russell, Grace Russell Norton stated that her grandmother taught music to augment the family's income. In a 15 February 1974 letter to William L. Russell, Norton also stated that her grandmother taught piano and had been educated at a select school in the eastern states.

147. Ava Leona Russell, Eureka Springs, AR, to Frank Norwood, 20 May 1881, William James Park Russell Family Letters.

148. Ava Leona Russell, Eureka Springs, AR, to Frank Norwood, Alexandria, LA, 18 December 1881, in ibid.

149. On the belief that spring water from the area had curative properties and on attempts to promote it as a curative, see May, "Eureka Springs." On the interest in hydropathic cures in the latter part of the nineteenth century, see Numbers, "Do-It-Yourself the Sectarian Way," pp. 92–93.

150. Ava Leona Russell, Eureka Springs, AR, to Frank Norwood, 6 January 1883, William James Park Russell Family Letters.

151. See *supra*, n. 147.

152. Ava Leona Russell, Eureka Springs, AR, to Frank Norwood, Alexandria, LA, 18 December 1881, William James Park Russell Family Letters.

153. Ava Leona Russell, Eureka Springs, AR, to Frank Norwood, 2 February 1883 (noting that the family had returned to Boonsboro), in ibid.

154. The date and place of death are written in Ava's Bible in her hand.

155. The dates of marriage and spouses are written in Ava's Bible, which says the couple married 8 March, while his letter to his parents about his marriage says that they married on the evening of 7 March. The latter is the date of the marriage in their marriage record in Washington Co., AR. The marriage of Seaborn Russell and Alcie Bachelor is in Franklin Co., AR, Marriage Bk. B, pp. 501–2; Frank Norwood and Ava Russell's marriage is in Washington Co., AR, Marriage Bk. G, p. 398; William Troutt and Sevie Russell's marriage is in Washington Co., AR, Marriage Bk. F, p. 568.

156. Ava Russell, Boonsboro, AR, to Ava Norwood, 29 April 1883, William James Park Russell Family Letters.

157. W. J. P. Russell, Arkadelphia, AR, to Frank Norwood, New Iberia, LA, 10 February 1883, in ibid.

158. Steven Teske, "Nashville (Howard County)," in *The Encyclopedia of*

Arkansas History and Culture, online at the website of the Butler Center for Arkansas Studies at http://www.encyclopediaofarkansas.net/encyclopedia/entry-detail.aspx?entryID=899 (accessed March 2017).

159. Ava Russell, Nashville, AR, to Ava Norwood, 3 December 1883, William James Park Russell Family Letters.

160. Ava Leona Russell, Eureka Springs, AR, to Frank Norwood, 15 February 1882, in ibid.

161. Death Certificate of Richard Delton [*sic*] Russell, 27 October 1928, Texas Death Certificate #45869, Van Zandt Co., TX, State Board of Health, Bureau of Vital Statistics. This document gives Richard's occupation as a cotton buyer.

162. See *supra*, n. 159.

163. See Betty DeBerg, *Ungodly Women: Gender and the First Wave of American Fundamentalism* (Macon: Mercer Univ. Press, 2000), pp. 23–24; Barbara Welter, *Dimity Convictions: The American Woman in the Nineteenth Century* (Athens, OH: Ohio Univ, Press, 1976), p. 126; Linda K. Kerber, "Separate Spheres, Female Worlds, Woman's Place: The Rhetoric of Women's History," *The Journal of American History* 75, no. 1 (1988), pp. 9–39; Michele Adams, "Divisions of Household Labor," in *The Concise Encyclopedia of Sociology*, ed. George Ritzer and J. Michael Ryan (Malden, MA: Wiley-Blackwell, 2011), pp. 156–57.

164. Mary Moore, Cowala, Indian Territory, to Ava Norwood, 14 February 1884, William James Park Russell Family Letters.

165. See Dorothy Bateman Barnes, "Wills Point, Texas," in *The Handbook of Texas Online* at the website of Texas State Historical Association at https://tshaonline.org/handbook/online/articles/hgw10 (accessed March 2017).

166. Seaborn Russell, Memphis, TN, to Ava Norwood, 31 August 1885, William James Park Russell Family Letters.

167. The card was with the collection of family letters given to William L. Russell by Sarah Lee Suttle, which now constitute the William James Park Russell Family Letters.

168. "State News, Morphined Himself," *Fort Worth Daily Gazette* (Fort Worth, TX), 1 January 1886, p. 5, col. 1.

169. Ava Russell, Dallas, TX, to Ava Norwood, 6 April 1886, William James Park Russell Family Letters.

170. "Execution Sale," *Fayetteville Weekly Democrat* (Fayetteville, AR), 25 May 1882, p. 3, col. 6.

171. *Morrison and Fourmy's General Directory of the City of Dallas 1886–87* (Galveston: Morrison & Fourmy, 1887), pp. 266, 350. There's a double listing with the same information. W. J. P. Russell and his son Ralph are both listed at 172 Elm Street. The directory erroneously gives W. J. P.'s initials as J. B.

172. Ava Russell, Dallas, TX, to Ava Norwood, 28 June 1886, William James Park Russell Family Letters.

173. The community's newspaper *Wills Point Chronicle* states in a 13 October 1887 article that the town's population was 1,200 and that it had four physicians. The article is cited by Kitty Wheeler, *Histories and Biographies of Van Zandt County*, vol. 2, *1848–1991* (Wills Point: Van Zandt County Genealogical Society,

1991). An excerpt from this volume entitled "Post Offices, Cities, Towns and People," is online at the website of the Van Zandt County Research Group at http://www.rootsweb.ancestry.com/~txvzcgrg/grgPO60.htm (accessed September 2017). This is the source for our citation of the 13 October 1887 issue of the *Wills Point Chronicle*. Seaborn's purchase of forty acres at Wills Point on 25 August 1886 is recorded in Van Zandt Co, TX, Deed Bk. 34, pp. 526–27.

174. See Russell's pension application cited *supra*, n. 3, and Ava Law Russell's widow's pension application cited *supra*, n. 33.

175. Ava Russell, Wills Point, TX, to Ava Norwood, 19 November 1886, William James Park Russell Family Letters.

176. The article is clipped and pasted into a scrapbook maintained by Ava Norwood and now in ibid.

177. W. J. P. Russell, Pine Bluff, AR, to Frank Norwood, 1 October 1887, William James Park Russell Family Letters.

178. W. J. P. Russell, Cumberland, MS, to Ava Norwood, 27 June 1888, in ibid.

179. See *supra*, n. 2.

180. See Russell's pension application, cited *supra*, n. 3. The claim application notes that he served in the US 3rd Infantry under Lieutenant Ward.

181. Index to Mexican War pension claims, Texas, NARA microfilm publication T317, claim 10579, certificate 9137.

182. W. J. P. Russell, Lake Charles, LA, to Ava Norwood, 4 June 1890, William James Park Russell Family Letters.

183. 30 May 1975 letter of Grace Russell Norton, Wills Point, TX, to William L. Russell, Maumelle, AR, in possession of William L. Russell.

184. See Ava's Bible, which records her husband's date and place of death; *Fort Worth Gazette* (Fort Worth, TX), 1 February 1892, p. 6, col. 4; *Times-Star* (Terrell, TX), 5 February 1892, p. 3. Ava's 14 April 1892 affidavit for a widow's pension for her husband's service also states that he died 25 January 1892 at Wills Point: see her widow's pension application cited *supra*, n. 33.

185. See Russell's pension application, cited *supra*, n. 3.

186. 1900 federal census, Van Zandt Co., TX; roll T623_1675, p. 12A, ED 129.

187. The date of Ava Law Russell's death was recorded in her family Bible by her daughter Ava. The 30 May 1975 letter of Grace Russell Norton to William L. Russell (see *supra*, n. 183) states that her grandmother Ava died at the home of daughter Ava Norwood in Stamps, AR.

188. 30 May 1975 letter of Grace Russell Norton to William L. Russell, see *supra*, n. 183.

Chapter 3

1. Diary of Seaborn Rentz Russell, 7 September 1922, original in possession of the Marvin Vaughter family. A transcription is in the William James Park Russell Family Letters.

2. George W. Russell, Allentown, PA, to William L. Russell, Maumelle, AR, March 1976; original in possession of William L. Russell and copy in William James Park Russell Family Letters.

3. Diary of Seaborn Russell, 13 July 1921.

4. See "Mrs. Russell's Death," *Arkansas Democrat* (Little Rock, AR), 7 May 1900, p. 3, col. 3.

5. Diary of Seaborn Russell, 11 March 1922.

6. See Bible of Ava Law Russell.

7. See 1860 federal census, Polk Co., GA, Militia District 1072, Van Wert Post Office; roll M653_134; p. 189. Congressman Seaborn Jones was the nephew of another noted Seaborn Jones who was first speaker of the Georgia House, for whom many Georgians named sons: see Anna Caroline Benning, "Seaborn Jones," in *Men of Mark in Georgia: A Complete and Elaborate History of the State from Its Settlement to the Present Time, Chiefly Told in Biographies and Autobiographies of the Most Eminent Men of Each Period of Georgia's Progress and Development*, ed. William J. Northen and John Temple Graves, vol. 2 (Atlanta: A. B. Caldwell, 1910), pp. 236–42; and Lucian Lamar Knight, *Georgia's Landmarks, Memorials, and Legends*, vol. 2 (Atlanta: Byrd, 1914), pp. 400–2. On Seaborn Jones of Van Wert, see Greg D. Sargent, *Polk County, Georgia* (Charleston, SC: Arcadia, 1998), p. 5, which notes that he was director of Polk's first railroad company, the Selma, Rome, and Dalton Co., and was instrumental in having the railroad extend from Van Wert to Rockmart. Several documents suggest connections between him and the Rentz family of Van Wert: on the federal census in 1870, Jones has in his household a family of African American servants with the surname Rentz; and a 21 March 1865 letter of David Clopton of Van Wert to his ward Fannie Franklin Hargrave suggests that as the Civil War ended, the Jones and Rentz families were actually living together—see 1870 federal census, Polk Co., GA; roll M593_170; page 266A; and Hargrave Family Papers, Annie Belle Weaver Special Collections, Irvine Sullivan Ingram Library, University of West GA.

8. Diary of Seaborn Russell, 28 July 1921.

9. George W. Russell, Allentown, PA, to William L. Russell, Maumelle, AR, March 1976: see *supra*, n. 2.

10. Franklin Co., AR, Marriage Bk. B, pp. 501–2.

11. Like the Russells, the Bachelor family prized education for both sons and daughters; Wilson Bachelor's diary indicates that he schooled all his children in the same subjects, with no distinctions based on gender: see Lindsey, *Fiat Flux*, pp. 46, 181–82, n. 58.

12. 1880 federal census, Washington Co., AR, Cane Hill Township, ED 211; roll: 58; p. 624C.

13. 1880 federal census, Productions of Agriculture, Sebastian-Woodruff, June 1880, Cane Hill Township, Washington Co., AR, pg. 7, reel MG04412, AR State Archives.

14. Franklin Co., AR, Tax Bk., 1882, p. 60; Franklin Co., AR, Tax Bk., Personal Property Assessed for Taxation, 1883, no pagination, School District 41 (Seaborn is taxed for horses and neat cattle); Franklin Co., AR, Tax Bk., 1884, p. 161; Franklin Co., AR, Real Estate Tax Bk., 1885, pg. 120, which shows S. R. Russell taxed for forty acres in Section 30, Township 9, Range 28. In both 1883–1884, Seaborn is delinquent. The tax lists indicate that the property was in Mill Creek Township, where Alcie's family lived.

15. Howard Co., AR, Personal Taxes, 1884, p. 40.

16. Seaborn R. Russell, Memphis, TN, to Ava Norwood, 31 August 1885, William James Park Russell Family Letters.

17. W. J. P. Russell, Dallas, TX, to Ava Norwood, 25 December 1885, in ibid.

18. Seaborn bought more land in June 1887 in concert with his mother: on both land purchases, see Van Zandt Co., TX, Deed Bk. 37, pp. 80–82, and 39, p. 314.

19. Ava Russell, Wills Point, TX, to Ava Norwood, 19 November 1886, William James Park Russell Family Letters.

20. *Wills Point Chronicle* (Wills Point, TX), 20 January 1887, p. 3, col. 5.

21. *Wills Point Chronicle*, 27 January 1887, p. 3, col. 3.

22. W. J. P. Russell, Wills Point, Texas, to Ava Norwood, 22 January 1887, William James Park Russell Family Letters.

23. See *supra*, p. 235, n. 176.

24. See *supra*, n. 18.

25. Franklin Co., AR, Deed Bk. XX, p. 1. Seaborn was taxed for the land in 1887: see Franklin Co., AR, List of Lands to be Assessed for Taxation in Franklin Co for 1887, p. 165.

26. *Wills Point Chronicle* (Wills Point, TX), 27 October 1887, p. 3, col. 5.

27. W. J. P. Russell, Wills Point, TX, to Frank Norwood, 28 October 1889, William James Park Russell Family Letters.

28. Van Zandt Co., TX, Deed Bk. 42, pp. 278–80.

29. The diary entries are transcribed in Lindsey, *Fiat Flux*, p. 76. On 24 December 1894, Wilson Bachelor noted that Alcie and her children were living near him (ibid., p. 77).

30. William L. Russell of Maumelle, AR, has a copy of the letter given to him in the 1970s by Maude Russell's nephew Clayton Russell of Fort Smith, AR, who had received a copy from Maude Russell's daughter Jamie Morris Walker of Lubbock, TX.

31. Van Zandt Co., TX, Deed Bk. 76, pp. 429–31.

32. Greene Co., AR, Personal Property Taxes Bk. 3, p. 67. In addition to a poll tax, Seaborn is taxed for a horse, a cow, and personal property evaluated at eighty dollars total.

33. Jackson Co., AR, Medical Register A, pp. 24–25, showing registration of the credentials of "S. R. Russell, age 33, April 4, 1892, Graduated 1880, Medical College of Philadelphia."

34. *Arkansas State Gazetteer Business Directories 1893–1894* (Detroit: R. L. Polk, 1894), p. 345.

35. "Lorado," in *Greene County, Arkansas: History and Families*, vol. 1, ed. Greene County Historical and Genealogical Society (Paducah, KY: Turner, 2001), p. 20. No author is given.

36. See Social Security file of Maybelle Emma Russell (#432096106), stating that she was born at Paragould, daughter of William Seaborn Russell and Emma O'Lear [*sic*].

37. Winnie Franklin, "Reminiscences of Early Lorado," *Greene County Historical Quarterly* 6, no. 4 (1971), p. 14.

38. Greene Co., AR, Personal Property Taxes Bk. 5, p. 64.

39. Greene Co., AR, Personal Property Taxes Bk. 1, p. 60.

40. Greene Co., AR, Mortgage Bk. 7, p. 236.

41. *Charlotte [NC] Medical Journal* 4, no. 2 (February 1894), p. 80.

42. Beebe Methodist Church Membership Roll, Beebe, AR (Chronological Roll of Full Membership), p. 247641, #353, 11–1899 (for Dr. W. S. R. Russell) and #354, 11–1899 (for Emma Russell). They were removed from membership in May 1900.

43. 1900 federal census, Franklin Co., AR, Mill Creek Township, ED 195; roll 58; p. 4B.

44. 1910 federal census, Franklin Co., AR, Mill Creek Township, ED 46; roll T624_50; p. 5A.

45. See *supra*, n. 5.

46. *Arkansas Democrat* (Little Rock, AR), 21 September 1900, p. 2, col. 4.

47. See "Mrs. Russell's Death."

48. *Nashville News* (Nashville, AR), 14 July 1900, p. 2.

49. Lounetta Hoobler Russell's Bible was published by P. W. Ziegler of Philadelphia and gives no publication date. It belonged to Seaborn and Lounetta's grandson Gary Frank Pack of North Little Rock, AR, until his death in 2012, and is now in possession of his widow, Sandy Pack. The marriage of Seaborn and Lounetta is recorded in Pulaski Co., AR, Marriage Bk. 39, p. 187.

50. *Arkansas Gazette* (Little Rock, AR), 24 April 1903, p. 1, col. 5.

51. Application for License to Practice Medicine in the State of Arkansas, W. S. R. Russell, Houston, Perry Co., AR, 8 July 1903, certificate 2655, State Medical Board of AR.

52. Robert S. Gillespie, "The Train Doctors: A Detailed History of Railway Surgeons," online at the website of RailwaySurgery.org at http://railwaysurgery .org/HistoryLong.htm (accessed October 2017).

53. See Steven Teske, "Houston (Perry County)," *Encyclopedia of Arkansas History and Culture*, online at website of Butler Center for Arkansas Studies at http://www.encyclopediaofarkansas.net/encyclopedia/entry-detail.aspx? entryID=7165 (accessed April 2017).

54. See George Kemper, "Houston," in *Perry County, Arkansas, Its Land and People*, ed. Perry County Historical and Genealogical Society (Marceline, MO: Walworth, 2004), p. 143–44.

55. Application for License to Practice Medicine in the State of Arkansas, W. S. R. Russell, Houston, Perry Co., AR, 8 July 1903, certificate 2655, State Medical Board of AR.

56. See College of Physicians and Surgeons, *Second Annual Catalogue and Announcement Session of 1907–1908* (Little Rock, AR, June 1907), unpaginated. Matriculants' names follow the title page. An extant copy is held by University of Arkansas for Medical Sciences Library, Historical Research Center, Little Rock, AR.

57. See "W. S. R. Russell," "United States Deceased Physician File (AMA), 1864–1968," American Medical Association, online at the FamilySearch website at https://familysearch.org/ark:/61903/3:1:3QSQ-G9QP-6GYW? cc=2061540&wc=M6Y8-XP6%3A353101901 (accessed April 2017). The AMA card appears to rely on information provided by the Arkansas Medical Board.

58. See Baird, *Medical Education in Arkansas*, pp. 53–55.

59. Perry Co., AR, Deed Bk. U, p. 418.

60. Perry Co., AR, Record of Mortgages of Personal Property Filed, 1904, p. 127, case file 2864, instrument dated 2 January 1904, filed 7 January 1904.

61. Pulaski Co., AR, List of Legal Voters, Persons Who Paid Poll Tax, 1904, Bk. 3, p. 314.

62. Pulaski Co., AR, List of Legal Voters, Persons Who Paid Poll Tax, Bk. 2, p. 49.

63. Diary of Seaborn Russell, 22 February 1922.

64. *Arkansas Gazette* (Little Rock, AR), 12 October 1960, p. 11A, col. 1.

65. Pulaski Co., AR, Medical Register, Bk. A, p. 6, 20 January 1904.

66. "Late Local News," *Arkansas Democrat* (Little Rock, AR), 23 September 1905, p. 7, col. 5.

67. Pulaski Co., AR, Deed Bk. 88, p. 324. The land was in Section 22, Township 1 North, Range 13 West.

68. See Pulaski Co., AR, Real Estate Taxes, Taxes Assessed and Extended against Real Property, 1906, p. 169; 1907, p. 181; 1908, p. 177; 1909, p. 175; 1910, p. 169; 1911, p. 175; 1912, p. 177; 1913, p. 176; 1914, p. 175; 1915, p. 190; 1916, p. 215; 1917, p. 203; 1918, p. 236; 1919, p. 244; 1920, p. 240; 1921, p. 240.

69. Perry Co., AR, Deed Bk. P, p. 520.

70. Diary of Seaborn Russell, 22 February 1922.

71. 1910 federal census, Pulaski Co., AR, Brodie Township, ED 106; roll T624_62; p. 3B. The street address is Upper Hot Springs Road.

72. "Same Judges and Clerks to Serve," *Arkansas Democrat* (Little Rock, AR), 20 March 1914, p. 12, col. 3.

73. *Polk's Southern Directory Co.'s Little Rock and Argenta City Directory 1914* (Little Rock: Polk's Southern Directory, 1914), p. 473 and 5a.

74. Diary of Seaborn Russell, 22 February 1922.

75. "Ruth Marie Powell," *Arkansas Democrat* (Little Rock, AR), 9 August 1918, p. 10, col. 2.

76. *Arkansas Democrat* (Little Rock, AR), 30 March 1918, p. 12, col. 3.

77. See *Polk's Southern Directory Co.'s Little Rock and North Little Rock City Directory 1919* (Little Rock: Polk's Southern Directory, 1919), p. 306.

78. "Is Fined $25 For Hitting Father In Law," *Arkansas Democrat* (Little Rock, AR), 16 April 1919, p. 7, col. 3.

79. See Michael Dougan, "Health and Medicine," *Encyclopedia of Arkansas History and Culture*, online at website of Butler Center for Arkansas Studies at http://www.encyclopediaofarkansas.net/encyclopedia/entry-detail.aspx?search=1&entryID=392 (accessed 17 January 2019).

80. See Michael Dougan, "Medical Malpractice," *Encyclopedia of Arkansas History and Culture*, online at website of Butler Center for Arkansas Studies at http://www.encyclopediaofarkansas.net/encyclopedia/entry-detail.aspx?search=1&entryID=5319 (accessed 7 February 2019).

81. See Melanie Welch, "Abortion", in *Encyclopedia of Arkansas History and Culture*, online at website of Butler Center for Arkansas Studies at http://www.encyclopediaofarkansas.net/encyclopedia/entry-detail.aspx?search=1&entryID=5324&media=print (accessed 7 February 2019).

82. Diary of Seaborn Russell, 7 July 1920.

83. See "Fords for Rent," *Arkansas Gazette* (Little Rock, AR), 17 Oct 1920, p. 10, col. 2.

84. Diary of Seaborn Russell, 25 July 1920.

85. Diary of Seaborn Russell, 21 September 1920.

86. This was William Steinkamp, born 16 April 1882 in Westphalia, Germany, according to his Social Security file, application #429286487. The 1920 federal census shows him and wife Sophie with a boarding house at 1120 W. 7th Street: See 1920 federal census, Little Rock, Pulaski Co., AR, Ward 5, ED 134; roll T625_79; p. 4B. The same census shows William H. Parsell, a furniture maker, with his family at 2723 W. 7th Street. He is aged fifty-six in 1920: See 1920 federal census, Little Rock, Pulaski Co., AR, Ward 4, ED 129; roll T625_78; p. 11A. On 3 September 1920, Seaborn's diary says he and "Uncle Tom Parsell" had attended the funeral of "poor Tom McDade," who had been murdered by his cousin James McDade—a "bad whiskey death": see Diary of Seaborn Russell, 3 September 1920.

87. Diary of Seaborn Russell, 12 January 1921.

88. Diary of Seaborn Russell, 13 January 1921.

89. Diary of Seaborn Russell, 22 January 1921.

90. Diary of Seaborn Russell, 26 January 1921.

91. Diary of Seaborn Russell, 22 November 1921.

92. Pulaski Co., AR, Marriage Bk. 62, p. 599. The couple divorced 16 October 1924: Arkansas Divorce Bk. 34, docket 32862.

93. Diary of Seaborn Russell, 29 January 1921. We can find no medical term equivalent to "tulymasis." Joseph Phineas Runyan (1869–1931) founded St. Luke in 1911 and operated it in conjunction with Dr. Henry Hodgen Kirby (1883–1922). Runyan was president of the Arkansas Medical Society in 1904 and founder, dean, and president of the College of Physicians and Surgeons in Little Rock from 1906 until this college merged with the medical depart-ment of University of Arkansas in 1912: see Dallas T. Herndon, *Centennial History of Arkansas*, vol. 2 (Chicago: S. J. Clarke, 1922), pp. 116–19; and Fay Hempstead, *Historical Review of Arkansas: Its Commerce, Industry and Modern Affairs*, vol. 2 (Chicago: Lewis, 1911), p. 712. Runyan's obituary is in *Journal of the Arkansas Medical Society* 27, no. 9 (February 1931), pp. 191–92. When the *Arkansas Democrat* announced the graduation of the first class of the College of Physicians and Surgeons on 1 May 1907, with Runyan as master of ceremo-nies, it noted that Dr. W. S. Russell of Halstead attended the graduation: see "Eleven Graduates in First Class of the College of P. & S.," *Arkansas Democrat* (Little Rock, AR), 1 May 1907, p. 6, col. 2. Seaborn and Runyan appear to have been close friends: Runyan was a pallbearer at Seaborn's funeral: See Seaborn's obituary, "Dr. William S. Russell," *Arkansas Gazette* (Little Rock, AR), 4 March 1928, p. 14, col. 4. Kirby was a noted surgeon: see Dallas T. Herndon, *Centennial History of Arkansas*, vol. 3 (Chicago: S. J. Clarke, 1922), pp. 159–60. He was the doctor in practice with Charles R. Shinault in 1905 when the *Arkansas Democrat* noted on 23 September that Dr. L. D. Wadley of Runyan & Shinault would relieve Dr. W. S. Russell in supervising a fumigating station on the Louisiana and Arkansas Railroad: see "Late Local News," *Arkansas Democrat* (Little Rock, AR), 23 September 1905, p. 7, col. 5.

94. Diary of Seaborn Russell, 26 June 1921.

95. "Around the City, the Condition of George Russell," *Arkansas Democrat* (Little Rock, AR), 27 June 1921, p. 6, col. 2.

96. Diary of Seaborn Russell, 27 June 1921.

97. Diary of Seaborn Russell, 28 June 1921.

98. Diary of Seaborn Russell, 29 June 1921 and 3 July 1921.

99. Diary of Seaborn Russell, 9–10 July 1921 (Seaborn has erroneously labeled the second entry as written on 10 June).

100. Diary of Seaborn Russell, 11–12 July 1921.

101. Diary of Seaborn Russell, 13 July 1921.

102. Diary of Seaborn Russell, 17, 20, 21, 22 July 1921.

103. Diary of Seaborn Russell, 28 July 1921.

104. Diary of Seaborn Russell, 9, 11, 12 August 1921.

105. Diary of Seaborn Russell, 14 and 21 August and 16 September 1921.

106. See *Polk's Southern Directory Co.'s Little Rock and North Little Rock City Directory 1920* (Little Rock: Polk's Southern Directory, 1920), p. 370.

107. Diary of Seaborn Russell, 4 October 1920.

108. Diary of Seaborn Russell, 6 October 1920.

109. Diary of Seaborn Russell, 7–8 September 1920.

110. Diary of Seaborn Russell, 20 and 27 March 1921. The phrase "the Feast of Reason and the Flow of Soul" is from Alexander Pope's *First Satire of the Second Book of Horace* (1733).

111. Diary of Seaborn Russell, 23 August 1921. Though Seaborn gives Eric's middle name as Alvin, his mother's Bible gives it as Allen. Allen also appears on the record of Eric's marriage to La Vera Burnett on 19 February 1894 (Van Zandt Co., TX, Marriage Bk. 6, p. 187) and on his death certificate, for which his widow was the informant (Death Certificate of Eric Allen Russell, Texas Death Certificate #21900, Dallas Co., TX, State Board of Health, Bureau of Vital Statistics).

112. Diary of Seaborn Russell, 7 November 1920.

113. Diary of Seaborn Russell, 4 and 5 January 1921.

114. Diary of Seaborn Russell, 8 January 1921.

115. William Kostlevy, *Holy Jumpers: Evangelicals and Radicals in Progressive Era America* (Oxford: Oxford Univ. Press, 2010), pp. 68–70. On 8 January 1921, the *Arkansas Democrat* reported about the revival Seaborn attended on 4 and 8 January, noting that Robinson was conducting a "coast-to-coast" evangelistic campaign, and would be preaching the following afternoon at Liberty Hall: see "Taught to Read by Using Bible as Text Book," *Arkansas Democrat* (Little Rock, AR), 8 January 1921, p. 10, col. 2.

116. Diary of Seaborn Russell, 24 April and 15 May 1921.

117. Diary of Seaborn Russell, 16 April 1922.

118. Diary of Seaborn Russell, 14 May 1922.

119. Diary of Seaborn Russell, 2 November 1920.

120. Diary of Seaborn Russell, 5 November 1920.

121. Diary of Seaborn Russell, 17 December 1920.

122. Diary of Seaborn Russell, 14 March 1922.

123. Dianne Dentice, "Ku Klux Klan (after 1900)," *Encyclopedia of Arkansas History and Culture*, online at website of Butler Center for Arkansas Studies

at http://www.encyclopediaofarkansas.net/encyclopedia/entry-detail.aspx?
search=1&entryID=2755 (accessed March 2017). On the Klan's organizing in the
1920s, see Linda Gordon's magisterial *The Second Coming of the KKK: The Ku
Klux Klan of the 1920s and the American Political Tradition* (New York: W. W.
Norton, 2017).

124. Charles C. Alexander, *The Ku Klux Klan in the Southwest* (Lexington:
Univ. of Kentucky Press, 1963), pp. 51–52. See also Carl Moneyhon, *Arkansas and
the New South, 1874–1929* (Fayetteville: Univ. of Arkansas Press, 1997), p. 142.

125. "Official Communication from the Knights of the Ku Klux Klan,
Addressed to the People of the State of Arkansas," *Arkansas Gazette* (Little
Rock, AR), 26 March 1922, p. 19 (full-page ad); "The Truth About the Knights
of the Ku Klux Klan," *Arkansas Gazette* (Little Rock, AR), 5 August 1922, p.
11 (full-page ad). On Knowles, see Herndon, *Centennial History of Arkansas*,
vol. 3, pp. 514–15. Other local pastors promoting the Klan at this time included
Rev. J. W. Coontz and Rev. P. C. Fletcher: see "Minister Praises the Ku Klux
Klan: Rev. J. W. Coontz in Sermon Says It Is to Protect American Homes,"
Arkansas Democrat (Little Rock, AR), 6 March 1922, p. 10, col. 2; and "Crowd
Fills Church to Hear Sermon on 'Klan,'" *Arkansas Democrat* (Little Rock, AR),
27 Feb. 1922, p. 10, col. 1–2. Coontz's sermon stated, "The Ku Klux Klan was born
out of the desire to preserve American government, American homes, and to
protect Protestantism," and Fletcher's called for turning immigrants away from
the US and for taking a "stand for the supremacy of the Aryan race."

126. Diary of Seaborn Russell, 11–12 March 1920.

127. Diary of Seaborn Russell, 14 March 1920.

128. Diary of Seaborn Russell, 13 July 1920.

129. Diary of Seaborn Russell, 6 April 1921.

130. On "old George W" and his accompanying his father on medical visits, see ibid., 22 February 1922. The observation about George's "metal" is from
Seaborn's diary entry of 21 February 1920.

131. Diary of Seaborn Russell, 4 October 1921.

132. William L. Russell made a written transcript of this interview on 21
July 1974; the transcript is in his possession.

133. Diary of Seaborn Russell, 1 January 1920.

134. Diary of Seaborn Russell, 7 March 1921.

135. Diary of Seaborn Russell, 13 July 1921.

136. Diary of Seaborn Russell, 5 August 1921.

137. The letter is in the William James Park Russell Family Letters.

138. See Goodspeed's *History of Benton, Washington, Carroll, Madison,
Crawford, Franklin, and Sebastian Counties, Arkansas*, p. 1223; and Lindsey, *Fiat
Flux*, p. 16.

139. The letter is in the William James Park Russell Family Letters. Sophia's
marriage is recorded in Franklin Co, AR, Marriage Bk. H, p. 283.

Chapter 4

1. Ralph Russell, Nashville, AR, to Ava Norwood, fall 1883, in William
James Park Russell Family Letters.

2. *Coosa River News* (Centre, AL), 3 November 1899, p. 5, col. 3.

3. *Passport Applications, 1795–1905*, NARA series, roll 441: *22 Apr 1895–30 Apr 1895*, Jefferson Co., AL, #22926.

4. See William James Park Russell Mexican War Enlistment Papers.

5. See Bible of Ava Law Russell.

6. Moore, *History of Alabama and Her People*, pp. 528–29.

7. Jefferson Co., AL, Death Certificates, vol. 20, #566.

8. See *supra*, n. 3.

9. Application for Certificate of Qualification to Practice Medicine, Ralph Morgan Russell, Etowah County, SG 6456, Alabama Board of Medical Examiners, 1879–2012, Government Records Collections, Alabama Department of Archives and History, Montgomery, AL.

10. Moore, *History of Alabama and Her People*, pp. 528–29.

11. See Ava Leona Russell, Eureka Springs, AR, to Frank Norwood, 20 May 1881, William James Park Russell Family Letters.

12. W. J. P. Russell to Frank Norwood, 27 December 1881, in ibid.

13. On Ralph's recognition that his uncle mentored him in business, see J. B. Cumming, Eulogy at Funeral of Ralph Russell, November 1916, in ibid.

14. See Ava Leona Russell, Eureka Springs, AR, to Frank Norwood, 17 October 1882, and Ava Russell, Boonsboro, AR to Ava Norwood, 29 April 1883, in ibid. A death notice in *Arkansas Democrat* (Little Rock, AR) on 23 October 1882 ("Arkansas State News," p. 2, col. 4) says that J. H. Law died on the seventeenth inst., while his obituary ("Sprays from Hot Springs") in the *Arkansas Gazette* (Little Rock, AR), 19 October 1882, says that he died on the eighteenth (p. 2, col. 1–2).

15. Ava Leona Russell, Eureka Springs, AR, to Frank Norwood, 17 October 1882, William James Park Russell Family Letters.

16. Mary Moore, Boonsboro, AR, to Ava Norwood, 8 April 1883, in ibid.

17. Ava Russell, Boonsboro, AR, to Ava Norwood, April 1883, in ibid.

18. Ava Russell, Boonsboro, AR, to Ava Norwood, 29 April 1883, in ibid.

19. Ralph mentions Walsh in a 10 September 1882 letter from Hot Springs to his sister Ava in Eureka Springs, and the law firm is mentioned in an 18 June 1883 letter to Ava: both are in ibid.

20. Mary Moore, Boonsboro, AR, to Ava Norwood, 17 June 1883, in ibid.

21. Ava Russell, Boonsboro, AR, to Ava Norwood, 18 June 1883, in ibid.

22. See *supra*, n. 1.

23. Ralph M. Russell, Nashville, AR, to Ava Norwood, fall of 1883, William James Park Russell Family Letters.

24. Ava Russell, Nashville, AR, to Ava Norwood, 3 December 1883, in ibid.

25. Mary Moore, Cowala, I.T., to Ava Norwood, 14 February 1884, in ibid.

26. W. J. P. Russell, Clinton, LA, to Ava Norwood, 17 March 1884, in ibid.

27. W. J. P. Russell, West Point, MS, to Ava Norwood, 2 July 1885, in ibid.

28. Ralph M. Russell, New York, NY, to Ava Norwood, 14 September 1885, in ibid.

29. P. B. F., "Domestic Correspondence," *Journal of the American Medical Association* 4, no. 13 (28 March 1885), p. 364; and Thomas M. Daniel, *Pioneers of Medicine and Their Impact on Tuberculosis* (Rochester: Univ. of Rochester Press, 2000), p. 110.

30. *Morrison and Fourmy's General Directory of the City of Dallas 1886–87*, pp. 266, 350.

31. Ava Russell, Dallas, TX, to Ava Norwood, 28 June 1886, William James Park Russell Family Letters.

32. Hall Co., GA, Marriage Bk. C, p. 314. The marriage license is signed by Ralph and Mollie's uncle James Franklin Law as county clerk.

33. See "They Will Go to Texas: From the *Cherokee, Ga., Advance*," *Atlanta Constitution* (Atlanta, GA), 28 August 1886, p. 8, col. 6. Another marriage notice is in *Montgomery Advertiser* (Montgomery, AL), 22 August 1886, p. 6, col. 1 ("Society, Gadsden").

34. Ava Norwood, Durham, NC, to Frank Norwood, 24 September 1886, William James Park Russell Family Letters.

35. W. J. P. Russell, Wills Point, TX, to Ava Norwood, 22 January 1887, in ibid.

36. Etowah Co., AL, Deed Bk. L, p. 595.

37. Certificate of Study and Moral Character, W. J. P. Russell for Ralph Morgan Russell, Bellevue Hospital Medical College, original in Bellevue archives, copy in William James Park Russell Family Letters.

38. Ralph M. Russell, New York, NY, to W. J. P. Russell, Willis Point, TX, 10 February 1888, William James Park Russell Family Letters.

39. See *Bellevue Hospital Medical College, Twenty-Seventh Annual Commencement* (12 March 1888), listing the graduates of this class.

40. See "Terrible Accident: Five Persons Killed and a Number Injured by an Accident on the Erie Railroad at Scio, N. Y.—A Greater Loss of Life Averted by a Seeming Miracle—The Victims," *Marion County Herald* (Palmyra, MO), 16 March 1888, p. 7, col. 1; and "The Thaw Causes a Bad Accident on the Erie Road at Scio, N. Y.," *The Eau Claire News* (Eau Claire, WI), 17 March 1888, p. 2, col. 5.

41. "Sleeping Cars Wrecked," *The Saint Paul Globe* (Saint Paul, MN), 12 March 1888, p. 5, col. 8.

42. *Gadsden Times* (Gadsden, AL), 26 April 1888, p. 3; "Gadsden's People," *Weekly Age* (Birmingham, AL), 2 May 1888, p. 6, col. 4.

43. "State Items," *Southern Star* (Newton, AL), 30 May 1888, p. 1, col. 4. *Hornellsville Weekly Tribune* (Hornellsville, NY), reported on 20 April 1888 ("Personal Mention," p. 5, col. 3) that Ralph and wife were at the Page House, where he had been confined following an accident with Train 5 at the Scio station.

44. Etowah Co., AL, Deed Bk. N, pp. 430–31, 24 April 1888.

45. The original application and license are on file at Alabama Department of Archives and History in Montgomery, AL, file #3078. See also State Board of Health, *Transactions of the Medical Association of the State of Alabama* (Montgomery: Brown, 1889), p. 101, noting that Ralph had been granted a license in Etowah County in 1888 and had a degree from Bellview [*sic*] Hospital Medical College.

46. *Gadsden Times* (Gadsden, AL), 24 January 1889, p. 3.

47. W. J. P. Russell, Lake Charles, LA, to Ava Norwood, 4 June 1890, William James Park Russell Family Letters.

48. Arthur Wayne Hafner, ed., *Directory of Deceased American Physicians, 1804–1929: A Genealogical Guide to Over 149,000 Medical Practitioners Providing*

*Brief Biographical Sketches Drawn from the American Medical Association's
Deceased Physician Masterfile* (Chicago: American Medical Association, 1993), p.
1347. This resource is also online at the FamilySearch website as "United States
Deceased Physician File (AMA), 1864–1968," a database maintained by AMA,
Chicago, with two file cards for Ralph, giving his date and cause of death, and
his educational background: see https://familysearch.org/ark:/61903/3:1:3QS7-
99QP-6PPM?i=1288&wc=M6Y8-XP6%3A353101901&cc=2061540.

    49. State Board of Health, *Transactions of the Medical Association of the State
of Alabama* (Montgomery: Brown, 1891), p. 206, noting that Ralph was not a
member of the Etowah County medical association.

    50. *Choctaw Herald* (Butler, AL), 23 December 1896, p. 4, col. 3.

    51. Ralph's 1891 Birmingham license is documented in "Medical Heritage"
in *The Heritage of Jefferson County, Alabama* (Clanton, AL: Heritage, 2002),
p. 189. It appears likely that Ralph was transferring his license from Etowah
to Jefferson County. See also *City Directory of Birmingham, Alabama, 1897*
(Maloney Directory, n.p., 1897), p. 626. The 1900 federal census also shows the
family living at this address: 1900 federal census, Birmingham, Ward 4, Jefferson
Co., AL, ED 0142; roll 22, p. 1B.

    52. "Successful Treatment of Consumption by a Birmingham (Ala.)
Physician," *Monroe Journal* (Claiborne, AL), 1 October 1896, p. 6, col. 5. The
same article appeared, with the title "Good News, Successful Treatment of
Consumption by a Birmingham (Ala.) Physician," in *The Randolph Toiler*
(Wedowee, AL), 21 August 1896, p. 4, col. 1.

    53. James Harvey Young, "Device Quackery in America," in *Sickness and
Health in America*, p. 97.

    54. Young, "Device Quackery in America," p. 97, citing Jacques M. Quen,
"Elisha Perkins, Physician, Nostrum-Vendor, or Charlatan?," *Bulletin of the
History of Medicine* 37 (1963),
pp. 159–66.

    55. Young, "Device Quackery," p. 97, citing Gerald Carson, *One for a Man,
Two for a Horse* (New York: Doubleday, 1961), pp. 33–35; and *Printers' Ink: Fifty
Years, 1888–1938* (New York: Printers' Ink, 1938), p. 84.

    56. Young, "Device Quackery," p. 97.

    57. Young, "Device Quackery," p. 97.

    58. Young, "Device Quackery," p. 97.

    59. "Mechanical Fakes: The Electropoise—Oxydonor—Oxygenor—
Oxygenator—Oxypathor—Oxytonor," in *Nostrums and Quackery: Articles on the
Nostrum Evil and Quackery Reprinted, with Additions and Modifications, from the
Journal of the American Medical Association*, ed. American Medical Association,
vol. 1 (Chicago: A. M. A., 1912), pp. 244, 247–49, 295–301.

    60. "Mechanical Fakes," p. 243.

    61. Young, "Device Quackery," p. 98.

    62. See *Wilda's Birmingham and Suburban Directory 1893* (Birmingham, AL:
RWA Wilda, 1893), p. 514.

    63. Church membership records show that "Mrs. R. M. Russell joined by
Cert 25 Nov 1894"; this information was sent to William L. Russell, Maumelle,
AR, by letter from Lucile Hanrick, church historian and archivist, on 10 June
2002. The letter is in William James Park Russell Family Letters.

64. *Birmingham Age-Herald* (Birmingham, AL), 14 February 1894, p. 3, col. 3; 14 March 1894, p. 6, col. 5.

65. See *supra*, n. 3.

66. "News of Society," *Fort Wayne Weekly Sentinel* (Fort Wayne, IN), 16 May 1895, p. 5, col. 6.

67. "Speaking of Society, Gadsden," *Montgomery Advertiser* (Montgomery, AL), 26 May 1895, p. 7, col. 3.

68. Patricia Methven, college archivist of King's College, to William L. Russell, North Little Rock, AR, 24 January 1982. The original letter is held by William L. Russell; a copy is in William James Park Russell Family Letters.

69. "News and Gossip of the Social World," *Atlanta Constitution* (Atlanta, GA), 14 July 1895, p. 6, col. 3.

70. *Maloney's 1900 Birmingham Directory* (Atlanta: Maloney Directory, 1900), p. 625.

71. *The Marion Times-Standard* (Marion, AL), 28 May 1896, p. 1, col. 2.

72. Ralph Morgan Russell, *Handbook of Home Medicine: Devoted Principally to the Latest and Most Approved Methods of Home Treatment of Diseases Peculiar to the South and West* (Chicago: Hammond, 1900–1911), pp. 371–77.

73. In addition to the sources already cited giving 404 18th Street as the Institute's address, the following sources also provide this address: an ad for Ralph's Vi-Be Ni liver pills carried in *Brevard News* (Brevard, NC) on 24 July 1914, p. 6, col. 1–2; and *Hayden v. Russell*, Jefferson Co., AL, Chancery Court, 5th Dist., Northwestern Chancery of Alabama (1916), a suit filed by Lucy Hayden against the estate of Ralph Russell following his death. The *Brevard News* ad ran again on 7 August 1914, p. 6, col. 1–2; 14 August, p. 6, col. 2–3; 21 August, p. 8, col. 4–5; 28 August, p. 8, col. 4–5; and 4 September 1914, p. 8, col. 4–5.

74. 1900 federal census, Birmingham, Ward 2, Jefferson Co., AL, ED 0135; roll 22, p. 4A.

75. 30 May 1975 letter of Grace Russell Norton, Wills Point, TX, to William L. Russell, Maumelle, AR, transcription in possession of William L. Russell.

76. US Patent Office, *Annual Report of the Commissioner of Patents* (D.C.: Government Printing Office, 1897), p. 452, trademark #28746, in Bk. 76, p. 958.

77. *Choctaw Herald* (Butler, AL), 17 March 1897, p. 4, col. 3, and 2 June 1897, p. 4, col. 3. The wording of the two ads differs slightly. We have transcribed the 2 June ad. Its phrasing, "Club, Reel," appears as "Club heel" in the 17 March ad. "Reel" is obviously a mistake.

78. *Choctaw Herald*, 2 June 1897, p. 4, col. 2.

79. The only extant copy yet found is in the Russell Plato Schwartz Orthopedics Collection (pamphlet box 1/19) in the Edward G. Miner Library, University of Rochester Medical Center, Rochester, NY.

80. US Letters Patent # 579,808. See United States Patent Office, *Official Gazette of the United States Patent Office* (Washington, D.C., Government Printing Office, 1897), vol. 78, p. 1990. The patent was issued 30 March 1897.

81. *People's Weekly Tribune* (Birmingham, AL), 26 March 1896, p. 8, col. 5–6, and 9 April 1896, p. 8, col. 5–6.

82. *Mountain Eagle* (Jasper, AL), 2 December 1896, p. 3, col. 6–7, and 25

August 1897, p. 4, col. 5–6. The ads in both issues are virtually the same, with the exception of the additional statement in August 1897 about the ability of Vi-Be Ni tonic to cure opium and morphine addiction. In the December 1896 issue, next to the ad, a report (p. 3, col. 4) states that Mrs. H. O. Babb and her two little daughters had just returned to Jasper from a stay at Dr. Russell's clinic, where little Annie Babb was being treated by Dr. Russell.

83. "X Rays and Skilled Surgeons," *Coosa River News* (Centre, AL), 3 June 1898, p. 1, col. 4.

84. No patent for this device has been located.

85. "Dr. Russell, of London: The Eminent Catarrh Specialist in the City," *Montgomery Advertiser* (Montgomery, AL), 6 November 1898, p. 5, col. 2.

86. *People's Party Advocate* (Ashland, AL), 15 December 1898, p. 3, col. 4.

87. *Tuscaloosa Weekly Times* (Tuscaloosa, AL), 2 Jun 1899, p. 1, col. 1–4.

88. See *supra*, n. 2.

89. The following libraries hold copies of the *Handbook of Home Medicine*, according to OCLC: Jefferson Co., AL Public Library, Birmingham (5th ed.) and Birmingham Botanical Gardens Library (5th ed.); Miner Library, University of Rochester Health Sciences Center (6th ed.); University of Alabama Libraries, Tuscaloosa (7th ed.); Auburn University Library, Auburn (7th ed., microfilm); Lister Hill Library of the Health Sciences, University of Alabama-Birmingham (11th ed.); and University of Arkansas for Medical Sciences Library, Little Rock (11th ed.).

90. Russell, *Handbook*, p. viii.

91. This information is on the title page of *Handbook*.

92. Russell, *Handbook*, pp. 64a and 64b.

93. Russell, *Handbook*, pp. vii-viii.

94. Russell, *Handbook*, pp. xi-xiii. A eulogy of Ralph by J. B. Cumming printed in an unidentified newspaper, a copy of which is in his sister Ava's scrapbook, stresses Ralph's strong religious convictions. The scrapbook is in William James Park Russell Family Letters.

95. Russell, *Handbook*, p. xiv.

96. Russell, *Handbook*, p. xv.

97. Russell, *Handbook*, pp. xii-xiii.

98. *Handbook* consistently uses the British spelling "focussing."

99. See Numbers, "Do-It-Yourself the Sectarian Way," pp. 89–90.

100. Anita Clair Fellman and Michael Fellman, *Making Sense of Self: Medical Advice Literature in Late Nineteenth-Century America* (Philadelphia: Univ. of Pennsylvania Press, 1981), pp. 9–10.

101. Russell, *Handbook*, p. 19.

102. James Harvey Young, "Patent Medicines and the Self-Help Syndrome," in *Medicine Without Doctors*, p. 111. pp. 95–116.

103. Russell, *Handbook*, p. 331.

104. Russell, *Handbook*, p. 331.

105. The two pages containing the list are unpaginated and are inserted between pp. 360–61 of *Handbook*, with a heading reading "Descriptions."

106. Binger, *Revolutionary Doctor*, p. 185.

107. Guenter B. Risse, "Introduction," in *Medicine Without Doctors*, p. 4.

108. Rosenberg, "Health in the Home," pp. 1–20, and "Preface," pp. xvii, in *Right Living*. Steven Stowe also argues that studies of how illness was treated at home in the nineteenth-century South have been far too limited and we still have much to learn about this topic: see "Conflict and Self-Sufficiency: Domestic Medicine in the American South," in *Right Living*, p. 147.

109. Rosenberg, "Health in the Home," pp. 4–5.

110. Christopher Hoolihan, "Every Man His Own Physician: Ephemera and Medical Self-Help," *The Ephemera Journal* 15, no. 3 (May 2013), pp. 3–4. As Thomas A. Horrocks notes, the emphasis on purging and puking in American medicine had much to do with theories that attributed illness to imbalance of the body's "humors": see "Rules, Remedies, and Regimens: Health Advice in Early American Almanacs," in *Right Living*, pp. 126–27.

111. Hoolihan, "Every Man His Own Physician," pp. 4–5. On the proliferation of domestic medical guides in the latter half of the 1800s, see Numbers, "Do-It-Yourself the Sectarian Way," p. 91.

112. Hoolihan, "Every Man His Own Physician," p. 5.

113. Hoolihan, "Every Man His Own Physician," pp. 7–8.

114. Hoolihan, "Every Man His Own Physician," p. 9.

115. Hoolihan, "Every Man His Own Physician." Hoolihan recommends viewing the collection held by the Edward C. Atwater Collection of American Popular Medicine at University of Rochester's Edward G. Miner Library.

116. Rosenberg, "Health in the Home," pp. 2–3. On Buchan's influence, see also John B. Blake, "From Buchan to Fishbein," in *Medicine Without Doctors*, pp. 12–16 (noting that Anthony Benezet's popular 1826 work *The Family Physician* marketed itself as an Americanization of Buchan); and Hoolihan, "Every Man His Own Physician," p. 4.

117. See the facsimile reprint edited by Charles E. Rosenberg: John C. Gunn's *Domestic Medicine, or, Poor Man's Friend* (Knoxville, 1830) (repr. Knoxville: Univ. of Tennessee Press, 1986).

118. Rosenberg, "Introduction," in ibid, p. v.

119. Thomas Johnson, *Every Man His Own Doctor; or the Poor Man's Family Physician: Prescribing Plain, Safe, and Easy Means to Cure Themselves, of the Most Disorders Incident to This Climate with Very Little Charge, the Medicines Being the Growth of This Country, and About Almost Every Man's Plantation* (Salisbury, NC, 1798). On Johnson's work, see Rosenberg, "Health in the Home," pp. 5–6.

120. James Ewell, *The Medical Companion, or Family Physician: Treating of the Diseases of the United States*, etc. (Philadelphia: John Bioren, 1807).

121. Thomas Ewell, *Letters to Ladies, Detailing Important Information, Concerning Themselves and Infants* (Philadelphia: W. Brown, 1817).

122. Robert Thomas and David Hosack, *A Treatise on Domestic Medicine: Pointing Out, in Plain Language, and as Free from Professional Terms as Possible, the Nature, Symptoms, Causes, Probable Terminations, and Treatment of All Diseases Incident to Men, Women, and Children, in Both Cold and Warm Climates*, etc. (New York: A. Paul, 1820).

123. Thomas Cooper, *A Treatise of Domestic Medicine, Intended for Families: In which the Treatment of Common Disorders are Alphabetically Enumerated*, etc.

(Reading, England: George Getz, 1824). On Cooper, see Blake, "From Buchan to Fishbein," p. 17.

124. William E. Horner, *The Home Book of Health and Medicine: Being a Popular Treatise on the Means of Avoiding and Curing Diseases, and of Preserving the Health and Vigour of the Body to the Latest Period, etc.* (Philadelphia: Key & Biddle, 1834).

125. William Matthews, *A Treatise on Domestic Medicine and Kindred Subjects: Embracing Anatomical and Physiological Sketches of the Human Body* (Indianapolis: John D. Defrees, 1848). On Matthews, see Blake, "From Buchan to Fishbein," pp. 17–18.

126. *Present Position of Medical Profession*, p. 15.

127. *Present Position of Medical Profession*, p. 15.

128. William H. Helfand, *Quack, Quack, Quack: The Sellers of Nostrums in Prints, Posters, Ephemera and Books* (New York: Grolier Club, 2002), pp. 11–12. The original 1784 report with Franklin's marginalia is now in the Library Company of Philadelphia.

129. Helfand, *Quack, Quack, Quack*, p. 14.

130. Helfand, *Quack, Quack, Quack*, p. 15.

131. Helfand, *Quack, Quack, Quack*, pp. 16–17.

132. Helfand, *Quack, Quack, Quack*, p. 20.

133. Helfand, *Quack, Quack, Quack*, pp. 18–19.

134. Helfand, *Quack, Quack, Quack*, pp. 19–21.

135. Helfand, *Quack, Quack, Quack*, p. 22.

136. Helfand, *Quack, Quack, Quack*, pp. 28–29.

137. Helfand, *Quack, Quack, Quack*, p. 32.

138. Helfand, *Quack, Quack, Quack*, p. 18.

139. Helfand, *Quack, Quack, Quack*, p. 26.

140. Helfand, *Quack, Quack, Quack*, p. 35.

141. Helfand, *Quack, Quack, Quack*, p. 37.

142. Helfand, *Quack, Quack, Quack*, p. 38.

143. Helfand, *Quack, Quack, Quack*, p. 41.

144. Helfand, *Quack, Quack, Quack*, pp. 41–42.

145. Helfand, *Quack, Quack, Quack*, p. 41.

146. Helfand, *Quack, Quack, Quack*, p. 50.

147. See *supra*, n. 59.

148. *Nostrums and Quackery*, vol. 1, "Preface," p. 7.

149. *Nostrums and Quackery*, vol. 1,, "Preface," p. 8.

150. "Medical Institutes," in *Nostrums and Quackery*, vol. 1,, pp. 260–310.

151. "Medical Institutes," in *Nostrums and Quackery*, vol. 1, p. 260.

152. "Medical Institutes," in *Nostrums and Quackery*, vol. 1, p. 284.

153. "Medical Institutes," in *Nostrums and Quackery*, vol. 1, pp.284–85.

154. "Medical Institutes," in *Nostrums and Quackery*, vol. 1, p. 285. Boston Medical Institute shared office space with a Bellevue Medical Institute, both headed by Dr. Edward Hibbard of Oak Park, IL. The name of one institute was on one side of the building, and the name of the other on the opposite side; however, when one went through either door, one reached the same offices. The

promotional literature of the two institutes indicates that Hibbard had a medical staff of eleven members, "including some of the most eminent physicians of America and Europe," but when he was prosecuted for fraud, it was found there were only two staff members, a Dr. Edmondson of mediocre ability and a Dr. Koehn: see ibid., pp. 280–82.

155. "Medical Institutes," in *Nostrums and Quackery*, vol. 1, p. 292.

156. "Medical Institutes," in *Nostrums and Quackery*, vol. 1, p. 294.

157. "Medical Institutes," in *Nostrums and Quackery*, vol. 1, pp. 296–97.

158. "Medical Institutes," in *Nostrums and Quackery*, vol. 1, pp. 300–1.

159. "Miscellaneous," in *Nostrums and Quackery*, vol. 1,, p. 480.

160. "Mail-Order Medical Concerns," in ibid., p. 216. Later efforts by the AMA and the government to contain quackery focused on use of radio stations in addition to the mail to defraud consumers. For example, Norman Baker, who did not even claim to be a physician, used a radio station to attract patients to his Iowa hospital for "cancer cures." The AMA convinced the Federal Radio Commission to shut down his station in 1931. After establishing another station in Mexico, Baker moved to Eureka Springs, Arkansas, where he was convicted in 1940 of sending fraudulent literature through the mail and was sentenced to three years in a federal prison—see Michael Dougan, "Norman Baker (1882–1958)," *Encyclopedia of Arkansas History and Culture*, online at the website of the Butler Center for Arkansas Studies at http://www.encyclopediaofarkansas.net/encyclopedia/entry-detail.aspx?search=1&entryID=4885 (accessed 19 January 2019).

161. *Nostrums and Quackery*, vol. 1, p. 229–30.

162. *Nostrums and Quackery*, vol. 1,, p. 231.

163. "Preface," in *Nostrums and Quackery*, vol. 1,, p. 9.

164. "Medical Waters," in *Nostrums and Quackery*, vol. 1,, pp. 471–72.

165. In 1899–1900, Ralph and Mollie were involved in ten land and mortgage transactions in Jefferson County: see Deed Book 210, p. 441, 18 September 1896; Deed Book 215, p. 397, 18 March 1897; Deed Book 219, pp. 75–79, 14 May 1897; Deed Book 247, p. 590, 13 January 1900; Deed Book 252, p. 456, 29 September 1899, and p. 470, 28 September 1899; Deed Book 254, p. 216, 7 November 1899; Deed Book 259, p. 241, 24 April 1900, and p. 271, 14 April 1900.

166. *Wiggins' Birmingham City Directory 1903* (Columbus, OH: Wiggins Directories), p. 715; *R. L. Polk & Co.'s Birmingham Directory 1904* (Birmingham: R. L. Polk, 1904), p. 839.

167. From 1904 to 1907, Birmingham city directories show the family living at 1306 Huntsville. In 1909, their address was 1320 Huntsville: see *R. L. Polk & Co.'s Birmingham Directory 1907*, vol. 22 (Birmingham: R. L. Polk, 1907), p. 974; and *R. L. Polk & Co.'s Birmingham Directory 1909*, vol. 24 (Birmingham: R. L. Polk, 1909), p. 771.

168. "Sim Strong," *Greensboro Watchman* (Greensboro, AL), 28 October 1915, p. 5, col. 4.

169. "Local Paragraphs," *Brevard News* (Brevard, NC), 23 August 1912, p. 5, col. 1.

170. The ad is in "Local Paragraphs," *Brevard News*, 24 July 1914, p. 6, col. 1–2.

171. See Susan Lefler, *Brevard Then and Now* (Charleston, SC: Arcadia, 2011), p. 10.

172. See *supra*, n. 7. The death certificate, his widow Mollie's appeal to probate his estate, the Alabama Death Index, and his tombstone state that he died on the fifth, while his biography in *History of Alabama and Her People* and *Directory of Deceased American Physicians* gives his death date as 4 November. Probate documents are in Jefferson Co., AL, Administrators' Records, vol. W-Y, 1915–1918, pp. 34–35. For the Alabama Death Index, see "Alabama Deaths, 1908–1974," citing Jefferson Co., AL, Death Certificates, vol. 20, #566, Department of Health, Montgomery; online at the FamilySearch website at https://familysearch.org/ark:/61903/1:1:JDXW-MMX (accessed June 2017).

173. "Dr. Russell To Be Buried Here," *Birmingham News* (Birmingham, AL), 6 November 1916, p. 3, col. 1.

174. *Hayden v. Russell* (1916): See *supra*, n. 73.

175. *Hayden v. Russell* (1916): See *supra*, n. 73.

176. See "Faithful Temperance Worker Passes," *Alabama Christian Advocate* (Birmingham AL), 1 February 1945, p. 10, col. 4; and "Well Known Church Worker Succumbs," *Birmingham News* (Birmingham, AL), 27 January 1945, p. 6, col. 2.

Chapter 5

1. "Uncle Sam Wants More Army Surgeons," *Lafayette County Democrat* (Stamps, AR), 1 October 1909, p. 6, col. 4. This article ran in newspapers around the US in the first week of October 1909.

2. George Seaborn Russell, foreword to an unpublished manuscript *Letters from the War*, which transcribes and annotates the correspondence of his parents George and Jeanette Roberts Russell during WWII.

3. The photo of George is in the 1941 yearbook of the University of Arkansas School of Medicine, *Arkansas Caduceus 1941* (Little Rock: UAMS, 1941) (unpaginated). Ben's graduation photo is in *The Volunteer*, vol. 16, *1912* (Knoxville: Univ. of Tennessee, 1912), p. 247.

4. Ben's birthplace is in his obituary: "Capt. B. F. Norwood, Navy Surgeon" in *Brooklyn Daily Eagle* (Brooklyn, NY), 14 January 1942, p. 13. See also his Social Security application (# 166288569), marriage registry of First Presbyterian Church, Philadelphia, 18 October 1933, and Ben's passenger listing of USS *Chaumont* when it sailed from Shanghai to San Francisco on 7 January 1926 (see "San Francisco Passenger Lists 1892–1953," #1410, RG 231, NARA).

5. G. W. Thompson, Kennedale, TX, to Frank Norwood, 13 January 1887, in William James Park Russell Family Letters.

6. See Sybil Creasy, *School Days in Van Zandt County, Tex*as, vol. 2 (Canton, TX: Van Zandt County Genealogical Society, 2002), pp. 65, 184.

7. Norwood, Benjamin Franklin 6261, US Department of Veterans Affairs, Records Management Center, NARA. Most of the reports are signed by the attending physician, and most signatures are not immediately legible.

8. These ships included the *Independence* (January–March 1904), *Solace* (March–June 1904), *Monterrey* (June–December 1904), *Rainbow* (December

1904–April 1905), *Frolic* (April 1905–April 1906), *Wilmington* (April 1906–December 1907), and *Denver* (December 1907–January 1908). The medical file contains documentation of all stages of Ben's naval career, supplementing other sources cited *infra*.

9. Norwood, Benjamin Franklin 6261.

10. Magnus Unemoa and William M. Shafer, "Antimicrobial Resistance in *Neisseria gonorrhoeae* in the 21st Century: Past, Evolution, and Future," *Clinical Microbiology Reviews* 27, no. 3 (July 2014), pp. 587–613.

11. See Norwood, Benjamin Franklin 6261.

12. See "Norwood, Benjamin Franklin," "United States Deceased Physician File (AMA), 1864–1968," American Medical Association, online at the FamilySearch website at https://www.familysearch.org/ark:/61903/3:1:3QS7-L9QP-V974-S?i=267&owc=waypoints&wc=M6Y8-XMW%3A353098001&cc=2061540 (accessed November 2017), which states that Ben studied at the Memphis school 1908–1912. A notice entitled "Local and Otherwise" in the *Lafayette County Democrat* (Stamps, AR) 17 September 1909 (p. 8, col. 4), reports that he had left that week for Memphis to attend medical college (for his second year).

13. Abraham Flexner, *Medical Education in the United States and Canada, a Report to the Carnegie Foundation for the Advancement of Teaching* (New York: Carnegie, 1910).

14. Flexner, *Medical Education*, pp. 187–88.

15. Flexner, *Medical Education*, p. 304.

16. Flexner, *Medical Education*, pp. 305–8.

17. Scrapbook of Ava Norwood in William James Park Russell Family Letters.

18. As noted *supra*, n. 3, Ben's graduation photo is in *The Volunteer*; biographical information is on p. 258.

19. See "Local Items," *Lafayette County Democrat* (Stamps, AR), 10 May 1912, p. 8, col. 4. Ben is listed as a 1912 graduate in "University of Tennessee Announcement, College of Medicine, Memphis, Tenn.," *University of Tennessee Bulletin* 3, no. 4 (June 1912), p. 44. "Degrees Conferred, 1911–1912," *University of Tennessee Record* 16, no. 4 (April 1913), p. 222, also lists him as a 1912 graduate with an M.D. degree. Ben's naval medical file indicates that he had diphtheria his final year of medical school.

20. See "Applicants Who Get License," *The Tennessean* (Nashville, TN), 6 June 1911, p. 3, col. 5, listing 278 applicants who had applied to practice medicine in Tennessee and had been interviewed on 2–3 May in Nashville by the state's Medical Board of Examiners. The list includes Ben F. Norwood of Memphis.

21. *Lafayette County Democrat* (Stamps, AR), 26 April 1912, p. 8.

22. See *Memphis City Directory 1909* (Detroit, Chicago, St. Louis: R. L. Polk, 1909), p. 1108; *1910*, p. 1138; *1911*, p. 1034; *1912*, p. 1102; *1914*, pp. 1050, 2019; *1915*, pp. 901, 1814; *1916*, pp. 867, 1773; and *1917*, p. 1874.

23. "Baby Welfare Week," *Arkansas Gazette* (Little Rock, AR), 6 May 1917, p. 30, col. 2; and "Making Comfort Bags," *Arkansas Gazette* (Little Rock, AR), 20 May 1917, p. 18, col. 4.

24. See Norwood, Benjamin Franklin 6261.

25. "Tennesseans Appointed," *The Tennessean* (Nashville, TN), 2 August 1917, p. 4, col. 7. On 25 November 1917, the *Arkansas Gazette* (Little Rock, AR) ("Soldiers from A.F.W.C. Homes—Stamps," p. 11, col. 5) carried a list of soldiers from A.F.W.C. homes in Camden District, in which Ben's name appears in the Stamps section.

26. Lincoln Humphreys, "Experiences of a Naval Medical Officer," *Journal of the Arkansas Medical Society* 17, no. 4 (September 1920), pp. 98–102.

27. See H. B. Jordan, "Beverly Wyly Dunn," *Sixty-Eighth Annual Report of Graduates of the United States Military Academy at West Point, New York* (Newburgh, NY: Moore, 1937), pp. 101–6; "Colonel Dies," *Biloxi Daily Herald* (Biloxi, MS), 12 May 1936, p. 3, col. 5; "Col. Dunn, Inventor of Explosives, Dies," *Tampa Times* (Tampa, FL), 11 May 1936, p. 2, col. 7; "High Explosive Inventor, Col. Beverly W. Dunn Dies," *Indianapolis Star* (Indianapolis, IN), 11 May 1936, p. 1, col. 1; and the Library of Congress, Harris and Ewing Collection, 1938, #LC-1422-D-4136.

28. See Bureau of Navigation, Navy Department, *Navy Directory, Officers of the United States Navy and Marine Corps* (Washington, D.C.: Government Printing Office, July 1918), p. 253; *Navy Directory, Officers of the United States Navy and Marine Corps* (Washington, D.C.: Government Printing Office, August 1918), p. 188; *Navy Directory, Officers of the United States Navy and Marine Corps* (Washington, D.C.: Government Printing Office, September 1918), p. 202; *Navy Directory, Officers of the United States Navy and Marine Corps* (Washington, D.C.: Government Printing Office, November 1918), p. 243; and US Naval Bureau of Naval Personnel, *Register of the Commissioned and Warrant Officers of the United States Navy and Marine Corps* (Washington, D.C.: Government Printing Office, 1918), pp. 144, 510, 634.

29. US Naval Bureau of Naval Personnel, *Register of the Commissioned and Warrant Officers of the United States Navy and Marine Corps* (Washington, D.C.: Government Printing Office, 1919), p. 212.

30. See US Naval Bureau of Naval Personnel, *Register of the Commissioned and Warrant Officers of the United States Navy and Marine Corps* (Washington, D.C.: Government Printing Office, 1920), pp. 152, 388; *Register of the Commissioned and Warrant Officers of the United States Navy and Marine Corps* (Washington, D.C.: Government Printing Office, 1921), pp. 146, 413; *Register of the Commissioned and Warrant Officers of the United States Navy and Marine Corps* (Washington, D.C.: Government Printing Office, 1922), pp. 124, 353; *Register of the Commissioned and Warrant Officers of the United States Navy and Marine Corps* (Washington, D.C.: Government Printing Office, 1923), pp. 128, 240; and "General Notes," *Bulletin of the Pan American Union* 52, no. 3 (March 1921), p. 312.

31. B. F. Norwood, "The Application of the Schick Reaction to 2,911 Naval Recruits and the Immunization of Susceptibles to Diphtheria with Toxin-Antitoxin," *United States Naval Medical Bulletin* 15, no. 2 (April 1921), pp. 485–91.

32. Norwood, "The Application of the Schick Reaction," p. 491.

33. B. F. Norwood, "A Case of Poisoning by Oil of Chenopodium," *United States Naval Medical Bulletin* 15, no. 4 (October 1921), pp. 818–23.

34. Norwood, "A Case of Poisoning," p. 818.

35. Norwood, "A Case of Poisoning," pp. 818–20.

36. Norwood, "A Case of Poisoning," pp. 821–22.

37. See Bureau of Navigation, Navy Department, *Navy Directory, Officers of the United States Navy and Marine Corps* (Washington, D.C.: Government Printing Office, September 1922), p. 56; *Navy Directory, Officers of the United States Navy and Marine Corps* (Washington, D.C.: Government Printing Office, November 1922), p. 55; *Army and Navy Register* 62,2180 (1 July 1922), p. 40; *Register of the Commissioned and Warrant Officers of the United States Navy and Marine Corps* (Washington, D.C.: Government Printing Office, 1922), pp. 124, 353; *Register of the Commissioned and Warrant Officers of the United States Navy and Marine Corps* (Washington, D.C.: Government Printing Office, 1923), pp. 128, 240; US Naval Bureau of Naval Personnel, *Register of the Commissioned and Warrant Officers of the United States Navy and Marine Corps* (Washington, D.C.: Government Printing Office, 1924), pp. 166, 368; and *Register of the Commissioned and Warrant Officers of the United States Navy and Marine Corps* (Washington, D.C.: Government Printing Office, 1925), pp. 170, 379.

38. See Bureau of Navigation, Navy Department, *Navy Directory, Officers of the United States Navy and Marine Corps* (Washington, D.C.: Government Printing Office, July 1925), p. 60; US Naval Bureau of Naval Personnel, *Register of the Commissioned and Warrant Officers of the United States Navy and Marine Corps* (Washington, D.C.: Government Printing Office, 1926), p. 178; *Register of the Commissioned and Warrant Officers of the United States Navy and Marine Corps* (Washington, D.C.: Government Printing Office, 1927), pp. 184, 318; and *Register of the Commissioned and Warrant Officers of the United States Navy and Marine Corps* (Washington, D.C.: Government Printing Office, 1928), pp. 190, 326.

39. B. F. Norwood, "Outbreak of Food Poisoning on Board the U.S.S. 'Cincinnati' Attributed to Corned-Beef Hash," *United States Naval Medical Bulletin* 24 (July 1926), pp. 680–82.

40. "USS *Chaumont* (AP-5), 1921-1948," online at the website of Naval Historical Center at https://www.ibiblio.org/hyperwar/OnlineLibrary/photos/sh-usn/usnsh-c/ap5.htm (accessed September 2019).

41. See Bureau of Navigation, Navy Department, *Navy Directory, Officers of the United States Navy and Marine Corps* (Washington, D.C.: Government Printing Office, October 1929), p. 64; and *Navy Directory, Officers of the United States Navy and Marine Corps* (Washington, D.C.: Government Printing Office, April 1930), p. 64.

42. On the marriage record, see *supra*, n. 4; and Philadelphia Co., PA, Clerk of Orphans' Court, Philadelphia Marriage License Index, 1885–1951, #628914. An announcement of the engagement is in the *Harrisburg Telegraph* (Harrisburg, PA), 30 September 1933, p. 4, col. 4, noting that Anne was the daughter of John Albert Robinson of Port Royal, PA, and Ben the son of Mrs. Benjamin Franklin Norwood and the late Mr. Norwood, Stamps, AR. The same announcement ran in the *Telegraph* on 3 October (p. 2).

43. See Bureau of Navigation, Navy Department, *Navy Directory, Officers of the United States Navy and Marine Corps* (Washington, D.C.: Government Printing Office, April 1934), p. 64; and *Navy Directory, Officers of the United States*

States Navy and Marine Corps (Washington, D.C.: Government Printing Office, July 1934), p. 67.

44. On 29 April 1936, Ben's sister Ruby Kitchens wrote her cousin Maude Russell that Ben was on his way to Balboa as a naval commander: see William James Park Russell Family Letters. See also *Charleston City Directory 1934* (Charleston: Southern Printing, 1934), p. 454, which shows him as an executive officer at the Navy Hospital in Charleston in that year; US Naval Bureau of Naval Personnel, *Register of the Commissioned and Warrant Officers of the United States Navy and Marine Corps* (Washington, D.C.: Government Printing Office, 1935), pp. 238, 372; Bureau of Navigation, Navy Department, *Navy Directory, Officers of the United States Navy and Marine Corps* (Washington, D.C.: Government Printing Office, April 1937), p. 73; US Naval Bureau of Naval Personnel, *Register of the Commissioned and Warrant Officers of the United States Navy and Marine Corps* (Washington, D.C.: Government Printing Office, 1940), pp. 272, 407.

45. 1940 federal census, Los Angeles, Los Angeles Co., California; roll T627_432; p. 10B; ED 60–1282; 13 April. For the listing of registered voters in Los Angeles precinct 2000-A in 1938, 1940, and 1942, see California State Library, *Great Register of Voters, 1900–1968* (1938: roll 45; 1940: roll 51; and 1942: roll 57). The 1942 listing postdates Ben's death. See also his and Anne's listing in *Los Angeles Directory Co.'s San Pedro and Wilmington City Directory 1940* (Los Angeles: Los Angeles Directory, 1940), p. 240.

46. See Bureau of Navigation, Navy Department, *Navy Directory, Officers of the United States Navy and Marine Corps* (Washington, D.C.: Government Printing Office, October 1941), p. 225.

47. On the obituary in *Brooklyn Daily Eagle*, see *supra*, n. 4. An obituary, "Captain Norwood Dies in N.Y. at 56," also appeared in *Philadelphia Inquirer* (Philadelphia, PA), 15 January 1942, p. 34, col. 1. See also US Naval Bureau of Naval Personnel, *Register of the Commissioned and Warrant Officers of the United States Navy and Marine Corps* (Washington, D.C.: Government Printing Office, 1942), p. 726.

48. Anne's legal victory was widely reported: see "Widow Awarded $21,131 Verdict," *The Gettysburg Times* (Gettysburg, PA), 25 February 1943, p. 4, col. 6; "Wins $21,131 Verdict in Husband's Death," *The Express* (Lock Haven, PA), 25 February 1943, p. 9, col. 5; "Insurance Companies Losers in Large Suit," *Warren Times Mirror* (Warren, PA), 25 February 1943, p. 11, col. 4; and "Awarded $21,131," *Wilkes-Barre Times Leader, the Evening News* (Wilkes-Barre, PA), 25 February 1943, p. 10, col. 1.

49. A copy of the original death certificate (Bureau of Medicine and Surgery, Navy Department, #1101804, US Naval Hospital, Brooklyn, NY) is in Ben's naval medical file. It was filed 12 January 1942 by attending physician H. L. Chasserot and gives the primary cause of death as hypertensive heart disease with edema of the brain and sclerosis of the cerebral arteries as the secondary cause. It notes Anne's report that Ben fell in the shower and complained of pain in his head and chest following the fall.

50. "Deaths Here," *Philadelphia Inquirer* (Philadelphia, PA), 9 September 1987, p. 57, col. 3.

51. Diary of Seaborn Russell, 22 February 1922.

52. George W. Russell, Allentown, PA, to William L. Russell, Maumelle, AR, March 1976, in William James Park Russell Family Letters.

53. The information provided here was shared with William L. Russell and Mary Ryan by George's children, George, Ann, and Paul, at a family meeting in Saylorsburg, PA, on 11 May 2017.

54. George Washington Russell birth certificate, Pulaski Co., AR, Registration District 6625, #2030.

55. On the CCC in Arkansas, see Patricia Paulus Laster, "Civilian Conservation Corps (CCC)," *Encyclopedia of Arkansas History and Culture*, online at website of Butler Center for Arkansas Studies at http://www.encyclopediaof arkansas.net/encyclopedia/entry-detail.aspx?entryID=2396 (accessed June 2017).

56. See George W. Russell's naval certificate now in possession of his son George S. Russell, Saylorsburg, PA.

57. 1940 federal census, Pulaski Co., AR, Big Rock Township, Little Rock; roll T627_167; p. 7B; ED 60–45; 6 April.

58. *Arkansas Caduceus 1941*, see *supra*, n. 3.

59. The original appointment letter is in possession of George S. Russell, Saylorsburg, PA, as is the statement of acceptance and oath of office dated 28 June 1941.

60. George W. Russell to Jeanette Roberts, 14 April 1945, in possession of George S. Russell, Saylorsburg, PA.

61. George W. Russell, Lieut. (MD) USN, US Naval Hospital, Memphis, Tennessee, to Jeanette Roberts, 14 April 1945, in possession of George S. Russell, Saylorsburg, PA.

62. The original nomination and appointment letters, both dated 23 September 1942, are in possession of George S. Russell, Saylorsburg, PA.

63. George received orders for detachment from the Naval Station in New Orleans on 28 March 1943, with orders to report to the US Naval Station at Moffett Field, CA. On 22 April, he was ordered from the Cub 9 Base Station in San Francisco to the USS *Pennsylvania*. The original detachment and order papers are in possession of George S. Russell, Saylorsburg, PA.

64. See Bill Russell, "William Leon Russell (1914–2000)," *Encyclopedia of Arkansas History and Culture*, online at the website of Butler Center for Arkansas Studies at http://www.encyclopediaofarkansas.net/encyclopedia/ entry-detail.aspx?entryID=8031 (accessed July 2017). On the USS *Pennsylvania* during the Second World War, see Christopher B. Havern Sr., "Pennsylvania III (Battleship No. 38) 1916–1946," online at the website of Naval History and Heritage Command at https://www.history.navy.mil/research/histories/ ship-histories/danfs/p/pennsylvania-ii.html (accessed July 2017).

65. The original appointment letter is in the possession of George S. Russell, Saylorsburg, PA, as is George's letter accepting the appointment dated 8 December 1943.

66. On *Letters from the War*, see *supra*, n. 2. All letters cited from this collection are in possession of George S. Russell, Saylorsburg, PA.

67. George Russell to Jeanette Roberts, 12 December 1943.

68. George Russell, USS *Pennsylvania*, c/o fleet postmaster in San Francisco, to Jeanette Roberts, 25 December 1943.

69. George Russell, USS *Pennsylvania*, c/o fleet postmaster in San Francisco, to Jeanette Roberts, 4 March and 12 March 1944.

70. This 7 February 1944 transfer document is in possession of George S. Russell, Saylorsburg, PA.

71. George Russell, USS *Pennsylvania*, c/o fleet postmaster in San Francisco, to Jeanette Roberts, 20 March 1944

72. See "Edward A. Strecker (1886–1959)," at the website of the Department of Psychiatry of the Perelman School of Medicine, University of Pennsylvania, at http://www.med.upenn.edu/psychiatry/streckerbio.html (accessed July 2017).

73. George Russell, 1817 Pine Street, Philadelphia, to Jeanette Roberts, 3 July, 8 July, and 8 September 1944.

74. See George's biography in *Who's Important in Medicine*, 2nd ed. (Hicksville, NY: Institute for Research in Biography, 1952), pp. 837–38, which also states that in 1944 he was assistant chief of the psychiatric staff at the US Naval Hospital in Memphis. George's appointment letter to the Memphis hospital, dated 13 September 1944, is in possession of George S. Russell, Saylorsburg, PA.

75. George Russell, Lieut. (MD) USN, US Naval Hospital, Memphis, TN, to Jeanette Roberts, Washington, D.C., 8 October 1944.

76. George Russell, Lieut. (MD) USN, US Naval Hospital, Memphis, TN, to Jeanette Roberts, Washington, D.C., 26 October 1944.

77. George Russell, Lieut. (MD) USN, US Naval Hospital, Memphis, TN, to Jeanette Roberts, Washington, D.C., 7 and 20 December 1944.

78. George Russell, Lieut. (MD) USN, US Naval Hospital, Memphis, TN, to Jeanette Roberts, Washington, D.C., 31 October 1944.

79. George Russell, Lieut. (MD) USN, US Naval Hospital, Memphis, TN, to Jeanette Roberts, Washington, D.C., 2 February 1945.

80. Jeanette Roberts, West Potomac Park, Barton Hall, Room 201-J, Washington, D.C., to George Russell, Memphis, TN, 7 February 1945.

81. George Russell, Lieut. (MD) USN, US Naval Hospital, Memphis, TN, to Jeanette Roberts, Washington, D.C., 22 February 1945.

82. George Russell, Lieut. (MD) USN, US Naval Hospital, Memphis, TN, to Jeanette Roberts, Washington, D. C., 12 March 1945; Jeanette Roberts, West Potomac Park, Barton Hall, Room 201-J, Washington, DC, to George Russell, Memphis, TN, 23 March 1945 and 3 April 1945.

83. Jeanette Roberts, Apt # 306, 1727 R Street NW, Washington, DC, to George Russell, Memphis, TN, 9 April 1945.

84. The couple's marriage license, dated 6 June 1945 (Cecil Co., MD application 62666, license 33889) is in possession of George S. Russell, Saylorsburg, PA. It shows them married on the day they received license.

85. Jeanette Russell, 1727 R Street NW, Washington, DC, to George Russell, Memphis, TN, 10 June and 13 June 1945.

86. George Russell, Lieut. (MD) USN, US Naval Hospital, Memphis, TN, to Jeanette Russell, 14 June 1945.

87. George's hospital admission papers dated 10 July 1945 are in possession of George S. Russell, Saylorsburg, PA.

88. The documents for these portions of George's naval career are in possession of George S. Russell, Saylorsburg, PA.

89. See George W. Russell's naval certificate in possession of George S. Russell, Saylorsburg, PA. George S. Russell also has the original commendation dated 15 January 1946.

90. George S. Russell, Saylorsburg, PA, has the original documentation of this process in George's naval career.

91. The trip is documented in reimbursement documents in possession of George S. Russell, Saylorsburg, PA.

92. See George W. Russell's naval certificate in possession of George S. Russell, Saylorsburg, PA.

93. The orders are in possession of George S. Russell, Saylorsburg, PA. The documents show that the Navy Retiring Board heard George's case and found him incapacitated on 3 May, with retirement officially approved on 26 October, and the retirement letter dated 22 November 1946.

94. The date is given on the certificate George received on completing his residency at Friends Hospital on 7 September 1947; this document is now in possession of George S. Russell, Saylorsburg, PA.

95. The teaching fellowship is noted in George's biography in *Who's Important in Medicine*, cited *supra*, n. 74.

96. The certificate of license is now in possession of George S. Russell, Saylorsburg, PA.

97. This information was communicated in a 6 April 2016 email to Mary Ryan from Timothy H. Horning of University of Pennsylvania Archives, who stated that the archival records show George earning this certificate in June 1948.

98. *Who's Important in Medicine*, cited *supra*, n. 74.

99. *Who's Important in Medicine*, cited *supra*, n. 74.

100. See obituary of Oliver Spurgeon English in *Journal News* (White Plains, NY) 7 Oct. 1993, p. 26/B2, col. 6, noting that he was one of the first psychotherapists to write about the connection between mental and physical health and that he co-authored *Psychosomatic Medicine* in the 1940s, "the first medical text to make the connection between stress and physical ailments."

101. A license dated 9 December 1958 also shows George licensed to practice medicine in Puerto Rico (original in possession of George S. Russell, Saylorsburg, PA).

102. See "Two New Mental Health Officials," *Daily Intelligencer* (Doylestown, PA), 14 January 1960, p. 1, col. 1–2 (with a photo of George); "Mental Health Unit Names Clinic Chiefs," *Daily Intelligencer* (Doylestown, PA), 15 January 1960, p. 2, col. 4–5; and "Center Appoints Two Psychiatrists," *The Bristol Daily Courier* (Bristol, PA), 18 January 1960, p. 4, col. 6.

103. See "Guidance Group Meets," *Daily Intelligencer* (Doylestown, PA), 7 April 1960, p. 1, col. 2; "Mental Clinics Open For 2 Nights A Week," *The Bristol Daily Courier* (Bristol, PA), 13 April 1960, p. 5, col. 1–2; "Officials of the Bucks County Mental Health Guidance Center," *Daily Intelligencer* (Doylestown, PA), 13 April 1960, p. 2, col. 5–6 (featuring a photo of the offi-

cials of Bucks County Mental Health Guidance Center, including George); "New Mental Health Program Offered in Bucks," *The Bristol Daily Courier* (Bristol, PA), 9 March 1961, p. 12, col. 1–7; "Bucks Clinic Adds to Staff," *The Bristol Daily Courier* (Bristol, PA), 10 August 1961, p. 18, col. 3–5; and "Two Psychologists Named to Serve Bucks Center," *Daily Intelligencer* (Doylestown, PA), 18 February 1963, p. 2, col. 4–5.

104. See "Mental Health Center Okays $96,000 Budget," *Daily Intelligencer* (Doylestown, PA), 20 June 1960, p. 2, col. 3; "Psychiatric Center 4 Years Old, Handles 10,000 Visits Yearly," *The Bristol Daily Courier* (Bristol, PA), 14 July 1962, p. 11; and "Psychiatric Center Ups Treatment," *Daily Intelligencer* (Doylestown, PA), 1 August 1963, p. 8, col. 8.

105. George's letterhead for the Allentown clinic shows it at 1536 Walnut Street.

106. The farmhouse into which the family moved in 1966 was built in 1754. George renovated the house and improved the property by having five ponds constructed on it. Later he bought a beach house at Long Beach Island, New Jersey. All property remains in possession of his children. This information was provided by George's children, George, Ann, and Paul, to William L. Russell and Mary Ryan at a family meeting in Saylorsburg, PA, on 11 May 2017.

107. This information was provided to William L. Russell and Mary Ryan by George S. Russell in a meeting in Saylorsburg, PA, on 12 May 2017.

108. The original incorporation document is in possession of George S. Russell, Saylorsburg, PA. William L. Russell has a copy.

109. James Bryce's famous summary of the goal of medical practice was made in New York at a dinner for General W. C. Gorgas in 1914: as cited, Dwight D. Eisenhower, "Address at Annual Meeting of American Medical Association" (June 1959), in *Public Papers of the Presidents of the United States, Dwight D. Eisenhower, 1959* (Washington, D.C.: Government Printing Office, 1999), p. 450.

BIBLIOGRAPHY

I. Monographs

Abbott, John S. C. *Comprising a Full and Impartial Account of the Origin and Progress of the Rebellion, of the Various Naval and Military Engagements, of the Heroic Deeds Performed by Armies and Individuals, and of Touching Scenes in the Field, the Camp, the Hospital, and the Cabin.* Vol. 2. New York: Henry Hill, 1866.

Adams, George Worthington. *Doctors in Blue: The Medical History of the Union Army in the Civil War.* Baton Rouge: Louisiana State Univ. Press, 1952.

Alexander, Charles C. *The Ku Klux Klan in the Southwest.* Lexington: Univ. of Kentucky Press, 1963.

Amato, Joseph A. *Jacob's Well: A Case for Rethinking Family History* (St. Paul: Minnesota Historical Soc., 2008).

American Medical Association, ed., *Nostrums and Quackery: Articles on the Nostrum Evil and Quackery Reprinted, with Additions and Modifications, from the Journal of the American Medical Association.* Vol. 1. Chicago: AMA, 1912.

Baird, W. David. *Medical Education in Arkansas 1879–1978.* Memphis: Memphis State Univ. Press, 1979.

Baptist, Edward. *The Half Has Never Been Told: Slavery and the Making of American Capitalism.* New York: Basic Books, 2014.

Barker, Jacob. *The Rebellion: Its Consequences, and the Congressional Committee, Denominated the Reconstruction Committee, with Their Action.* New Orleans: Commercial Print, 1866.

Battle, Kemp Plummer. *History of the University of North Carolina:.* Vol. 1, *From its Beginning to the Death of President Swain, 1789–1868.* Raleigh, NC: Edwards & Broughton, 1907.

Bergeron, Paul H. *Andrew Johnson's Civil War and Reconstruction.* Knoxville: Univ. of Tennessee Press, 2011.

Billingsley, Carolyn Earle. *Communities of Kinship: Antebellum Families and the Settlement of the Cotton Frontier.* Athens: Univ. of Georgia Press, 2004.

Binger, Carl. *Revolutionary Doctor, Benjamin Rush, 1746–1813.* New York: W. W. Norton & Company, 1966.

Blume, Clarence F., and Mabel Rumple Blume. *Historic Rocky River Church Buildings and Burying Grounds: Cabarrus County, Concord, North Carolina, 1751–1958.* N.p.: Rocky River Historical Foundation, 1958.

Boland, Frank Kells. *The First Anesthetic: The Story of Crawford Long.* Athens: Univ. of Georgia Press, 1950.

Bracken, Sharon, ed. *Historic McLennan County: An Illustrated History.* San Antonio: Lammert, 2010.

Buchan, William. *Domestic Medicine, or a Treatise on the Prevention and Cure of Diseases, by Regimen and Simple Medicines: with An Appendix Containing a Dispensatory for the Use of Private Practitioners.* London: Strahan, 1803.

Bulloch, Joseph Gaston Baillie. *A History and Genealogy of the Habersham Family.* Columbia, SC: R. L. Bryan, 1901.

Capers, Ellison. *Confederate Military History.* Vol. 5. Atlanta: Confederate, 1899.

Carson, Gerald. *One for a Man, Two for a Horse.* New York: Doubleday, 1961.

Churchill, Edward D., ed. *To Work in the Vineyard of Surgery: The Reminiscences of J. Collins Warren (1842–1927).* Cambridge: Harvard Univ. Press, 1958.

Cooper, Thomas. *A Treatise of Domestic Medicine, Intended for Families: In which the Treatment of Common Disorders are Alphabetically Enumerated,* etc. Reading, England: George Getz, 1824.

Cozzens, Peter. *The Darkest Days of the War: The Battles of Iuka and Corinth.* Chapel Hill: Univ. of North Carolina Press, 1997.

Craig, Tom Moore, ed. *Upcountry South Carolina Goes to War: Letters of the Anderson, Brockman, and Moore Families, 1853–1865.* Columbia: Univ. of South Carolina Press, 2009.

Creasy, Sybil. *School Days in Van Zandt County, Texas.* Vol. 2. Canton, TX: Van Zandt County Genealogical Society, 2002.

Daniel, Thomas M. *Pioneers of Medicine and Their Impact on Tuberculosis.* Rochester: Univ. of Rochester Press, 2000.

Dary, David. *Frontier Medicine.* New York: Knopf, 2008.

DeBerg, Betty. *Ungodly Women: Gender and the First Wave of American Fundamentalism.* Macon: Mercer Univ. Press, 2000.

Druitt, Robert. *The Principles and Practice of Modern Surgery.* Philadelphia: Lea and Blanchard, 1844.

Elliott, J. H. *Spain, Europe and the Wider World, 1500–1800.* New Haven: Yale Univ. Press, 2009.

Elrod, Frary. *Historical Notes on Jackson County, Georgia.* Jefferson, GA: n.p., 1967.

Eve, Paul D. *The Present Position of the Medical Profession in Society: An Introductory Lecture Delivered in the Medical College of Georgia, November 5, 1849.* Augusta: James McCafferty, 1849.

Ewell, James. *The Medical Companion, or Family Physician: Treating of the Diseases of the United States,* etc. Philadelphia: John Bioren, 1807.

Ewell, Thomas. *Letters to Ladies, Detailing Important Information, Concerning Themselves and Infants.* Philadelphia: W. Brown, 1817.

Feis, William B. *Grant's Secret Service.* Lincoln: Univ. of Nebraska Press, 2002.

Fellman, Anita Clair, and Michael Fellman. *Making Sense of Self: Medical Advice Literature in Late Nineteenth-Century America.* Philadelphia: Univ. of Pennsylvania Press, 1981.

Finger, John R. *Tennessee Frontiers: Three Regions in Transition.* Bloomington: Indiana Univ. Press, 2001.

Finger, Stanley. *Origins of Neuroscience: A History of Explorations into Brain Function.* Oxford: Oxford Univ. Press, 2001.

Fischer, David Hackett. *Albion's Seed.* New York: Oxford Univ. Press, 1989.

Fitch, John. *Annals of the Army of the Cumberland.* Philadelphia: J. B. Lippincott, 1863.

Flanigan, James C. *History of Gwinnett County, Georgia, 1818–1943*. Vol. 1, *1818–1943*. Hapeville, GA: Tyler, 1943.

———. *History of Gwinnett County, Georgia*. Vol. 2, *1818–1960*. Hapeville, GA: Tyler, 1943.

Flexner, Abraham. *Medical Education in the United States and Canada*. New York: Carnegie, 1910.

Foote, William Henry. *Sketches of North Carolina: Historical and Biographical, Illustrative of the Principles of a Portion of Her Early Settlers*. New York: Robert Carter, 1846.

Fountain, Sarah M. ed. *Sisters, Seeds and Cedars: Rediscovering Nineteenth-Century Life Through Correspondence from Rural Arkansas and Alabama*. Conway, AR: Univ. of Central Arkansas Press, 1995.

Garrett, Franklin M. *Atlanta and Environs: A Chronicle of Its People and Events, 1820s-1870s*. Vol. 1. Athens: Univ. of Georgia Press, 1969.

Garrett, Mary Lou Stewart. *History of Fairview Presbyterian Church of Greenville County, South Carolina*. Fountain Inn, SC: Fairview Presbyterian Church Session, 1986.

Garrison, Fielding H. *An Introduction to the History of Medicine*. 4th ed. Philadelphia: W. B. Saunders Company, 1929.

Gibson, William. *Institutes and Practice of Surgery: Being Outlines of a Course of Lectures*. Philadelphia: Edward Parker, 1824.

Gillespie, Michele, and Sally G. McMillen, ed. *North Carolina Women: Their Lives and Times*. Athens: Univ. of Georgia Press, 2014.

Goodspeed's *History of Benton, Washington, Carroll, Madison, Crawford, Franklin, and Sebastian Counties, Arkansas* (Chicago: Goodspeed, 1889).

Goodspeed's *A Reminiscent History of the Ozark Region* (Chicago: Goodspeed, 1894).

Gordon, Linda. *The Second Coming of the KKK: The Ku Klux Klan of the 1920s and the American Political Tradition*. New York: W. W. Norton, 2017.

Graf, Leroy P., and Ralph W. Haskins, ed. *The Papers of Andrew Johnson*. Vol. 6, *1862–1864*. Knoxville: Univ. of Tennessee Press, 1983.

Greene County [AR] Historical and Genealogical Society, ed. *Greene County, Arkansas: History and Families*. Vol. 1. Paducah, KY: Turner, 2001.

Gross, Samuel D. *A System of Surgery*. Philadelphia: Blanchard and Lea, 1862.

Gunn, John C. *Domestic Medicine, or, Poor Man's Friend*. Edited by Charles E. Rosenberg. Madisonville: Johnston and Edwards, 1830. Reprinted Knoxville: Univ. of Tennessee Press, 1986.

Gwinnett County Historical Society. *Gwinnett County: It All Started Here*. Dacula, GA: Dacula Rapid Press, 1978.

Hamilton, Frank H. *Introductory Lecture before the Surgical Class of Geneva Medical College*. Geneva: Merrel, 1840.

Hannan, Caryn, ed. *Georgia Biographical Dictionary*. Vol. 1, *A-J*. St. Clair Shores, MI: Somerset, 1999.

Harris, William S. *Historical Sketch of Poplar Tent Church, Cabarrus County, North Carolina*. Concord, NC: Times Book and Jobs Press, 1924.

Helfand, William H. *Quack, Quack, Quack: The Sellers of Nostrums in Prints, Posters, Ephemera and Books*. New York: Grolier Club, 2002.

Hempstead, Fay. *Historical Review of Arkansas: Its Commerce, Industry and Modern Affairs*. Vol. 1–3. Chicago: Lewis, 1911.

Herbert, William Chapman. *A Brief History of Medicine in the Spartanburg Region and the Spartanburg County Medical Society, 1700–1990*. Spartanburg: Spartanburg Medical Society, 1992.

Herman, Arthur. *The Scottish Enlightenment: The Scots' Invention of the Modern World*. New York: Random House, 2001.

Herndon, Dallas T. *Centennial History of Arkansas*. Vol. 2. Chicago: S. J. Clarke, 1911.

———. *Centennial History of Arkansas*. Vol. 3. Chicago: S. J. Clarke, 1922.

Hill, Samuel S. ed. *Encyclopedia of Religion in the South*. Macon: Mercer Univ. Press, 1984.

Hillhouse, Albert M. *A History of Burke County, Georgia, 1777–1950*. Swainsboro, GA: Magnolia, 1985.

Huff, Frederick Ware. *Four Families, Winn, Thomas, Ware, Garrett of the Southern United States from 1600s to 1993*. Kennesaw, GA: priv. publ., 1993.

Hunter, C. L. *Sketches of Western North Carolina Illustrating Principally the Revolutionary Period of Mecklenburg, Rowan, Lincoln and Adjoining Counties*. Raleigh, 1877.

Jefferson County Heritage Book Committee, ed. *The Heritage of Jefferson County, Alabama*. Clanton, AL: Heritage, 2002.

Johnson, Thomas. *Every Man His Own Doctor; or the Poor Man's Family Physician: Prescribing Plain, Safe, and Easy Means to Cure Themselves, of the Most Disorders Incident to This Climate with Very Little Charge, the Medicines Being the Growth of This Country, and About Almost Every Man's Plantation*. Salisbury, NC, 1798.

Jordan, Mary Alice. *Cotton to Kaolin: A History of Washington County, Georgia*. Milledgeville: Boyd, 1989.

Kelley, Dayton. *The Handbook of Waco and McLennan County, Texas*. Waco: Texian, 1972.

Knight, Lucian Lamar. *Georgia's Bi-centennial Memoirs and Memories: A Tale of Two Centuries, Reviewing the State's Marvelous Story of Achievement, Since Oglethorpe's Landing in 1733*. Vol. 1. Atlanta: priv. publ., 1931.

———. *Georgia's Landmarks, Memorials, and Legends*. Vol. 2. Atlanta: Byrd, 1914.

Kostlevy, William. *Holy Jumpers: Evangelicals and Radicals in Progressive Era America*. Oxford: Oxford Univ. Press, 2010.

Landrum, J. B. O. *History of Spartanburg County*. Atlanta: Franklin, 1900.

Laslett, Peter. *The World We Have Lost: England Before the Industrial Age*. London: Methuen, 1965.

Lass, William E. *A History of Steamboating on the Upper Missouri River*. Lincoln: Univ. of Nebraska Press, 1962.

Leavitt, Judith Walzer, and Ronald L. Numbers, ed. *Sickness and Health in America: Readings in the History of Medicine and Public Health*. Madison: Univ. of Wisconsin Press, 1978.

Lefler, Susan. *Brevard Then and Now*. Charleston, SC: Arcadia, 2011.

Leyburn, James C. *The Scotch-Irish: A Social History*. Chapel Hill: Univ. of North Carolina Press, 1962.

Lindsey, William D., ed. *Fiat Flux: The Writings of Wilson R. Bachelor, Nineteenth-Century Country Doctor and Philosopher.* Fayetteville: Univ. of Arkansas Press, 2013.

Liston, Robert. *Elements of Surgery.* Philadelphia: Ed. Barrington & Geo. D. Hasswell, 1842.

———. *Practical Surgery, with Notes and Additional Illustrations by George W. Norris.* Philadelphia: James Crissey, 1838.

Livingston, John. *Portraits of Eminent Americans Now Living: With Biographical and Historical Memoirs of Their Lives and Actions.* Vol. 3. New York: R. Craighead, 1854.

Long, Dorothy, ed. *Medicine in North Carolina: Essays in the History of Medical Science and Medical Service, 1524–1960.* Vol. 1, *Development of Medical Science, Medical Administrative Agencies, and Medical Service Facilities in North Carolina.* Raleigh: North Carolina Med. Soc., 1972.

———, ed. *Medicine in North Carolina: Essays in the History of Medical Science and Medical Service, 1524–1960.* Vol. 2, *Medical Education and Medical Service in North Carolina.* Raleigh: North Carolina Med. Soc., 1972.

McAllister, J. T. *Virginia Militia in the Revolutionary War.* Hot Springs, VA: McAllister, 1913.

McCabe, Alice Smythe, ed. *Gwinnett County, Georgia, Families, 1818–1968.* Atlanta: Cherokee, 1980.

McClellan, George. *Principles and Practice of Surgery.* Philadelphia: Grigg & Elliott, 1848.

McManners, John, ed. *The Oxford Illustrated History of Christianity.* New York: Oxford Univ. Press, 1990.

Matthews, William. *A Treatise on Domestic Medicine and Kindred Subjects: Embracing Anatomical and Physiological Sketches of the Human Body.* Indianapolis: John D. Defrees, 1848.

Meriwether, Robert L., ed., *Papers of John C. Calhoun.* Vol. 5, *1820–1821.* Columbia: Univ. of South Carolina Press, 1959.

Miller, James David. *South by Southwest: Planter Emigration and Identity in the South and Southwest.* Charlottesville: Univ. of Virginia, 2002.

Moneyhon, Carl. *Arkansas and the New South, 1874–1929* (Fayetteville: Univ. of Arkansas Press, 1997).

Moore, Albert Burton. *History of Alabama and Her People.* Vol. 2. Chicago: American Historical Society, 1927.

Moore, David G. *William S. Rosecrans and the Union Victory: A Civil War Biography.* Jefferson, NC: McFarland, 2014.

Morgan, John. *A Discourse upon the Institution of Medical Schools in America.* Philadelphia: 1765. Reprinted Baltimore: Johns Hopkins Press, 1937.

Moss, Bobby Gilmer. *The Patriots at the Cowpens.* Blacksburg, SC: Moss, 1985.

Northen, William J., and John Temple Graves, ed. *Men of Mark in Georgia: A Complete and Elaborate History of the State from Its Settlement to the Present Time, Chiefly Told in Biographies and Autobiographies of the Most Eminent Men of Each Period of Georgia's Progress and Development.* Vol. 2. Atlanta: A. B. Caldwell, 1910.

Norwood, William Frederick. *Medical Education in the United States Before the Civil War.* Philadelphia: Univ. of Pennsylvania Press, 1944.

Numbers, Ronald L., ed. *The Education of American Physicians: Historical Essays.* Berkeley: Univ. of California Press, 1980.

Pendleton District Historic and Recreation Commission. *Pendleton Historic District: A Survey.* Pendleton, SC: Pendleton Dist. Historic and Recreation Commission, 1973.

Perry County Historical and Genealogical Society. *Perry County, Arkansas, Its Land and People.* Marceline, MO: Walworth, 2004.

Phillips, A. L. *An Historical Sketch of the Presbyterian Church of Fayetteville, North Carolina.* Fayetteville, NC: J.E. Garrett, 1889.

Pitts, Lulie. *History of Gordon County, Georgia.* Calhoun, GA: Calhoun Times Press, 1933.

Porter, Roy, ed. *The Cambridge History of Science.* Vol. 4, *Eighteenth-Century Science.* Cambridge: Cambridge Univ. Press, 2003.

Powell, William S., ed. *Dictionary of North Carolina Biography,* 6 vols. Chapel Hill: Univ. of North Carolina Press, 1988–1996.

Rankin, Harriet Sutton. *History of First Presbyterian Church, Fayetteville, North Carolina: From Old Manuscripts and Addresses.* Fayetteville, NC: First Presbyterian Church, 1928.

Risse, Guenter B., Ronald L. Numbers, and Judith Walzer Leavitt, ed. *Medicine Without Doctors: Home Health Care in American History.* New York: Science History Publications, 1977.

Ritzer, George, and J. Michael Ryan, ed. *The Concise Encyclopedia of Sociology.* Malden, MA: Wiley-Blackwell, 2011.

Rohrbough, Malcolm J. *The Trans-Appalachian Frontier: People, Societies, and Institutions 1775–1850.* New York: Oxford Univ. Press, 1978.

Rosenberg, Charles E., ed. *Right Living: An Anglo-American Tradition of Self-Help Medicine and Hygiene.* Baltimore: Johns Hopkins, 2003.

Runes, Dagobert, ed. *The Selected Writings of Benjamin Rush.* New York: Philosophical Library, 1947.

Rush, Benjamin. *The Autobiography of Benjamin Rush: His "Travels Through Life" Together with His Commonplace Book for 1789–1813.* Edited by George W. Corner. Princeton: Princeton Univ. Press, 1948.

Russell, Ralph Morgan. *Handbook of Home Medicine: Devoted Principally to the Latest and Most Approved Methods of Home Treatment of Diseases Peculiar to the South and West.* Chicago: Hammond, 1900–1911.

Russo, David J. *Families and Communities: A New View of American History.* Nashville: American Assoc. for State and Local History, 1977.

Sargent, Greg D. *Polk County, Georgia.* Charleston, SC: Arcadia, 1998.

Schroeder-Lein, Glenna R. *Confederate Hospitals on the Move: Samuel H. Stout and the Army of Tennessee.* Columbia: Univ. of South Carolina Press, 1994.

Sherrod, Ricky Lee, and Annette Pierce Sherrod. *Plain Folk, Planters, and the Complexities of Southern Society.* Nacogdoches: Stephen F. Austin Univ. Press, 2014.

Shryock, Richard Harrison. *American Medical Research Past and Present.* New York: Commonwealth Fund, 1947.

Smith, Merril D. *Women's Roles in Eighteenth-Century America*. Santa Barbara, CA: Greenwood, 2010.

Spencer, Thomas Morris, ed. *The Other Missouri History: Populists, Prostitutes, and Regular Folk*. Columbia: Univ. of Missouri Press, 2004.

Sprague, William B., ed. *Annals of the American Pulpit*. Vol. 4, *Presbyterian*. New York: Robert Carter & Brothers, 1859.

Stowe, Steven M. *Doctoring the South: Southern Physicians and Everyday Medicine in the Mid-Nineteenth Century*. Chapel Hill: Univ. of North Carolina Press, 2004.

Sweet, William Warren. *Religion on the American Frontier*. Vol. 1, *The Baptists, 1783–1830*. New York: Henry Holt, 1931.

———. *Religion on the American Frontier*. Vol. 4, *The Methodists, 1783–1840*. New York: Cooper Square, 1964.

———. *Religion on the American Frontier*. Vol. 2, *The Presbyterians, 1783–1840*. New York: Cooper Square, 1964.

Thomas, Robert, and David Hosack. *A Treatise on Domestic Medicine: Pointing Out, in Plain Language, and as Free from Professional Terms as Possible, the Nature, Symptoms, Causes, Probable Terminations, and Treatment of All Diseases Incident to Men, Women, and Children, in Both Cold and Warm Climates, etc*. New York: A. Paul, 1820.

Thomson, Samuel. *New Guide to Health, or Botanic Family Physician*. Boston: House, 1825.

Tompkins, Daniel Augustus. *History of Mecklenburg County and the City of Charlotte: From 1740 to 1903*. Vol. 1. Charlotte: Observer, 1903.

Towne, Stephen E. *Surveillance and Spies in the Civil War: Exposing Confederate Conspiracies in America's Heartland*. Athens, OH: Ohio Univ. Press, 2014.

Trefousse, Hans L. *Andrew Johnson: A Biography*. New York: W. W. Norton, 1989.

Velpeau, Alfred. *New Elements of Operative Surgery*. New York: Henry G. Langley, 1845–1847.

Welter, Barbara. *Dimity Convictions: The American Woman in the Nineteenth Century*. Athens, OH: Ohio Univ. Press, 1976.

Wheeler, John Hill. *Historical Sketches of North Carolina: From 1584 to 1851*. Philadelphia: Lippincott, 1851.

Wheeler, Kitty. *Histories and Biographies of Van Zandt County*. Vol. 2, *1848–1991*. Wills Point: Van Zandt County Genealogical Society, 1991.

Wickes, Stephen. *History of Medicine in New Jersey and of Its Medical Men, from the Settlement of the Province to A. D. 1800*. Newark: Martin R. Dennis, 1879.

Wills, Gregory A. *Democratic Religion: Freedom, Authority, and Church Discipline in the Baptist South, 1785–1900*. New York: Oxford Univ. Press, 1997.

Wilson, Charles Reagan, and William Ferris, ed. *Encyclopedia of Southern Culture, 1473–1476*. Chapel Hill: Univ. of North Carolina Press, 1989.

Wyatt-Brown, Bertram. *Honor and Violence in the Old South*. New York: Oxford Univ. Press, 1986.

Winters, John D. *The Civil War in Louisiana*. Baton Rouge: Louisiana State Univ. Press. 1963.

II. Published Articles and Essays

Abrahams, Harold J. "Extinct Medical Schools of Nineteenth Century Philadelphia: (II) The Philadelphia College of Medicine." *Transactions and Studies of the College of Physicians of Philadelphia* 30 (1963): pp. 163–178.

Adams, Michele. "Divisions of Household Labor." In *The Concise Encyclopedia of Sociology*, edited by George Ritzer and J. Michael Ryan, pp. 156–157. Malden, MA: Wiley-Blackwell, 2011.

Andrews, Gregg. "The Racial Politics in Ralls County, 1865–1870." In *The Other Missouri History: Populists, Prostitutes, and Regular Folk*, edited by Thomas Morris Spencer, pp. 8–30. Columbia: Univ. of Missouri Press, 2004.

Ayers, Edward L. "Honor." In *Encyclopedia of Southern Culture*, edited by Charles Reagan Wilson and William Ferris, pp. 1483–1484. Chapel Hill: Univ. of North Carolina Press, 1989.

Bailey, David T. "Frontier Religion." In *Encyclopedia of Southern Culture*, edited by Charles Reagan Wilson and William Ferris, pp. 1286–1288. Chapel Hill: Univ. of North Carolina Press, 1989.

Benning, Anna Caroline. "Seaborn Jones." In *Men of Mark in Georgia: A Complete and Elaborate History of the State from Its Settlement to the Present Time, Chiefly Told in Biographies and Autobiographies of the Most Eminent Men of Each Period of Georgia's Progress and Development*. Vol. 2, edited by William J. Northen and John Temple Graves, pp. 236–242. Atlanta: A. B. Caldwell, 1910.

Berman. Alex. "The Heroic Approach in 19th-Century Therapeutics." In *Sickness and Health in America: Readings in the History of Medicine and Public Health*, edited by Judith Walzer Leavitt and Ronald L. Numbers, pp. 77–85. Madison: Univ. of Wisconsin Press, 1978.

Bevan, A. D. "The Study and Teaching and the Practice of Surgery." *Annals of Surgery* 98 (1933): pp. 481–494.

Blackburn, George T. "Harris, Charles Wilson." In *Dictionary of North Carolina Biography*. Vol. 3, *H–K*, edited by William S. Powell, pp. 50–51. Chapel Hill: Univ. of North Carolina Press, 1988.

Blake, John B. "From Buchan to Fishbein." In *Medicine Without Doctors: Home Health Care in American History*, edited by Guenter B. Risse, Ronald L. Numbers, and Judith Walzer Leavitt, pp. 11–30. New York: Science History Publications, 1977. Brieger, Gert H. "Surgery." In *The Education of American Physicians: Historical Essays*, edited by Ronald Numbers, pp. 175–204. Berkeley: Univ. of California Press, 1980.

Broman, Thomas H. "The Medical Sciences." In *The Cambridge History of Science*. Vol. 4, *Eighteenth-Century Science*, edited by Roy Porter, pp. 463–485. Cambridge: Cambridge Univ. Press, 2003.

Bruce, Dickson D., Jr. "Frontier, Influence of." In *Encyclopedia of Religion in the South*, edited by Samuel S. Hill, pp. 273–275. Macon: Mercer Univ. Press, 1984.

Buckley, Thomas E. "Placed in the Power of Violence: The Divorce Petition of Evelina Gregory Roane, 1824." *Virginia Magazine of History and Biography* 110, no. 1 (January 1992): pp. 29–78.

Cassedy, James H. "Why Self-Help? Americans Alone with Their Diseases 1800–1840." In *Medicine Without Doctors: Home Health Care in American History*, edited by Guenter B. Risse, Ronald L. Numbers, and Judith Walzer Leavitt, pp. 31–48. New York: Science History Publications, 1977.

Clower, George W. "Thomas Winn (c. 1741–1797) and His Remarkable Connection with Atlanta Through His Descendants." *Atlanta Historical Bulletin* 12, no. 4 (1967): pp. 38–46.

Detlefsen, Nancy Roberts: "Bosqueville." In *Historic McLennan County: An Illustrated History*, edited by Sharon Bracken, p. 19. San Antonio: Lammert, 2010.

Duffy, John. "The Changing Image of the American Physician." In *Sickness and Health in America: Readings in the History of Medicine and Public Health*, edited by Judith Walzer Leavitt and Ronald L. Numbers, pp. 131–137. Madison: Univ. of Wisconsin Press, 1978.

Ebert, Myrl. "The Rise and Development of the American Medical Periodical, 1797–1850." *Bulletin of the Medical Library Association* 40 (1952): pp. 243–276.

Edwards, Laura F. "Gender and the Changing Roles of Women." In *A Companion to 19th-Century America*, edited by William Barney, pp. 225–226. Malden, MA: Wiley-Blackwell, 2001.

Feis, William B. "'There Is a Bad Enemy in This City': Colonel William Truesdail's Army Police and the Occupation of Nashville, 1862–1863." *North and South* 8, no. 2 (March 2005): pp. 34–45.

Fountain, Sarah M. "Introduction." In *Sisters, Seeds and Cedars: Rediscovering Nineteenth-Century Life Through Correspondence from Rural Arkansas and Alabama*, edited by Sarah M. Fountain, p. xiii–xvi. Conway, AR: Univ. of Central Arkansas Press, 1995. Franklin, Winnie. "Reminiscences of Early Lorado." *Greene County [AR] Historical Quarterly* 6, no. 4 (1971): pp. 14–15.

Furches, D. M. "Judge Harris, of Iredell." *North Carolina Journal of Law* 2, no. 6 (June 1905): pp. 267–270.

Gastil, Raymond D. "Violence, Crime, and Punishment." In *Encyclopedia of Southern Culture, 1473–1476*, edited by Charles Reagan Wilson and William Ferris, pp. 1473–1476. Chapel Hill: Univ. of North Carolina Press, 1989.

"General Notes." *Bulletin of the Pan American Union* 52, no. 3 (March 1921): pp. 303–316.

Gordon, James M. "Contributions to Practical Midwifery, with Cases Occurring in Obstetrical Practice." *Southern Medical and Surgical Journal* 3, no. 12 (December 1847): pp. 703–717.

———. "Letter." *Southern Medical and Surgical Journal* 5, no. 2 (February 1849): pp. 120–121.

———. "Observations on Ranula: with Cases, Treatment and Cure." *Southern Medical and Surgical Journal* 5, no. 2 (February 1849): pp. 65–69.

———. "A Remarkable Case of Volvulus and Strangulation of the Intestines Within the Abdomen." *Boston Medical and Surgical Journal* 33, no. 2 (August 1845): pp. 39–41.

———. "A Remarkable Case of Volvulus and Strangulation of the Intestines Within the Abdomen." *Southern Medical and Surgical Journal* 1, no. 8, new series (August 1845): pp. 444–447.

Green, Edith Huff, and Mildred Huff Breedlove. "John Huff." In *Gwinnett County, Georgia, Families, 1818–1968*, edited by Alice Smythe McCabe, pp. 245–255. (Atlanta: Cherokee, 1980).

Griesemer, A. D., W. D. Widmann, K. A. Forde, and M. A. Hardy. "John Jones, M.D.: Pioneer, Patriot, and Founder of American Surgery." *World Journal of Surgery* 34, no. 4 (April 2010): pp. 605–609.

Helfand, William H. "Advertising Health to the People: The Early Illustrated Posters." In *Right Living: An Anglo-American Tradition of Self-Help Medicine and Hygiene*, edited by Charles E. Rosenberg, pp. 170–185. Baltimore: Johns Hopkins, 2003.

Hoolihan, Christopher. "Every Man His Own Physician: Ephemera and Medical Self-Help." *The Ephemera Journal* 15, no. 3 (May 2013): pp. 3–9.

Horn, Stanley F. "Dr. John Rolfe Hudson and the Confederate Underground in Nashville." *Tennessee Historical Quarterly* 22, no. 1 (March 1964): pp. 38–52.

Horrocks, Thomas A. "Rules, Remedies, and Regimens: Health Advice in Early American Almanacs." In *Right Living: An Anglo-American Tradition of Self-Help Medicine and Hygiene*, edited by Charles E. Rosenberg, pp. 112–146. Baltimore: Johns Hopkins, 2003.

"Howell, Evan Park." *Georgia Biographical Dictionary*. Vol. 1, *A–J*, edited by Caryn Hannan, pp. 423–424. St. Clair Shores, MI: Somerset, 1999.

Hoyt, William R. "Presbyterianism." *Encyclopedia of Religion in the South*, edited by Samuel S. Hill, pp. 607–611. Macon: Mercer Univ. Press, 1984.

Humphreys, Lincoln. "Experiences of a Naval Medical Officer." *Journal of the Arkansas Medical Society* 17, no. 4 (September 1920): pp. 98–102.

Johnson, Lucie Miller. "John Robinson." *Dictionary of North Carolina Biography*. Vol. 5, *P–S*, edited by William S. Powell, pp. 236–237. Chapel Hill: Univ. of North Carolina Press, 1994).

Jordan, H. B. "Beverly Wyly Dunn." *Sixty-Eighth Annual Report of Graduates of the United States Military Academy at West Point, New York*, pp. 101–106. Newburgh, NY: Moore, 1937.

"Joseph P. Runyan Obituary." *Journal of the Arkansas Medical Society* 27, no. 9 (February 1931): pp. 191–192.

Kaufman, Martin. "American Medical Education." In *The Education of American Physicians: Historical Essays*, edited by Ronald L. Numbers, pp. 7–28. Berkeley: Univ. of California Press, 1980.

Kemper, George. "Houston." In *Perry County, Arkansas, Its Land and People*, edited by Perry County Historical and Genealogical Society, pp. 143–144. Marceline, MO: Walworth, 2004.

Kent, Annie Mae, and Edith Huff Green. "Dr. William James Russell." In *Gwinnett County, Georgia, Families, 1818–1968*, edited by Alice Smythe McCabe, pp. 431–432. Atlanta: Cherokee, 1980.

Kerber, Linda K. "Separate Spheres, Female Worlds, Woman's Place: The Rhetoric of Women's History." *The Journal of American History* 75, no. 1 (1988): pp. 9–39.

"Last Roll: L. A. Whatley," *Confederate Veteran* 19, no. 10 (October 1911): p. 488.

"Last Roll: Mrs. Araminta Claiborne Hudson," *Confederate Veteran* 12, no. 4 (1904): p. 194.

Lindsey, William D. "Introduction." In *Fiat Flux: The Writings of Wilson R. Bachelor, Nineteenth-Century Country Doctor and Philosopher,* edited by Lindsey, pp. 3–37. Fayetteville: Univ. of Arkansas Press, 2013.

Livingston, John. "William J. Russell, M.D., of Lawrenceville, Gwinnett County, Georgia." *Portraits of Eminent Americans Now Living: With Biographical and Historical Memoirs of Their Lives and Actions.* Vol. 3, pp. 281–284. New York: R. Craighead, 1854.

"Lorado." In *Greene County, Arkansas: History and Families.* Vol. 1, edited by Greene County Historical and Genealogical Society, p. 20. Paducah, KY: Turner, 2001.

Marty, Martin. "North America." In *The Oxford Illustrated History of Christianity,* edited by John McManners, pp. 384–419. New York: Oxford Univ. Press, 1990.

McLendon, William M. "Edenborough Medical College: North Carolina's First Chartered School of Medicine." In *Medicine in North Carolina: Essays in the History of Medical Science and Medical Service, 1524–1960.* Vol. 2, *Medical Education and Medical Service in North Carolina,* edited by Dorothy Lang, pp. 351–363. Raleigh: North Carolina Med. Soc., 1972.

"Mechanical Fakes: The Electropoise—Oxydonor—Oxygenor—Oxygenator— Oxypathor—Oxytonor." In *Nostrums and Quackery: Articles on the Nostrum Evil and Quackery Reprinted, with Additions and Modifications, from the Journal of the American Medical Association.* Vol. 1, edited by American Medical Association, pp. 243–257. Chicago: AMA, 1912.

"Medical Heritage." *The Heritage of Jefferson County, Alabama,* edited by Jefferson County Heritage Book Committee, pp. 186–206. Clanton, AL: Heritage, 2002.

"Medical Intelligence." *The Southern Medical and Surgical Journal* 1, no. 4 (1845): 224.

Morrison, Alfred J. "Militia Officers, Prince Edward County, 1777–1781." *Virginia Magazine of History and Biography* 21 (1913): pp. 201–202.

Morrison, Robert H. "John Robinson." In *Annals of the American Pulpit.* Vol. 4, *Presbyterian,* edited by William B. Sprague, pp. 113–117. New York: Robert Carter & Brothers, 1859.

Norwood, B. F. "The Application of the Schick Reaction to 2,911 Naval Recruits and the Immunization of Susceptibles to Diphtheria with Toxin-Antitoxin." *United States Naval Medical Bulletin* 15, no. 2 (April 1921): pp. 485–491.

———. "A Case of Poisoning by Oil of Chenopodium." *United States Naval Medical Bulletin* 15, no. 4 (October 1921): pp. 818–823.

———. "Outbreak of Food Poisoning on Board the U.S.S. 'Cincinnati' Attributed to Corned-Beef Hash." *United States Naval Medical Bulletin* 24 (July 1926): pp. 680–682.

Norwood, William Frederick. "Medical Education and the Rise of Hospitals: II: The Nineteenth Century." *JAMA* 186, no. 11 (December 1963): pp. 134–138.

Numbers, Ronald L. "Do-It-Yourself the Sectarian Way." In *Sickness and Health in America: Readings in the History of Medicine and Public Health,* edited by

Judith Walzer Leavitt and Ronald L. Numbers, pp. 87–96. Madison: Univ. of Wisconsin Press, 1978.

P. B. F. "Domestic Correspondence," *Journal of the American Medical Association* 4, no. 13 (28 March 1885): pp. 362–364.

Pentecost, C. L., and Aldyne Maltbie. "William Maltbie." In *Gwinnett County, Georgia, Families, 1818–1968*, edited by Alice Smythe McCabe, pp. 319–321. Atlanta: Cherokee, 1980.

Risse, Guenter B. "Introduction." In *Medicine Without Doctors: Home Health Care in American History*, edited by Guenter B. Risse, Ronald L. Numbers, and Judith Walzer Leavitt, pp. 1–10. New York: Science History Publications, 1977.

Robbins, Angela. "Alice Morgan Person: 'My Life Has Been Out of the Ordinary Run of Woman's Life.'" *North Carolina Women: Their Lives and Times*, edited by Michele Gillespie and Sally G. McMillen, pp. 152–173. Athens: Univ. of Georgia Press, 2014.

Rogers, Blair O. "Surgery in the Revolutionary War, Contributions of John Jones, M.D. (1729–1791)." *Plastic and Reconstructive Surgery* 49, no. 1 (January 1972): pp. 1–13.

Rosenberg, Charles E. "Health in the Home: A Tradition of Print and Practice." In *Right Living: An Anglo-American Tradition of Self-Help Medicine and Hygiene*, edited by Charles E. Rosenberg, pp. 1–20. Baltimore: Johns Hopkins, 2003.

———. "Introduction." In *Domestic Medicine, or, Poor Man's Friend*, edited by Rosenberg, pp. v–xxi. Knoxville, 1830. Reprinted Knoxville: Univ. of Tennessee Press, 1986.

———. "Preface." *Right Living: An Anglo-American Tradition of Self-Help Medicine and Hygiene*, edited by Rosenberg, pp. vii–ix. Baltimore: Johns Hopkins, 2003.

Runes, Dagobert D. "Preface." In *The Selected Writings of Benjamin Rush*, edited by Runes, pp. vii–ix. New York: Philosophical Library, 1947.

Silveus, Marian. "Churches and Social Control on the Western Pennsylvania Frontier." *Western Pennsylvania Historical Magazine* 19 (1936): pp. 123–134.

Smith, Stephen. "Union of Didactic and Clinical Instruction." *American Medical Times* 9 (1864): pp. 119–122.

Smith, Timothy B. "A Siege from the Start: The Spring 1862 Campaign against Corinth, Mississippi." *Journal of Mississippi History* 66, no. 4 (2004): pp. 403–424.

Stowe, Steven. "Conflict and Self-Sufficiency: Domestic Medicine in the American South." In *Right Living: An Anglo-American Tradition of Self-Help Medicine and Hygiene*, edited by Charles E. Rosenberg, pp. 148–169. Baltimore: Johns Hopkins, 2003.

Taylor, Orville W. "Arkansas." In *Encyclopedia of Religion in the South*, edited by Samuel S. Hill, pp. 50–69. Macon: Mercer Univ. Press, 1984.

Unemoa, Magnus, and William M. Shafer. "Antimicrobial Resistance in *Neisseria gonorrhoeae* in the 21st Century: Past, Evolution, and Future." *Clinical Microbiology Reviews* 27, no. 3 (July 2014): pp. 587–613.

Waite, Frederick C. "The Professional Education of Pioneer Ohio Physicians." *Ohio State Archaeological and Historical Society* 48 (1939): pp. 189–197.

Wilson, Charles Reagan. "Religion and Education." In *Encyclopedia of Southern Culture, 1473–1476*, edited by Charles Reagan Wilson and William Ferris, pp. 261–263. Chapel Hill: Univ. of North Carolina Press, 1989.

Young, James Harvey. "Device Quackery in America." In *Sickness and Health in America: Readings in the History of Medicine and Public Health*, edited by Judith Walzer Leavitt and Ronald L. Numbers, pp. 97–102. Madison: Univ. of Wisconsin Press, 1978.

———. "Patent Medicines and the Self-Help Syndrome." In *Medicine Without Doctors: Home Health Care in American History*, edited by Guenter B. Risse, Ronald L. Numbers, and Judith Walzer Leavitt, pp. 95–116. New York: Science History Publications, 1977.

III. Published Catalogs, Biographical Directories, City Directories, Gazetteers, Legislative Documents, Yearbooks

Acts and Resolutions of the General Assembly of the State of Georgia Passed in Milledgeville at an Annual Session in November and December 1837. Milledgeville: P. L. Robinson, 1838.

Acts Passed by the General Assembly of the State of Georgia, Passed in Milledgeville, at a Biennial Session in November, December, and January, 1851–2. Macon: Samuel J. Ray, 1852.

Arkansas Caduceus 1941. Little Rock: Univ. of Arkansas Medical School, 1941.

Arkansas State Gazetteer Business Directories 1893–1894. Detroit: R. L. Polk, 1894.

Army and Navy Register 62,2180 (1 July 1922).

Bellevue Hospital Medical College, Twenty-Seventh Annual Commencement. 12 March 1888.

Bureau of Navigation, Navy Department. *Navy Directory, Officers of the United States Navy and Marine Corps.* Washington, D.C.: Government Printing Office, July 1918.

———. *Navy Directory, Officers of the United States Navy and Marine Corps.* Washington, D.C.: Government Printing Office, August, September, November 1918; December 1919; September, November 1922; July 1925; October 1929; April 1930; April, July 1934; April 1937; October 1941.

Cameron, Mabel Ward. *The Biographical Cyclopedia of American Women.* Vol. 2, *American Biographical Notes.* New York: Halvord, 1924.

Catalogue of the Classes and Graduates of the Philadelphia College of Medicine for 1849–'50, and 1850. Philadelphia: Hughes & Gaskill, 1850.

Charleston City Directory 1934. Charleston, SC: Southern Printing, 1934.

City Directory of Birmingham, Alabama, 1897. N.p.: Maloney Directory, 1897.

College of Physicians and Surgeons. *Second Annual Catalogue and Announcement Session of 1907–1908.* Little Rock, AR, June 1907.

Daniell, Lewis E. *Personnel of the Texas State Government: With Sketches of Distinguished Texans, Embracing the Executive and Staff, Heads of the Departments, United States Senators and Representatives, Members of the XXth Legislature.* Austin: City Printing, 1887.

"Degrees Conferred, 1911–1912." *University of Tennessee Record* 16, no. 4 (April 1913): 221–223.

Hafner, Arthur Wayne, ed., *Directory of Deceased American Physicians, 1804–1929: A Genealogical Guide to Over 149,000 Medical Practitioners Providing Brief Biographical Sketches Drawn from the American Medical Association's Deceased Physician Masterfile*. Chicago: American Medical Association, 1993.

Hammond, N. J. *Reports of Cases in Law and Equity, Argued and Determined in the Supreme Court of the State of Georgia, at Milledgeville, June Term 1867, and Part of December Term 1867*. Vol. 36. Macon: J. W. Burke, 1868.

Los Angeles Directory Co.'s San Pedro and Wilmington City Directory 1940. Los Angeles: Los Angeles Directory, 1940.

Martin, B. Y. *Reports of Cases in Law and Equity, Argued and Determined in the Supreme Court of the State of Georgia from November Term, 1859, at Milledgeville, to June Term, 1860, at Macon, Inclusive*. Vol. 30. Atlanta: Franklin, 1862.

Maloney's 1900 Birmingham Directory. Atlanta: Maloney Directory, 1900.

Morrison and Fourmy's General Directory of the City of Dallas 1886–87. Galveston: Morrison & Fourmy, 1887.

Polk's Little Rock and North Little Rock Directory 1925. Little Rock: R. L. Polk, 1925, 1926, 1928.

Polk's Memphis City Directory 1909. Detroit: R. L. Polk, 1909, 1910, 1911, 1912, 1914, 1915, 1916., 1917.

Polk's Southern Directory Co.'s Little Rock and Argenta City Directory 1914. Little Rock: Polk's Southern Directory, 1914.

Polk's Southern Directory Co.'s Little Rock and North Little Rock City Directory 1919. Little Rock: Polk's Southern Directory, 1919, 1920.

R. L. Polk & Co.'s Birmingham Directory 1904 (Birmingham: R. L. Polk, 1904, 1907, 1909).

Seventeenth Annual Announcement of the Medical College of Georgia. Augusta: Jas. McCafferty, 1848.

Southern Directory Co.'s Little Rock City Directory 1922. Little Rock: Southern Directory, 1922.

State Board of Health. *Transactions of the Medical Association of the State of Alabama* Montgomery: Brown, 1889, 1891, 1917.

Third Session, Forty-First Congress, Executive Documents Printed by Order of the House of Representatives 1870–'1. United States Congressional Serial Set 1453. Washington, D.C.: Government Printing Office, 1871.

"University of Tennessee Announcement, College of Medicine, Memphis, Tenn." *University of Tennessee Bulletin* 3, no. 4 (June 1912): 1–47.

US Letters Patent #579,808.

US Naval Bureau of Naval Personnel. *Register of the Commissioned and Warrant Officers of the United States Navy and Marine Corps* (Washington, D.C.: Government Printing Office, 1918, 1919, 1920, 1921, 1922, 1923, 1924, 1925, 1926, 1927, 1935, 1940, 1942).

US Patent Office. *Annual Report of the Commissioner of Patents*. Washington, D.C.: Government Printing Office, 1897.

US Patent Office. *Official Gazette of the United States Patent Office*. Vol. 78. Washington, D.C., Government Printing Office, 1897.

The Volunteer. Vol. 16, *1912*. Knoxville: Univ. of Tennessee, 1912.

The War of the Rebellion: A Compilation of the Official Records of the Union and Confederate Armies. Series 2, vol. 5, serial 118, *Correspondence, Orders, etc., Relating to Prisoners of War and State, Dec. 1, 1862–June 10, 1863.* Washington: Government Printing Office, 1899.

Who's Important in Medicine, 2nd ed. Hicksville, NY: Institute for Research in Biography, 1952.

Wiggins' Birmingham City Directory 1903. Columbus, OH: Wiggins Directories, 1903.

Wilda's Birmingham and Suburban Directory 1893. Birmingham, AL: RWA Wilda, 1893.

IV. Newspaper Articles and Published Transcripts of Newspaper Articles

Accident of Andrew J. Shaffer. *Weekly Gwinnett Herald* (Lawrenceville, GA), 19 March 1873, p. 3.

Advertisement for Electrozone and Russell Medical Institute. *People's Party Advocate* (Ashland, AL), 15 December 1898, p. 3, col. 4.

Advertisement for Maltbie Chemical Company's Acetaniled and Caffeine Compound. Voucher by W. S. R. Russell. *Charlotte [NC] Medical Journal* 4, no. 2 (February 1894): 80.

Advertisement for Maurice & Co. *Beaumont Banner* (Beaumont, TX), 8 January 1861, p. 3.

Advertisement for Medical Services of Drs. Adams and Potts. *Times-Picayune* (New Orleans, LA), 3 February 1872, p. 2.

Advertisement for Medical Services of John J. Boring. *Atlanta Constitution* (Atlanta, GA), 1 July 1868, p. 1.

Advertisement for Medical Services of Dr. Carr. *Semi-Weekly Mississippian* (Jackson, MS), 11 September 1860, p. 1.

Advertisement for Medical Services of Drs. Choppin, Beard, Brickell, and Bruns. *The South-Western* (Shreveport, LA), 17 November 1889, p. 3.

Advertisement for Medical Services of E. Collins. *Arkansas Gazette* (Little Rock, AR), 22 February 1870, p. 2

Advertisement for Medical Services of Dr. Connaughton. *Arkansas Gazette* (Little Rock, AR), 3 April 1878, p. 6.

Advertisement for Medical Services of Dr. Hartman and Dr. Miller. *Times Democrat* (New Orleans, LA), 4 March 1884, p. 8.

Advertisement for Medical Services of J. W. McClure. *Arkansas Gazette* (Little Rock, AR), 8 July 1871, p. 4.

Advertisement for Medical Services of A. J. Miller. *Times-Picayune* (New Orleans, LA), 17 December 1884, p. 4.

Advertisement for Medical Services of S. H. Mitchell. *Hinds County Gazette* (Raymond, MS), 23 March 1853, p. 3.

Advertisement for Medical Services of C. W. Parker. *The Meridional* (Abbeville, LA), 14 May 1892, p. 1.

Advertisement for Medical Services of Dr. Prentice. *Times-Picayune* (New Orleans, LA), 28 April 1884, p. 2.

Advertisement for Medical Services of Ralph Morgan Russell. *Tuscaloosa Weekly Times* (Tuscaloosa, AL), 2 June 1899, p. 1, col. 1–4.

Advertisement for Medical Services of William James Park Russell. *Arkansas Gazette* (Little Rock, AR), 13 October 1868, p. 3, col. 5; 15–16 October 1868, p. 2, col. 5; 21 October 1868, p. 3, col. 2; 13 November 1868, p. 3, col. 3.

Advertisement for Medical Services of William James Park Russell. *Southern Banner* (Athens, GA), 1 July 1858, p. 3, col. 2.

Advertisement for Medical Services of William James Park Russell. *Tuskegee Republican* (Tuskegee, AL), 3 June 1858, p. 2, col. 1.

Advertisement for Medical Services of William James Park Russell. *Tuskegee Republican* (Tuskegee, AL), 10 June 1858, p. 2, col. 6.

Advertisement for Medical Services of Wedon Smith. *Richland Beacon* (Rayville, LA), 4 May 1889, p. 3.

Advertisement for Medical Services of J. S. Stewart and J. B. Chess. *Dallas Daily Herald* (Dallas, TX), 4 January 1876, p. 3.

Advertisement for Medical Services of Surgeons of Central Surgical Infirmary of Indianapolis. *Arkansas Gazette* (Little Rock, AR), 5 February 1880, p. 1.

Advertisement for Medical Services of Surgeons of Surgical Institutes of Atlanta and Indianapolis. *The Times* (Shreveport, LA), 11 March 1884, p. 4.

Advertisement for Perry Davis' Vegetable Pain Killer. *Red Bluff Independent* (Red Bluff, CA), 23 January 1867, p. 4, col. 3.

Advertisement for Russell Medical Institute. *Birmingham Age-Herald* (Birmingham, AL), 14 February 1894, p. 3, col. 3; 14 March 1894, p. 6, col. 5.

Advertisement for Russell Medical Institute *Choctaw Herald* (Butler, AL), 17 March 1897, p. 4, col. 3; 2 June 1897, p. 4, col. 2–3.

Advertisement for Russell Medical Institute. *Mountain Eagle* (Jasper, AL), 2 December 1896, p. 3, col. 6–7.

Advertisement for Russell Medical Institute. *Mountain Eagle* (Jasper, AL), 25 August 1897, p. 4, col. 5–6.

Advertisement for Russell Medical Institute. *People's Weekly Tribune* (Birmingham, AL), 26 March 1896, p. 8, col. 5–6.

Advertisement for Russell Medical Institute. *People's Weekly Tribune* (Birmingham, AL), 9 April 1896, p. 8, col. 5–6.

Advertisement for Vi-Be Ni Liver Pills. *Brevard News* (Brevard, NC), 24 July 1914, p. 6, col. 1–2; 7 August 1914, p. 6, col. 1–2; 14 August, p. 6, col. 2–3; 21 August, p. 8, col. 4–5; 28 August, p. 8, col. 4–5; 4 September 1914, p. 8, col. 4–5.

Advertisement for Vi-Be Ni Malt Tonic. *Coosa River News* (Centre, AL), 3 November 1899, p. 5, col. 3.

Announcement of Business Trip of Wm. S. Russell, Representing D. Appleton & Co. *Nashville News* (Nashville, AR), 14 July 1900, p. 2.

Announcement of Engagement of Benjamin Franklin Norwood and Anne Parker Robinson. *Harrisburg Telegraph* (Harrisburg, PA), 30 September 1933, p. 4, col. 4.

Announcement of Guardianship of Rebecca Park by William James Russell. *The Athenian* (Athens, GA), 14 December 1827, p. 1.

Announcement of Medical Trip of Drs. William James Park Russell and

Seaborn Rentz Russell. *Wills Point Chronicle* (Wills Point, TX), 27 January 1887, p. 3, col. 3.

Announcement of Opening of Medical Practice, Seaborn Rentz Russell. *Wills Point Chronicle* (Wills Point, TX), 20 January 1887, p. 3, col. 5.

Announcement of Return of Seaborn Rentz Russell to Wills Point, TX, Following Medical Trip. *Wills Point Chronicle* (Wills Point, TX), 27 October 1887, p. 3, col. 5.

Announcement of William James Park Russell as Officer in Johnson Club. *Van Buren Press* (Van Buren, AR), 7 September 1866, p. 2, col. 4.

"Applicants Who Get License." *The Tennessean* (Nashville, TN), 6 June 1911, p. 3, col. 5,

"Around the City, the Condition of George Russell." *Arkansas Democrat* (Little Rock, AR), 27 June 1921, p. 6, col. 2.

"Awarded $21,131." *Wilkes-Barre Times Leader, the Evening News* (Wilkes-Barre, PA), 25 February 1943, p. 10, col. 1.

"Baby Welfare Week." *Arkansas Gazette* (Little Rock, AR), 6 May 1917, p. 30, col. 2.

"Bucks Clinic Adds to Staff." *The Bristol Daily Courier* (Bristol, PA), 10 August 1961, p. 18, col. 3–5.

"Capt. A. L. Woodliff of Birmingham, Dead." *Montgomery Times* (Montgomery, AL), 24 December 1904, p. 8, col. 2.

"Capt. B. F. Norwood, Navy Surgeon." *Brooklyn Daily Eagle* (Brooklyn, NY), 14 January 1942, p. 13, col. 3.

"Captain Norwood Dies in N.Y. at 56." *Philadelphia Inquirer* (Philadelphia, PA), 15 January 1942 p. 34, col. 1.

"A Card, Dardanelle, Yell Co., Ark, October 16, 1868 [Advertisement for Medical Services of William James Park Russell]." *Arkansas Gazette* (Little Rock, AR), 20 October 1868, p. 2, col. 2.

"Center Appoints Two Psychiatrists." *The Bristol Daily Courier* (Bristol, PA), 18 January 1960, p. 4, col. 6.

"City News, Vaughter—Russell." *Arkansas Gazette* (Little Rock, AR), 10 April 1921, p. 10, col. 3.

"Col. Dunn, Inventor of Explosives, Dies." *Tampa Times* (Tampa, FL), 11 May 1936, p. 2, col. 7.

"Colonel Dies." *Biloxi Daily Herald* (Biloxi, MS), 12 May 1936, p. 3, col. 5.

"The Cotton Crop in Illinois." *Alton Telegraph* (Alton, IL), 24 November 1865, p. 6, col. 4.

"Cotton in Union County." *Ottawa Free Trader* (Ottawa, IL), 3 February 1866, p. 2, col. 1.

"Cotton Speculators—Singular Reports." *Nashville Daily Union* (Nashville, TN), 12 Sept 1863, p. 1, col. 7.

"Crowd Fills Church to Hear Sermon on 'Klan.'" *Arkansas Democrat* (Little Rock, AR), 27 February 1922, p. 10, col. 1–2.

"Death of Dr. Shaffer." *Atlanta Constitution* (Atlanta, GA), 27 May 1887, p. 3, col. 4.

"Death of Dr. W. J. Russell." *Gwinnett Herald* (Lawrenceville, GA), 9 October 1872, p. 3, col. 2.

Death of Infant Child of Dr. W. S. R. Russell. *Arkansas Democrat* (Little Rock, AR), 21 September 1900, p. 2, col. 4.

Death of Joseph H. Law. "Arkansas State News." *Arkansas Democrat* (Little Rock, AR), 23 October 1882, p. 2, col. 4.

Death of Joseph H. Law. "Sprays from Hot Springs." *Arkansas Gazette* (Little Rock, AR), 19 October 1882, p. 2, col. 1–2.

Death of Thomas W. Alexander. *Southern Recorder* (Milledgeville, GA), 9 March 1847, p. 3, col. 6.

Death of William James Park Russell. *Fort Worth Gazette* (Fort Worth, TX), 1 February 1892, p. 6, col. 4.

Death of William James Park Russell. *Times-Star* (Terrell, TX), 5 February 1892, p. 3.

"Deaths Elsewhere." *The Tennessean* (Nashville, TN), 23 December 1904, p. 6, col. 6.

"Deaths Here (Death of Anne Parker Robinson Norwood)." *Philadelphia Inquirer* (Philadelphia, PA), 9 September 1987, p. 57, col. 3.

"Dr. J. F. Alexander Breathes His Last." *Atlanta Constitution* (Atlanta, GA), 15 November 1901, p. 7, col. 4–5.

"Dr. Russell, of London: The Eminent Catarrh Specialist in the City." *Montgomery Advertiser* (Montgomery, AL), 6 November 1898, p. 5, col. 2.

"Dr. Russell to be Buried Here." *Birmingham News* (Birmingham, AL), 6 November 1916, p. 3, col. 1.

"Dr. William S. Russell." *Arkansas Gazette* (Little Rock, AR), 4 March 1928, p. 14, col. 4.

"Eleven Graduates in First Class of the College of P. & S." *Arkansas Democrat* (Little Rock, AR), 1 May 1907, p. 6, col. 2.

Endorsement of Hugh Lawson White as Presidential Nominee. *Columbus Enquirer* (Columbus, GA), 13 May 1836, p. 3, col. 3.

"Execution Sale." *Fayetteville Weekly Democrat* (Fayetteville, AR), 25 May 1882, p. 3, col. 6.

"Faithful Temperance Worker Passes." *Alabama Christian Advocate* (Birmingham, AL), 1 February 1945, p. 10, col. 4.

"Fall of Rosecrans." *Shelby Volunteer* (Shelbyville, IN), 5 November 1863, p. 1, col. 3–5.

"Fords for Rent." *Arkansas Gazette* (Little Rock, AR), 17 Oct 1920, p. 10, col. 2.

Formation of Lawrenceville Manufacturing Company. *Southern Banner* (Athens, GA), 24 April 1851, p. 4, col. 2.

"From the West: The Cotton Business." *New York Times* (New York, NY), 4 December 1864, p. 3, col. 6.

"Frozen to Death." *Concord Weekly Gazette* (Concord, NC), 31 January 1857, p. 2.

"Gadsden's People." *Weekly Age* (Birmingham, AL), 2 May 1888, p. 6, col. 4.

"Good News, Successful Treatment of Consumption by a Birmingham (Ala.) Physician." *The Randolph Toiler* (Wedowee, AL), 21 August 1896, p. 4, col. 1.

"Guidance Group Meets." *Daily Intelligencer* (Doylestown, PA), 7 April 1960, p. 1, col. 2.

"High Explosive Inventor, Col. Beverly W. Dunn Dies." *Indianapolis Star* (Indianapolis, IN), 11 May 1936, p. 1, col. 1.

"Insurance Companies Losers in Large Suit." *Warren Times Mirror* (Warren, PA), 25 February 1943, p. 11, col. 4.

"Is Fined $25 For Hitting Father in Law." *Arkansas Democrat* (Little Rock, AR), 16 April 1919, p. 7, col. 3.

"Late Local News." *Arkansas Democrat* (Little Rock, AR), 23 September 1905, p. 7, col. 5.

"Latest News." *Nashville Daily Union* (Nashville, TN), 15 August 1863, p. 3, col. 2.

"A Letter from the Great Western Canal Survey." *Atlanta Constitution* (Atlanta, GA), 8 February 1872, p. 1, col. 2.

"List of Arrivals." *Corinth War Eagle* (Corinth, MS), 7 August 1862, p. 2, col. 2.

"Local and Commercial, Further Arrests." *Nashville Daily Union* (Nashville, TN), 15 April 1863, p. 3, col. 1.

"Local and Otherwise." *Lafayette County Democrat* (Stamps, AR), 17 September 1909, p. 8, col. 4.

"Local Items." *Lafayette County Democrat* (Stamps, AR), 10 May 1912, p. 8, col. 4.

"Local Paragraphs." *Brevard News* (Brevard, NC), 23 August 1912, p. 5, col. 1.

"Making Comfort Bags." *Arkansas Gazette* (Little Rock, AR), 20 May 1917, p. 18, col. 4.

"A MAN WITHOUT FEELING. Subject of a Clinic by Dr. Russell. NOTHING SEEMS TO HURT HIM. He Can Be Stabbed and Shot without Pain and Eats Glass with a Relish—A Wonder." *The Marion Times-Standard* (Marion, AL), 28 May 1896, p. 1, col. 2.

Marriage of Ralph Morgan Russell and Mollie Woodliff. "Society, Gadsden." *Montgomery Advertiser* (Montgomery, AL), 22 August 1886, p. 6, col. 1.

Marriage of William J. Russell and Iantha Huff. *Southern Recorder* (Milledgeville, GA), 6 May 1845, p. 3, col. 6.

Massey, R. J. "Atlanta's Leading Physicians—Aided in Establishing Atlanta College of Physicians and Surgeons." *Atlanta Constitution* (Atlanta, GA), 25 February 1906, p. 8A, col. 2–4.

"Mental Clinics Open For 2 Nights A Week." *The Bristol Daily Courier* (Bristol, PA), 13 April 1960, p. 5, col. 1–2.

"Mental Health Center Okays $96,000 Budget." *Daily Intelligencer* (Doylestown, PA), 20 June 1960, p. 2, col. 3.

"Mental Health Unit Names Clinic Chiefs." *Daily Intelligencer* (Doylestown, PA), 15 January 1960, p. 2, col. 4–5.

"Methodist Minister Dies: Dr. J. J. Boring Passes Away After a Long Illness at Americus." *Atlanta Constitution* (Atlanta, GA) 11 December 1897, p. 3, col. 3.

"Minister Praises the Ku Klux Klan: Rev. J. W. Coontz in Sermon Says It Is to Protect American Homes." *Arkansas Democrat* (Little Rock, AR), 6 March 1922, p. 10, col. 2.

"Mrs. Russell's Death." *Arkansas Democrat* (Little Rock, AR), 7 May 1900, p. 3, col. 3.

"New Mental Health Program Offered in Bucks." *The Bristol Daily Courier* (Bristol, PA), 9 March 1961, p. 12, col. 1–7.

"News and Gossip of the Social World." *Atlanta Constitution* (Atlanta, GA), 14 July 1895, p. 6, col. 3.

"News of Society." *Fort Wayne Weekly Sentinel* (Fort Wayne, IN), 16 May 1895, p. 5, col. 6.

Notice of A. Tabor about William J. P. Russell. *Southern Banner* (Athens, GA), 23 September 1858, p. 3, col. 2.

Notice of Medical School Graduation of Benjamin Franklin Norwood. *Lafayette County Democrat* (Stamps, AR), 10 May 1912, p. 8.

Obituary of Bessie Russell Vaughter. *Arkansas Gazette* (Little Rock, AR), 12 October 1960, p. 11A, col. 1.

Obituary of John Alexander. *The Athenian* (Athens, GA), 14 May 1830, p. 3, col. 3–4.

Obituary of Mrs. Sophia P. Russell. *Southern Recorder* (Milledgeville, GA), 9 April 1844, p. 3, col. 6–7.

Obituary of O. Spurgeon English. *Journal News* (White Plains, NY) 7 October 1993, p. 26/B2, col. 6.

Obituary of Ralph Morgan Russell. *Birmingham News* (Birmingham, AL), 6 November 1916, p. 3, col. 1.

"Obituary [of William Watts Montgomery]." *Augusta Chronicle* (Augusta, GA), 15 September 1843, p. 3.

"Official Communication from the Knights of the Ku Klux Klan, Addressed to the People of the State of Arkansas." *Arkansas Gazette* (Little Rock, AR), 26 March 1922, p. 19. Full-page ad.

"Officials of the Bucks County Mental Health Guidance Center." *Daily Intelligencer* (Doylestown, PA), 13 April 1960, p. 2, col. 5–6.

"An Old Land Mark Is Being Removed." *Gwinnett News-Herald* (Lawrenceville, GA), 7 February 1910.

"Personal Mention." *Hornellsville Weekly Tribune* (Hornellsville, NY), 20 April 1888, p. 5, col. 3.

"Proceedings of the Anti-Van Buren Convention." *Southern Recorder* (Milledgeville, GA), 10 May 1836, p. 2, col. 4.

"Psychiatric Center 4 Years Old, Handles 10,000 Visits Yearly." *The Bristol Daily Courier* (Bristol, PA), 14 July 1962, p. 11, col. 1–3.

"Psychiatric Center Ups Treatment." *Daily Intelligencer* (Doylestown, PA), 1 August 1963, p. 8, col. 8.

Railway Accident of Dr. W. S. Russell. *Arkansas Gazette* (Little Rock, AR), 24 April 1903, p. 1, col. 5.

Report of Benjamin Franklin Norwood Receiving Position in New York. *Lafayette County Democrat* (Stamps, AR), 26 April 1912, p. 8.

Report of Ralph Morgan Russell Receiving Payment for Railroad Injuries. *Gadsden Times* (Gadsden, AL), 26 April 1888, p. 3.

Report of Ralph Morgan Russell Returning to Gadsden. *Gadsden Times* (Gadsden, AL) 24 January 1889, p. 3.

"Roundabout in Georgia." *Atlanta Constitution* (Atlanta, GA), 29 June 1877, p. 3, col. 4.

"Ruth Marie Powell." *Arkansas Democrat* (Little Rock, AR), 9 August 1918, p. 10, col. 2.

"Same Judges and Clerks to Serve." *Arkansas Democrat* (Little Rock, AR), 20 March 1914, p. 12, col. 3.

"Sim Strong." *Greensboro Watchman* (Greensboro, AL), 28 October 1915, p. 5, col. 4.

"Sleeping Cars Wrecked." *The Saint Paul Globe* (Saint Paul, MN), 12 March 1888, p. 5, col. 8.

"Soldiers from A.F.W.C. Homes—Stamps." *Arkansas Gazette* (Little Rock, AR), 25 November 1917, p. 11, col. 5.

"Speaking of Society, Gadsden." *Montgomery Advertiser* (Montgomery, AL), 26 May 1895, p. 7, col. 3.

"State Items." *Southern Star* (Newton, AL), 30 May 1888, p. 1, col. 4.

"State News, Morphined Himself." *Fort Worth Daily Gazette* (Fort Worth, TX), 1 January 1886, p. 5, col. 1.

Statistics of Wills Point, TX, 1887. *Wills Point Chronicle* (Wills Point, TX), 13 October 1887; as cited, Kitty Wheeler, "Post Offices, Cities, Towns and People," at the website of the Van Zandt County Research Group. https://sites.rootsweb.com/~txvzcgrg/grgPO60.htm. Accessed September 2019.

"Successful Treatment of Consumption by a Birmingham (Ala.) Physician." *Monroe Journal* (Claiborne, AL), 1 October 1896, p. 6, col. 5.

"Taught to Read by Using Bible as Text Book." *Arkansas Democrat* (Little Rock, AR), 8 January 1921, p. 10, col. 2.

"Telegraphic Intelligence." *The Daily Delta* (New Orleans, LA), 8 August 1860, p. 2.

"Tennesseans Appointed." *The Tennessean* (Nashville, TN), 2 August 1917, p. 4, col. 7.

"Terrible Accident: Five Persons Killed and a Number Injured by an Accident on the Erie Railroad at Scio, N. Y.—A Greater Loss of Life Averted by a Seeming Miracle—The Victims." *Marion County Herald* (Palmyra, MO), 16 March 1888, p. 7, col. 1.

Testimonial of Mrs. H. O. Babb, Jasper, AL, on Behalf of Russell Medical Institute. *Mountain Eagle* (Jasper, AL), 2 December 1896 p. 3, col. 4.

"The Thaw Causes a Bad Accident on the Erie Road at Scio, N. Y." *The Eau Claire News* (Eau Claire, WI), 17 March 1888, p. 2, col. 5.

"A Trip to Murfreesboro." *Nashville Daily Union* (Nashville, TN), 8 April 1863, p. 3, col. 1.

"The Truth About the Knights of the Ku Klux Klan." *Arkansas Gazette* (Little Rock, AR), 5 August 1922, p. 11. Full-page ad.

"They Will Go to Texas: From the *Cherokee, Ga., Advance.*" *Atlanta Constitution* (Atlanta, GA), 28 August 1886, p. 8, col. 6.

"Two New Mental Health Officials." *Daily Intelligencer* (Doylestown, PA), 14 January 1960, p. 1, col. 1–2.

"Two Psychologists Named to Serve Bucks Center." *Daily Intelligencer* (Doylestown, PA), 18 February 1963, p. 2, col. 4–5.

Unclaimed Letter Notice for Dr. W. J. P. Russell, New Orleans Post Office. *Times-Picayune* (New Orleans, LA), 21 December 1860, p. 4.

"Uncle Sam Wants More Army Surgeons." *Lafayette County Democrat* (Stamps, AR), 1 October 1909, p. 6, col. 4.

"Well Known Church Worker Succumbs." *Birmingham News* (Birmingham, AL), 27 January 1945, p. 6, col. 2.

"Widow Awarded $21,131 Verdict." *The Gettysburg Times* (Gettysburg, PA), 25 February 1943, p. 4, col. 6.

"Wins $21,131 Verdict in Husband's Death." *The Express* (Lock Haven, PA), 25 February 1943, p. 9, col. 5.

Wynn, Bob. "Ramshackle House Holds Slice of History." *Gwinnett Daily News* (Lawrenceville, GA), 6 November 1986, p. C-1.

"X Rays and Skilled Surgeons." *Coosa River News* (Centre, AL), 3 June 1898, p. 1, col. 4.

"The Yellow Fever." *Baltimore Sun* (Baltimore, MD), 12 September 1854, p. 2, col. 1.

"The Yellow Fever." *Richmond Dispatch* (Richmond, VA), 15 September 1854, p. 2, col. 2.

V. Online Sources, Articles, and Documents

"Alabama Deaths, 1908–1974." Department of Health, Montgomery. FamilySearch. https://familysearch.org/ark:/61903/1:1:JDXW-MMX. Accessed June 2017.

Allison, Julanne S. "Cane Hill (Washington County)." *The Encyclopedia of Arkansas History and Culture*. Butler Center for Arkansas Studies. http://www.encyclopediaofarkansas.net/encyclopedia/entry-detail.aspx?entryID=2705#. Accessed February 2017.

American Medical Association. "United States Deceased Physician File (AMA), 1864–1968." FamilySearch https://familysearch.org/ark:/61903/3:1:3QSQ-G9QP-6GYW?cc=2061540&wc=M6Y8-XP6%3A353101901. Accessed April 2017.

Barnes, Dorothy Bateman. "Wills Point, Texas." *The Handbook of Texas Online*. Texas State Historical Association. https://tshaonline.org/handbook/online/articles/hgw10. Accessed March 2017.

Dentice, Dianne. "Ku Klux Klan (after 1900)." *Encyclopedia of Arkansas History and Culture*. Butler Center for Arkansas Studies. http://www.encyclopediaofarkansas.net/encyclopedia/entry-detail.aspx?search=1&entryID=2755. Accessed March 2017.

Dougan, Michael. "Health and Medicine." *Encyclopedia of Arkansas History and Culture*. Butler Center for Arkansas Studies. http://www.encyclopediaofarkansas.net/encyclopedia/entry-detail.aspx?search=1&entryID=392. Accessed 17 January 2019.

———. "Medical Malpractice." *Encyclopedia of Arkansas History and Culture*. Butler Center for Arkansas Studies. http://www.encyclopediaofarkansas.net/encyclopedia/entry-detail.aspx?search=1&entryID=5319. Accessed 7 February 2019).

———. "Norman Baker (1882–1958)." *Encyclopedia of Arkansas History and Culture*. Butler Center for Arkansas Studies. http://www.encyclopediaofarkansas.net/encyclopedia/entry-detail.aspx?search=1&entryID=4885. Accessed 19 January 2019.

"Dr. J. R. Hudson, List of Military Prisoners." Files of Union Provost Marshal 4348 (Jackson, 1863). Tennessee State Library and Archives. http://share.tn.gov/tsla/UnionProvostPDFs/4348.pdf. Accessed February 2017.

"Dr. J. R. Hudson, Smuggling and Other Offences." Files of Union Provost
    Marshal 4275 (Nashville, 1863), Tennessee State Library and Archives.
    http://share.tn.gov/tsla/UnionProvostPDFs/4275.pdf. Accessed February
    2017.
"Edward A. Strecker (1886–1959)." Department of Psychiatry of the Perelman
    School of Medicine. University of Pennsylvania. http://www.med.upenn
    .edu/psychiatry/streckerbio.html. Accessed July 2017.
Fairview Presbyterian Church. "Fairview Presbyterian Church History."
    Fairview Presbyterian Church. http://www.fairviewpres.org/historyfull
    .html. Accessed June 2017.
Gillespie, Robert S. "The Train Doctors: A Detailed History of Railway
    Surgeons." Railway Surgery. http://railwaysurgery.org/HistoryLong.htm.
    Accessed October 2017.
Gracey, Brittani Baldwin, and Hillary R. Hunt. "Mental Health." *Encyclopedia
    of Arkansas History and Culture*, Butler Center for Arkansas Studies. http://
    www.encyclopediaofarkansas.net/encyclopedia/entry-detail.aspx?entry
    ID=5196. Accessed July 2017.
Guide to Charles Wilson Harris Papers, collection 315. Southern Historical
    Collection. Louis Round Wilson Library, Univ. of NC. http://finding-aids
    .lib.unc.edu/00315. Accessed November 2016.
Havern, Christopher B., Sr., "Pennsylvania III (Battleship No. 38) 1916–1946."
    Naval History and Heritage Command. https://www.history.navy.mil/
    research/histories/ship-histories/danfs/p/pennsylvania-ii.html. Accessed
    July 2017.
Hughes, Phyllis, and Marvin Hughes. "National Register Narrative, Isaac
    Adair House, c. 1827." National Register of Historic Places Registration
    Form. National Park Service. 20 October 2000. https://focus.nps.gov/
    GetAsset?assetID=4c81ecfc-55ae-48e8-ac3a-f36443df5180. Accessed January
    2017.
Laster, Patricia Paulus. "Civilian Conservation Corps (CCC)." *Encyclopedia of
    Arkansas History and Culture*. Butler Center for Arkansas Studies. http://
    www.encyclopediaofarkansas.net/encyclopedia/entry-detail.aspx?
    entryID=2396. Accessed June 2017.
"List of Persons Adjudged Insane and Ordered to Be Committed to the
    Insane Asylum at Milledgeville from the *Atlanta Constitution* Newspaper
    1870–1914." Baldwin Co., GA, GenWeb page, maintained by Eileen Babb
    McAdams. http://theusgenweb.org/ga/baldwin/cshinmates.html. Accessed
    August 2019).
May, Bethany. "Eureka Springs." *The Encyclopedia of Arkansas History and
    Culture*. Butler Center for Arkansas Studies. http://www.encyclopedia
    ofarkansas.net/encyclopedia/entry-detail.aspx?entryID=843. Accessed
    February 2017.
Minutes of the Medical College of Georgia Board of Trustees Meetings,
    1829–1892. Original at Medical College of Georgia. Online at Augusta
    University's Open Repository website. http://augusta.openrepository.com/
    augusta/handle/10675.2/965. Accessed February 2017.
"Norwood, Benjamin Franklin," "United States Deceased Physician File
    (AMA), 1864–1968," American Medical Association. FamilySearch.

https://www.familysearch.org/ark:/61903/3:1:3QS7-L9QP-V974-S?i=
267&owc=waypoints&wc=M6Y8-XMW%3A353098001&cc=2061540.
Accessed November 2017.

Record Book 1. Faculty of the Medical College of Georgia, October 1833–
November 1852. Augusta University's Open Repository. http://augusta
.openrepository.com/augusta/handle/10675.2/966. Accessed January 2017.

Russell, Bill. "William Leon Russell (1914–2000)." *Encyclopedia of Arkansas
History and Culture*. Butler Center for Arkansas Studies. http://www
.encyclopediaofarkansas.net/encyclopedia/entry-detail.aspx?entryID
=8031. Accessed July 2017.

Smyrl, Vivian Elizabeth. "Bosqueville, Texas." *The Handbook of Texas Online*.
Texas State Historical Association. https://tshaonline.org/handbook/
online/articles/hnb63. Accessed January 2017.

Spurgeon, John. "Trail of Tears National Historic Trail." *The Encyclopedia of
Arkansas History and Culture*. Butler Center for Arkansas Studies. http://
www.encyclopediaofarkansas.net/encyclopedia/entry-detail.aspx?
search=1&entryID=4887. Accessed November 2017.

Teske, Steven. "Houston (Perry County)." *Encyclopedia of Arkansas History and
Culture*. Butler Center for Arkansas Studies. http://www.encyclopedia
ofarkansas.net/encyclopedia/entry-detail.aspx?entryID=7165. Accessed
April 2017.

———. "Nashville (Howard County)." *The Encyclopedia of Arkansas History and
Culture*. Butler Center for Arkansas Studies. http://www.encyclopedia
ofarkansas.net/encyclopedia/entry-detail.aspx?entryID=899. Accessed
March 2017.

Twenty-Fifth Annual Announcement of the Medical College of Georgia. Augusta:
Medical College of Georgia, 1850. Augusta University's Open Repository.
http://augusta.openrepository.com/augusta/handle/10675.2/319890.
Accessed February 2017.

"USS *Chaumont* (AP-5), 1921-1948." Naval Historical Center. https://www
.ibiblio.org/hyperwar/OnlineLibrary/photos/sh-usn/usnsh-c/ap5.htm .
Accessed September 2019.

"W. J. Russell of Gwinnett County, Georgia." Prints and Photographs
Department. Boston Athenæum. http://cdm.bostonathenaeum.org/cdm/
singleitem/collection/p13110coll5/id/2507/rec/94. Accessed January 2017.

"W. S. R. Russell." "United States Deceased Physician File (AMA), 1864–1968."
American Medical Association (Chicago). FamilySearch.https://family
search.org/ark:/61903/3:1:3QSQ-G9QP-6GYW?cc=2061540&wc=M6Y8
-XP6%3A353101901. Accessed April 2017.

Welch, Melanie. "Abortion." *Encyclopedia of Arkansas History and Culture*. Butler
Center for Arkansas Studies. http://www.encyclopediaofarkansas.net/
encyclopedia/entry-detail.aspx?search=1&entryID=5324&media=print.
Accessed 7 February 2019.

Wheeler, Kitty. "Post Offices, Cities, Towns and People." Van Zandt County
Research Group. http://www.rootsweb.ancestry.com/~txvzcgrg/grgPO60
.htm. Accessed September 2017.

VI. Unpublished Sources

Application for Certificate of Qualification to Practice Medicine, Ralph
    Morgan Russell, Etowah County, SG 6456, Alabama Board of Medical
    Examiners, 1879–2012, Government Records Collections, Alabama
    Department of Archives and History, Montgomery, AL.
Application for License to Practice Medicine in the State of Arkansas, W. S. R.
    Russell, Houston, Perry Co., AR, 8 July 1903, certificate 2655, State Medical
    Board of Arkansas.
Arkansas Divorce Bk. 34.
Arkansas Marriage Records, Vital Records Division of Arkansas Department of
    Health, Bk. 109.
Army Register of Enlistments, January 1847–June 1849, MIUSA1798_102882, roll
    23, RG 94, NARA.
Avarilla Law Russell Pension Application for William James Park Russell's
    Mexican War service, application 10579, certificate 9137.
Avarilla Law Russell Scrapbook, in the William James Park Russell Family
    Letters, 1820–1989, Small Manuscript Collection S4082, University of
    Arkansas for Medical Sciences Library, Historical Research Center, Little
    Rock, AR.
Beebe Methodist Church Membership Roll (Chronological Roll of Full
    Membership, in possession of First United Methodist Church, Beebe, AR).
Benjamin Franklin Norwood, Social Security File, Application #166288569.
Bible of Avarilla Octavia Dunn Parks Russell, in possession of Hurley family,
    Terrell, Texas.
Bible of Lounetta Hoobler Russell (Philadelphia: P. W. Ziegler, n.d.), in posses-
    sion of Sandy Pack, North Little Rock, AR.
Birth Certificate of George Washington Russell, Pulaski Co., AR, Registration
    District 6625, #2030.
Cabarrus Co., NC, Court of Pleas and Quarter Sessions, Minutes Bk. 1,
    1797–1805.
California State Library, *Great Register of Voters, 1900–1968.*
Carded Records Showing Military Service of Soldiers Who Fought in
    Confederate Organizations, Compiled 1903–1927, Documenting the Period
    1861–1865, M266, roll 532, RG 109 NARA.
"Case of Elisha H. Forsyth, Citizen, Tried in September 1863," Records of the
    Office of the Judge Advocate General, Army Court Martial Case Files,
    1809–1894, box 2025, file 778, RG 153, NARA.
Certificate of Completion of Psychiatric Residency, George Washington
    Russell, Friends Hospital, Philadelphia, PA, 7 September 1947 (in posses-
    sion of George S. Russell, Saylorsburg, PA).
Certificate of License, George Washington Russell, Medical Board of Puerto
    Rico, 9 December 1958, in possession of George S. Russell, Saylorsburg, PA.
Certificate of License, George Washington Russell, State Board of Medical
    Education and Licensure to practice medicine in the Commonwealth
    of Pennsylvania, 11 March 1948 (in possession of George S. Russell,
    Saylorsburg, PA).

Certificate of Study and Moral Character, W. J. P. Russell for Ralph Morgan
    Russell, Bellevue Hospital Medical College, original in Bellevue archives,
    copy in the William James Park Russell Family Letters, 1820–1989, Small
    Manuscript Collection S4082, University of Arkansas for Medical Sciences
    Library, Historical Research Center, Little Rock, AR.
Crawford Co., AR, Marriage Bk. A.
Death Certificate of Eric Allen Russell, Texas Death Certificate #21900, Dallas
    Co., TX, State Board of Health, Bureau of Vital Statistics
Death Certificate of Ralph Morgan Russell, Alabama Death Certificates vol.
    20, #566, Jefferson Co., AL.
Death Certificate of Richard Delton [sic] Russell, 27 October 1928, Texas Death
    Certificate #45869, Van Zandt Co., TX, State Board of Health, Bureau of
    Vital Statistics.
Diary of Seaborn Rentz Russell, 1920, original in possession of the Marvin
    Vaughter family, North Little Rock, AR; transcribed (in part) in the
    William James Park Russell Family Letters, 1820–1989, Small Manuscript
    Collection S4082, University of Arkansas for Medical Sciences Library,
    Historical Research Center, Little Rock, AR.
Diary of Seaborn Rentz Russell, 1921, original in possession of Ann Russell
    Zorn, Philadelphia, PA; transcribed in the William James Park Russell
    Family Letters, 1820–1989, Small Manuscript Collection S4082, University
    of Arkansas for Medical Sciences Library, Historical Research Center,
    Little Rock, AR.
Diary of Seaborn Rentz Russell, 1922, original in possession of George S.
    Russell, Saylorsburg, PA; transcribed in the William James Park Russell
    Family Letters, 1820–1989, Small Manuscript Collection S4082, University
    of Arkansas for Medical Sciences Library, Historical Research Center,
    Little Rock, AR.
"Dr. Russell's Account," Handwritten Ledger of Unidentified Fayetteville
    Attorney, Fayetteville Public Library. Fayetteville, AR. Emailed commu-
    nication, Sarah Braswell, historical research coordinator, Office of Medical
    Historian in Residence, Augusta University, to Mary Ryan, Little Rock,
    AR, July 2017.
Emailed communication, William Feis, professor of history, Buena Vista Univ.,
    Storm Lake, IA, to William L. Russell, Maumelle, AR, 8 August 2017.
Emailed communication, Timothy H. Horning, University of Pennsylvania
    Archives, to Mary Ryan, Little Rock, AR, 6 April 2016.
Etowah Co., AL, Deed Bks. L and N.
Fairview Presbyterian Church (Lawrenceville, GA) Session Minutes and
    Register, 1823–1835, 1835–1880.
First Presbyterian Church, Philadelphia, PA, Marriage Registry.
First United Methodist Church, Birmingham, AL, Membership Records.
Forsyth Co., GA, Marriage Bk. C.
Franklin Co., AR, List of Lands to be Assessed for Taxation for 1887.
Franklin Co., AR, Marriage Bk. B.
Franklin Co., AR, Real Estate Tax Bk. 1885.
Franklin Co., AR, Tax Bks., 1882, 1883, 1884.

George Washington Russell and Jeanette Laverne Roberts, *Letters from the War*, unpublished collection of WWII correspondence owned and transcribed by George S. Russell, Saylorsburg, PA, with foreword by George S. Russell.

Greene Co., AR, Mortgage Bk. 7.

Greene Co., AR, Personal Property Taxes Bks. 1, 3, and 5.

Greene Co., GA, Deed Bk. 1.

Greene Co., GA, Marriage Bk. 1829–1849.

Greene Co., GA, Superior Court Minutes, Bk. 6.

Greene Co., GA, Will Bk. 4.

Gwinnett Co., GA Deed Bk. N.

Gwinnett Co., GA, Marriage Bk. 4, 1843–1864.

Gwinnett Co., GA, Marriage Bk. 4, #2, 1871–1882.

Gwinnett Co., GA, Tax Digest, 1864.

Gwinnett Co., GA, Will Bk. D.

Hall Co., GA, Deed Bks. G and I.

Hall Co., GA, Marriage Bks. A and C.

Hall Co., GA, Will Bk. A.

Hargrave Family Papers, Annie Belle Weaver Special Collections, Irvine Sullivan Ingram Library, Univ. of West GA.

Harris and Ewing Collection, Library of Congress.

Hayden v. Russell, Jefferson Co., AL, Chancery Court, 5th Dist., Northwestern Chancery of Alabama (1916).

Howard Co., AR, Personal Taxes, 1884.

Incorporation of Pocono Abstract Agency, 10 March 1981, original document in possession of George S. Russell, Saylorsburg, PA.

Index to Mexican War Pension Claims, Texas, NARA microfilm publication T317.

Jackson Co., AR, Medical Register A.

Jackson Co., GA, Superior Ct. Minutes, 1801–1803, 1814–1822, 1822–1831, 1832–1843.

Jefferson Co., AL, Administrators' Records, vol. W-Y.

Jefferson Co., AL, Death Certificates, vol. 20.

Jefferson Co., AL, Deed Bks. 210, 215, 219, 247, 252, 254 259.

Letter of George W. Russell, Allentown, PA, to William L. Russell, Maumelle, AR, March 1976; original in possession of William L. Russell and copy in William James Park Russell Family Letters, 1820–1989, Small Manuscript Collection S4082, University of Arkansas for Medical Sciences Library, Historical Research Center, Little Rock, AR.

Letter of Grace Russell Norton, Wills Point, TX, to William L. Russell, Maumelle, AR, 15 February 1974, in possession of William L. Russell.

Letter of Grace Russell Norton, Wills Point, TX, to William L. Russell, Maumelle, AR, 30 May 1975, in possession of William L. Russell.

Letter of Lelia Graham Marsh, Salem College alumnae secretary (Winston-Salem, NC), to Mrs. W. L. (Ruby Norwood) Kitchens, 2 March 1959, in possession of William L. Russell, Maumelle, AR.

Letter of Lucile Hanrick, church historian and archivist, First United Methodist Church, Birmingham, AL, to William L. Russell, Maumelle, AR, 10 June 2002, in possession of William L. Russell.

Letter of Patricia Methven, college archivist of King's College, London, England, to William L. Russell, North Little Rock, AR, 24 January 1982; in possession of William L. Russell, Maumelle, AR, with a copy held by William James Park Russell Family Letters, 1820–1989, Small Manuscript Collection S4082, University of Arkansas for Medical Sciences Library, Historical Research Center, Little Rock, AR.

Letter of Ralph Morgan Russell, Birmingham, AL, to Prof. J. M. Page, University of Virginia, 11 September 1906; original on file at Office of the Registrar, University of Virginia, copy placed by William L. Russell, Maumelle, AR, in William James Park Russell Family Letters, 1820–1989, Small Manuscript Collection S4082, University of Arkansas for Medical Sciences Library, Historical Research Center, Little Rock, AR.

Letter of Ruby Norwood Kitchens to Maude Russell, 29 April 1936, original in possession of descendants of Jamie Morris Walker, Lubbock TX, copy in possession of William L. Russell, Maumelle, AR.

Letter of William J. Russell to Governor Joseph E. Brown, in Governor Joseph Emerson Brown correspondence file, 1861–1865, Georgia Archives, Series 245, Governors Subject Correspondence, 3335–16, unit 93–1219A.

Letter of William L. Russell, Maumelle, AR, to William D. Lindsey, Little Rock, AR, 8 April 1996, in possession of William D. Lindsey.

"List of Mail Scouts and Police Vouchers cashed by Col. Taylor Chief Quarter Master Department of the Cumberland from November 1st 1862 to May 1st 1863," Records of the Provost Marshal General's Bureau, entry 41, "Correspondence, Reports and Other Records Relating to Policemen," RG 110, NARA.

Maybelle Emma Russell, Social Security File, Application #432096106.

Medical College of Georgia Register of Students 1832–1861.

Morgan Co., GA, Marriage Bk. 1855–1854.

"Norwood, Benjamin Franklin," US Department of Veterans Affairs, Records Management Center, 6261, NARA.

Oral interview of George S. Russell, Ann Russell Zorn, and Paul Russell, Saylorsburg, PA, by William L. Russell and Mary Ryan, Maumelle and Little Rock, AR, 11–12 May 2017.

Oral Interview of Grace Russell Norton, Wills Point, TX, by William L. Russell, Maumelle, AR, 4 January 1974; transcript in possession of William L. Russell.

Oral Interview of Lavetta Russell Pack by William L. Russell, Maumelle, AR, 20 August 1973; transcript in possession of William L. Russell.

Oral Interview of Marvin Earl Vaughter, Little Rock, AR, by William L. Russell, Maumelle, AR, 15 August 1973; transcript in possession of William L. Russell.

Passport Applications, 1795–1905, NARA series, roll 441: *22 Apr 1895–30 Apr 1895*.

Paulding Co., GA, Marriage Bk.1.

Perry Co., AR, Deed Bks. P and U.

Perry Co., AR, Record of Mortgages of Personal Property Filed, 1904.

Philadelphia Co., PA, Clerk of the Orphans' Court, Philadelphia Marriage License Index, 1885–1951.

Polk Co., GA, Deed Bk. A.

"Proceedings of the Military Commission in the Case of Elisha H. Forsyth," RG 153, NARA.

"Provost Marshal, Letters and Telegrams Sent 1863," Department of the Cumberland, pt. 1, RG 393, NARA.

"Provost Marshal, Register of Letters Received, January 1863–December 1864," Department of the Cumberland, pt. 1, RG 393, NARA.

Pulaski Co., AR, Deed Bk. 88.

Pulaski Co., AR, List of Legal Voters, Persons Who Paid Poll Tax, 1904, Bks. 2 and 3.

Pulaski Co., AR, Marriage Bks. 39, 55, 62.

Pulaski Co., AR, Medical Register, Bk. A.

Pulaski Co., AR, Real Estate Taxes, Taxes Assessed and Extended against Real Property, 1906–1921.

Ralph Morgan Russell, *An Illustrated Lecture on Deformities of the Human Frame, Their Cause, Means of Prevention, and Method of Cure,* in Russell Plato Schwartz Orthopedics Collection (pamphlet box 1/19), Edward G. Miner Library, University of Rochester Medical Center, Rochester, NY.

"Rediscovering a Landmark: The William J. Russell House," ms. in Russell file, Gwinnett County Historical Society.

Richard Dickson Winn, unpublished and untitled manuscript re: Winn family history, November 1885; in possession of C. L. Pentecost, 1980.

Salem College (Winston-Salem, NC) File Card Register of Students, 1840–1842, transcribed by Lelia Graham Marsh, Salem Alumnae secretary, March 1959.

"San Francisco Passenger Lists 1892–1953," RG 231, NARA.

Union Citizens' File, Union Provost Marshals' File of Papers Relating to Individual Civilians, 1861–1867, file 22632.

Union Co., IL, Deed Bks. 19 and 21.

Van Zandt Co., TX, Deed Bks. 34, 37, 39, 42, 76.

Van Zandt Co., TX, Marriage Bk. 6.

Washington Co., AR, Deed Bk. R.

Washington Co., AR, Marriage Bks. C, F, G.

Washington Co., AR Personal Property Tax, 1870.

Washington Co., AR, Real Estate Tax Record, 1878.

William James Park Russell Family Letters, 1820–1989, Small Manuscript Collection S4082, University of Arkansas for Medical Sciences Library, Historical Research Center, Little Rock, AR.

William James Park Russell File, Union Citizens' File, Union Provost Marshals' File of Papers Relating to Individual Civilians, 1861–1867, file 22632, M345, RG 109, NARA.

William James Park Russell Mexican War Enlistment Papers, 1st Series, 1798–1894, box 675, Entry 91, NARA.

William James Park Russell Mexican War Pension Application 21053, certificate 18030.

William Steinkamp, Social Security File, Application #429286487.

William Truesdail to William Rosecrans, 15 January 1863, Records of the United States Army Continental Command, part I, entry 925, box 20, RG 393, NARA.

INDEX

WILLIAM D. LINDSEY is a former academic and university administrator and the winner of the Booker Worthen Literary Prize for *Fiat Flux: The Writings of Wilson R. Bachelor, Nineteenth-Century Country Doctor and Philosopher.*

WILLIAM L. RUSSELL is a retired colonel in the U.S. Army and media-relations specialist who is descended from the Russell physicians.

MARY L. RYAN worked in health sciences libraries at Tulane University and the Texas Medical Center and was director of the University of Arkansas for Medical Sciences Library for seventeen years.